DEMENTIA

Dementia

DEMENTIA

Volume 1:

History and Incidence

Patrick McNamara, Editor

Brain, Behavior, and Evolution
Patrick McNamara, Series Editor

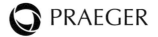 PRAEGER

AN IMPRINT OF ABC-CLIO, LLC
Santa Barbara, California • Denver, Colorado • Oxford, England

Library of Congress Cataloging-in-Publication Data

Dementia / Patrick McNamara, editor.
    p. cm.—(Brain, behavior, and evolution)
  Includes bibliographical references and index.
    ISBN 978-0-313-38434-9 (hard copy : alk. paper)—ISBN 978-0-313-38435-6 (ebook)
    1. Dementia. 2. Alzheimer's disease. I. McNamara, Patrick, 1956– II. Series: Brain,
behavior, and evolution
    [DNLM: 1. Dementia. WM 220]
    RC521.D4524   2011
    616.8'3—dc22   2010041082

ISBN 978-0-313-38434-9
EISBN 978-0-313-38435-6

15   14   13   12   11   1   2   3   4   5

This book is also available on the World Wide Web as an eBook.
Visit www.abc-clio.com for details.

Praeger
An Imprint of ABC-CLIO, LLC

ABC-CLIO, LLC
130 Cremona Drive, P.O. Box 1911
Santa Barbara, California 93116-1911

This book is printed on acid-free paper ∞

Manufactured in the United States of America

Contents

Series Foreword

Beginning in the 1990s, behavioral scientists—that is, people who study mind, brain, and behavior—began to take the theory of evolution seriously. They began to borrow techniques developed by the evolutionary biologists and apply them to problems in mind, brain, and behavior. Now, of course, virtually all behavioral scientists up to that time had claimed to endorse evolutionary theory, but few used it to study the problems they were interested in. All that changed in the 1990s. Since that pivotal decade, breakthroughs in the behavioral and brain sciences have been constant, rapid, and unremitting. The purpose of the Brain, Behavior, and Evolution series of titles published by ABC-CLIO is to bring these new breakthroughs in the behavioral sciences to the attention of the general public.

In the past decade, some of these scientific breakthroughs have come to inform the clinical and biomedical disciplines. That means that people suffering from all kinds of diseases and disorders, particularly brain and behavioral disorders, will benefit from these new therapies. That is exciting news indeed, and the general public needs to learn about these breakthrough findings and treatments. A whole new field called evolutionary medicine has begun to transform the way medicine is practiced and has led to new treatments and new approaches to diseases, like the dementias, sleep disorders, psychiatric diseases, and developmental disorders that seemed intractable to previous efforts. The series of books in the Brain, Behavior, and Evolution series seeks both to contribute to this new evolutionary approach to brain and behavior and to bring the insights emerging from the new evolutionary approaches to psychology, medicine, and anthropology to the general public.

The Brain, Behavior, and Evolution series was inspired by and brought to fruition with the help of Debora Carvalko at ABC-CLIO. The series editor,

Dr. Patrick McNamara, is the director of the Evolutionary Neurobehavior Laboratory in the Department of Neurology at Boston University School of Medicine. He has devoted most of his scientific work to development of an evolutionary approach to problems of sleep medicine and to neuro-degenerative diseases. Titles in the series will focus on applied and clinical implications of evolutionary approaches to the whole range of brain and behavioral disorders. Contributions are solicited from leading figures in the fields of interest to the series. Each volume will cover the basics, define the terms, and analyze the full range of issues and findings relevant to the clinical disorder or topic that is the focus of the volume. Each volume will demonstrate how the application of evolutionary modes of analysis leads to new insights on causes of disorder and functional breakdowns in brain and behavior relationships. Each volume, furthermore, will be aimed at both popular and professional audiences and will be written in a style appropriate for the general reader, the local and university libraries, and graduate and undergraduate students. The publications that become part of this series will therefore bring the gold discovered by scientists using evolutionary methods to understand brain and behavior to the attention of the general public, and ultimately, it is hoped, to those families and individuals currently suffering from those most intractable of disorders—the brain and behavioral disorders.

Preface: Hopeful Trends in Meeting the Challenge of the Dementias

Patrick McNamara

It is estimated that 24.3 million people around the world have dementia and that, with an estimated 4.6 million new cases every year, we can expect about 43 million people and their families to face the challenge of dementia by 2020. There are several forms of dementia, with the most common being Alzheimer's disease (40% of cases), vascular dementia with or without Alzheimer features (25%), and dementia with Lewy bodies (25%), the latter being related to the increasingly important form of dementia associated with Parkinson's disease. The annual healthcare costs for Alzheimer's disease alone is estimated at about $155 billion in the United States. A substantial portion of these costs is due to behavioral and neuropsychiatric disturbances associated with the dementing process—yet these neuropsychiatric and behavioral problems have only recently become the focus of study and treatment in the biomedical communities.

The successes of neuropsychiatric approaches to the dementias is measured in reduced suffering for patients and their families and reduced healthcare costs for the system as a whole. The authors of the chapters in these three volumes, devoted to emerging trends in dementia studies, have virtually all emphasized identification, study, and treatment of behavioral and neuropsychiatric problems of patients and their families. The reason they have done so is the dawning realization in both the biomedical and caregiving communities that targeting behavioral and neuropsychiatric problems of dementia leads to some pretty effective scientific studies of mechanisms and very effective and low-cost treatment programs that act to alleviate both patients' suffering and caregivers' burdens.

Although the standard, it has long been established that dementia most commonly occurs in older people, and that primary symptoms are memory impairment (both short- and long-term), deficits in executive functions, and impairments of abstract thinking and judgment. It has now become crystal clear that some of the best and earliest predictors of dementia risk are mood and personality changes, which all too often are misdiagnosed as depression or some other common mood disorder. Family members may express concern to a primary care physician, but these concerns too often get ignored or shunted aside as a standard mood disorder. It is vitally important to take reports of significant behavioral changes seriously as identification of cognitive components of a dementing process—may be a later-occurring symptom than the behavioral changes. Although the three-step diagnostic process (single question about memory, MMSE, neuropsychological testing) has high positive predictive value, it only detects 18% of future dementia cases. It is the behavioral and neuropsychiatric disturbances, along with incipient cognitive changes, that may yield better detection rates for dementia.

Tremendous progress has been made in identification of biomarkers for dementia. The use of functional imaging, proteomic, genetic, biochemical and electrophysiological markers, including sleep polysomnographic techniques, has meant that our ability to detect dementia early on has vastly improved. In addition, the new appreciation of the importance of behavioral and psychiatric problems in dementia as well as validated assessment tools to measure these behavioral problems suggests that it is time to deploy all these new techniques to identify those at risk for dementia so as to prevent or to slow onset of the disorder in these individuals. What is needed are large-scale, multisite, comparative studies that can evaluate optimal use and validity of these various techniques for detecting and selecting asymptomatic people at risk for dementia.

The recent Leon Thal Symposium 2009 in Las Vegas, Nevada, explored algorithms, biomarkers, and assessment tools for identifying asymptomatic individuals at elevated risk for dementia. The consensus recommendations of symposium participants included:

1. Establishment of a National Database for Longitudinal Studies as a shared research core resource;
2. Launch of a large collaborative study that will compare multiple screening approaches and biomarkers to determine the best method for identifying asymptomatic people at risk;

3. Initiation of a Global Database that extends the concept of the National Database for Longitudinal Studies for longitudinal studies beyond the United States; and

4. Development of an educational campaign that will promote healthy brain aging. (Khachaturian et al. 2010)

These are all laudable recommendations. But behavioral and neuropsychiatric assessment tools must be included in these large multisite studies of at-risk individuals.

A perusal of the essays in these volumes (volume 1 focuses on epidemiologic, descriptive, historical, and diagnostic innovations in dementia; volume 2 focuses on biobehavioral mechanisms of dementia; and volume 3 focuses on emerging treatment strategies including treatments for behavioral problems of dementia) leaves one with a sense of hope and confidence that the daunting challenges of the dementias, both for patients and for families, are finally being effectively addressed.

REFERENCE

Khachaturian, Z. S., D. Barnes, R. Einstein, et al. 2010. Developing a national strategy to prevent dementia: Leon Thal Symposium 2009. *Alzheimer's and Dementia* 6 (2): 89–97.

Chapter 1

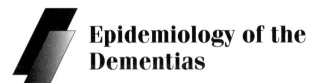

Epidemiology of the Dementias

Chengxuan Qiu and Laura Fratiglioni

Dementia is defined as a clinical syndrome characterized by progressive deterioration in multiple cognitive domains which is severe enough to interfere with daily functioning. Epidemiology deals with the distribution, determinants, and prevention of a disease in the population. Since the 1980s, numerous community-based prospective studies of aging and health have been implemented in the world; many of which have focused on dementia and its main subtypes of Alzheimer's disease (AD) and vascular dementia (VaD). These studies have significantly contributed to the understanding of epidemiology of the dementias, including occurrence, determinants, and prevention. In this chapter, we review the literature of epidemiological research in the dementias by focusing on the most recent studies.

OCCURRENCE

The occurrence of a disease can be measured as the proportion of people affected by the disease in a defined population at a specific time point (prevalence), or as the number of new cases that occur during a specific time period in a population at risk for developing that disease (incidence). The prevalence reflects the public health burden of the disease, whereas the incidence indicates the risk of developing that disease. The prevalence is determined by both incidence and duration of the disease, and in certain circumstances the prevalence may be estimated as incidence × average disease duration.

Prevalence

In a consensus report in 2005, it was estimated that more than 25 million people in the world were affected by dementia, most suffering from AD, with around 5 million new cases occurring every year (Ferri et al. 2005). As the population ages, the number of patients with dementia is anticipated to double every 20 years. In Europe, the number of dementia cases has reached more than 6 million in 2010; this number is projected to be 14 million in 2050 (Mura et al. 2010). In the United States, there were 4.5 million AD patients in the year 2000; the number is projected to reach 13.2 million by 2050 (Hebert et al. 2003). In the Asia Pacific region, the number of dementia cases will increase from 13.7 million in 2005 to 64.6 million by 2050 (Access Economics 2006). The global prevalence of dementia was estimated to be 3.9 percent in people aged 60+ years, with the regional prevalence being 1.6 percent in Africa, 4.0 percent in China and the western Pacific region, 4.6 percent in Latin America, 5.4 percent in Western Europe, and 6.4 percent in North America (Ferri et al. 2005). Figure 1.1 shows the age-specific prevalence of dementia across different regions. The prevalence of dementia is very low in persons under 60; after age 65, the rate doubles almost every five years until very old ages; nearly half of the oldest old (i.e., 90 years and older) become demented (von Strauss et al. 1999; Corrada et al. 2008). Thus, the overall prevalence and burden of the dementias depend largely on age structure of the population.

The prevalence of dementia appears to vary by regions across the world, but this may be due to variation in age structure of the populations, diagnostic accuracy, and disease duration or survival. In Europe, the pooling data suggest that the age-standardized prevalence in people aged 65 years or older is 6.4 percent for dementia and 4.4 percent for AD (Lobo et al. 2000). A systematic review of studies from developing countries reported that the overall prevalence in people aged 65 years or over was 5.3 percent for dementia and 3.4 percent for AD (Kalaria et al. 2008). The 10/66 Dementia Research Group found that the prevalence of dementia (DSM-IV criteria) in people aged 65+ years in seven developing nations varied widely from less than 0.5 percent to more than 6 percent (Llibre Rodriguez et al. 2008). The prevalence of dementia in India and Sub-Saharan Africa was about half of other regions (Ferri et al. 2005).

The proportion of subtype dementias also differs across continents. In Europe and North America, AD and VaD account for up to 70 percent and 20–30 percent, respectively, of all dementia cases (Lobo et al. 2000), whereas earlier studies from Asia showed a relatively high proportion for VaD (Chiu and Zhang 2000; Ikeda et al. 2001). The difference may be due

Figure 1.1

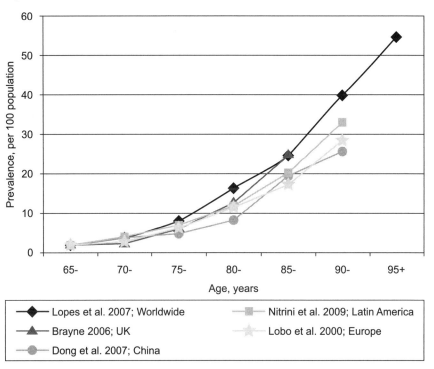

Age-specific prevalence rates of dementia (per 100 population) across the world. (Lobo et al. 2000; Brayne 2006; Dong et al. 2007; Lopes et al. 2007; Nitrini et al. 2009).

to variations in diagnostic criteria, ascertainment procedure of the cases, selective survival, and geographical distribution of vascular diseases such as stroke (Matthews and Brayne 2005). Indeed, the large-scale community-based surveys and meta-analysis in Asian countries have yielded the proportion of major dementia subtypes (e.g., AD and VaD) largely comparable with those in Western countries (Zhang et al. 2005; Kalaria et al. 2008). In addition, population-based neuropathological studies reveal that dementia often occurs with concomitant AD pathologies and cerebrovascular lesions (Schneider et al. 2007).

Incidence

Over the past decades, many incidence studies of dementia have become available; the majority of which are conducted among developed nations (Fratiglioni et al. 2008; Qiu, Kivipelto, et al. 2009). Pooling data in Europe suggested that the overall incidence of dementia in people aged 65 years or older was 19.4 per 1,000 person-years (Fratiglioni, Launer, et al. 2000), and the incidence was 13.6 per 1,000 person-years in Brazil (Kalaria et al. 2008). Figure 1.2 shows the age-specific incidence of dementia across the world. The incidence rates of dementia increase steeply with advancing age. In Europe, approximately two per 1,000 person-years become demented among people aged 65–69 years, and the incidence increases to 70 to 80 per 1,000 person-years for people 90 years or over (Fratiglioni, Launer, et al. 2000). The age-specific pattern of incidence for AD is similar to that of all-cause dementia, but the age-specific pattern for VaD is less stable. It remains debatable regarding whether the incidence of dementia continues to increase even in the oldest-old or reaches a plateau at a certain age. The Cache County Study found that the incidence of dementia increased with age, peaked, and then started to decline at extreme old ages for both men and women (Miech et al. 2002). But some meta-analyses and large-scale studies in Europe provided no evidence for the potential decline in the incidence of dementia among the oldest old (Fratiglioni et al. 2008; Matthews and Brayne 2005). The apparent decline seen in some studies may be an artifact due to poor response rate and survival effect in the very old. Several studies in Europe observed a higher incidence rate of dementia and AD in women than in men, especially among the oldest-old (Fratiglioni, Launer, et al. 2000), whereas studies in North America found no gender difference (Kawas et al. 2000; Kukull et al. 2002).

Mortality and Case-Fatality

Dementia is one of the leading causes of death in older people. However, death certificates grossly underreport its cause (Jin et al. 2004), even when multiple underlying causes of death are taken into account (Ganguli and Rodriguez 1999). The community-based follow-up studies could provide reliable data on mortality. In the Swedish Kungsholmen Project of people aged 75 years or over, the mortality rate of dementia was 2.4 per 100 person-years; 70 percent of incident dementia cases died within five years following the diagnosis (Agüero-Torres et al. 1999). A follow-up study of nursing home residents with advanced dementia suggested that 55 percent of the patients died over eighteen months; pneumonia, febrile episodes, and eating problems are the most frequent complications that significantly contribute to the six-month mortality (Mitchell et al. 2009).

Several community-based studies have shown that dementia increases the risk of death by two to five times (Agüero-Torres et al. 1999; Jagger

Figure 1.2

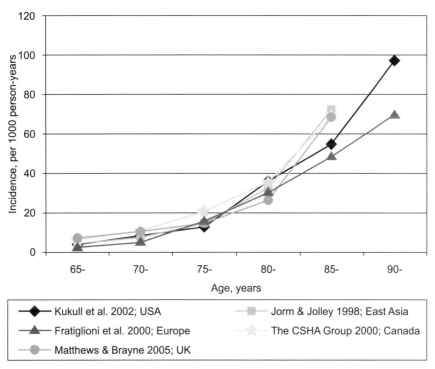

Age-specific incidence rates of dementia (per 1,000 person-years) across the world. (Jorm and Jolley 1998; Fratiglioni, Launer, et al. 2000; Canadian Study of Health and Aging Working Group 2000; Kukull et al. 2002; Matthews and Brayne 2005).

et al. 2000; Wolfson et al. 2001), supporting the malignancy of dementia. The median survival time of patients with dementia ranges from two to five years after the diagnosis depending on demographic features and comorbidity (Helzner et al. 2008; Xie et al. 2008). After the age of 85, although dementia still shortens life expectancy, the extent is somehow less than in younger-old people (Tschanz et al. 2004). Older age, male gender, low education, morbidities, and functional disability contribute to a shorter survival in patients with dementia (Helmer et al. 2001; Xie et al. 2008).

DETERMINANTS

The dementias are multifactorial disorders that are determined by genetic and environmental factors as well as their interactions.

Population-based prospective study is the major epidemiological approach to identifying influential factors for chronic multifactorial diseases such as dementia, in which the life-course approach should be taken into consideration (Whalley et al. 2006). Age is the most powerful determinant of dementia, and gene mutations contribute to a small proportion of all cases. Two groups of modifiable factors for late-life dementias have been established, that is, the "vascular risk factors" that have been strongly associated with an increased risk of dementia, and the "psychosocial factors" that may contribute to the delay of dementia onset. Evidence supporting these etiological profiles has been fully summarized elsewhere (Qiu, Kivipelto, et al. 2009; Qiu, Xu, and Fratiglioni 2010), which also provide a complete list of references when not otherwise specified herein.

Gene Mutations and Genetic Risk Factors

Mutations in amyloid precursor protein, presenilin-1, and presenilin-2 genes can cause early-onset familial AD that accounts for no more than 5 percent of all cases (Blennow et al. 2006). The majority of AD cases are sporadic, with considerable heterogeneity in their risk profiles and neuropathological features. First-degree relatives of AD patients have a higher lifetime risk for developing AD than relatives of nondemented people or the general population (Green et al. 2002; Seshadri and Wolf 2007). It is likely that shared genetic and environmental factors contribute to the familial aggregation; twin studies can address this issue. The Swedish Twin Study estimated that the heritability of AD ranged from 0.58 to 0.74, with other variance being attributable to environmental factors (Gatz et al. 2006). However, familial aggregation of AD can only be partially explained by known genetic factors such as APOE ε4 allele, indicating that other susceptibility genes may be involved in AD (Huang et al. 2004; Hayden et al. 2009).

The APOE ε4 allele is the only established genetic risk factor for both early and late-onset AD; it is a *susceptibility* gene, being neither necessary nor sufficient for the development of AD. The risk of AD increases with increasing number of the ε4 alleles in a dose-dependent manner (Qiu, Kivipelto, et al. 2004), but the risk effect decreases with increasing age. Overall, approximately 15 to 20 percent of AD cases are attributable to the APOE ε4 allele (Slooter et al. 1998; Qiu et al. 2004). Other candidate genes for AD, such as angiotensin-I converting enzyme gene, cholesterol 24-hydroxylase gene, and insulin degrading enzyme gene, remains to be clearly identified (Bertram et al. 2007).

Vascular Risk Factors

A number of vascular risk factors and disorders have been linked to dementia and AD as well, but some factors have a differential association with the risk of dementia depending on the age when the exposure is assessed. The age-dependent association is likely due to the pathophysiological and metabolic changes with age in vascular factors such as blood pressure, body mass index (BMI), and total serum cholesterol.

High Blood Pressure

An association of elevated blood pressure in midlife with an increased risk of dementia and AD later in life has been reported in several population-based studies (Qiu et al. 2005; Alonso et al. 2009); such an association was particularly evident for blood pressure levels of 160/95 mm Hg or higher, and for people who had high blood pressure but who were not treated with blood pressure–lowering drugs. It is plausible that long-term hypertension can be linked to the dementias by causing cerebral atherosclerosis and microvascular lesions (e.g., white-matter lesions, silent infarcts, and microbleeds). Furthermore, the postmortem and neuroimaging studies have directly linked midlife high blood pressure to the brain pathologies and imaging markers of AD such as neuritic plaques, neurofibrillary tangles, and more severe atrophy of the hippocampus (Korf et al. 2004; Launer et al. 2008).

Follow-up studies of late-life blood pressure and risk of dementia yield mixed results, largely depending on the length of follow-up. The short-term follow-up studies (e.g., less than 3 years) often found no association or even an inverse association between blood pressure and risk of dementia and AD (Qiu et al. 2005). Because dementia has a long latent period and blood pressure may start to decline a few years before the onset of the dementia syndrome due to ongoing brain aging and degenerative process, the inverse or lack of association has been interpreted as a consequence of the disease. However, studies of very old people (e.g., 75 years or older) with a longer follow-up period (e.g., more than 6 years) also revealed an increased risk of dementia associated with low blood pressure (Qiu, Winblad, et al. 2009), suggesting that among very old people low blood pressure may also contribute to the development of dementia, possibly by influencing cerebral blood perfusion.

Use of antihypertensive drugs has been associated with a decreased incidence of dementia and AD in several observational studies (Qiu et al. 2005); recent studies further suggest that the beneficial effect is more evident for young-old people, for angiotensin receptor blockers, and for long-term treatment (Peila et al. 2006; Haag et al. 2009; Li et al. 2010). Neuropathological data also showed fewer neuritic plaques and neurofibrillary tangles in medicated hypertensives than nonhypertensive groups, suggesting a possible effect of antihypertensive therapy against AD pathologies (Hoffman et al. 2009). However, systematic review and meta-analysis of major randomized controlled clinical trials conducted in hypertensive individuals have only shown a marginal beneficial effect of antihypertensive therapy against the dementias (Peters, Beckett, et al. 2008; McGuinness, Todd, et al. 2009).

Diabetes Mellitus

Diabetes has often been associated with VaD, but the association with AD is also reported in systematic reviews (Biessels et al. 2006; Lu et al. 2009; Kopf and Frölich 2009). Pooled analysis of eight follow-up studies has shown that diabetes is associated with a nearly 50 percent increased risk of dementia independent of cardiovascular factors and comorbidities (Lu et al. 2009). Neuropathological data from the Honolulu-Asia Aging Study indicated that diabetes, especially diabetes in combination with APOE ε4 allele, was associated with a substantially increased risk of dementia and a heavier burden of Alzheimer pathologies (Peila et al. 2002), although other studies remain uncertain whether diabetes is associated with AD pathologies (Arvanitakis et al. 2006; Sonnen et al. 2009). Furthermore, long-term follow-up studies show that midlife diabetes is more strongly associated with an elevated risk of dementia (Alonso et al. 2009; Xu et al. 2009), suggesting that long duration and more severe diabetes play a crucial role in determining the disease risk. In addition, a higher HbA1c is associated with lower cognitive function in individuals with diabetes (Cukierman-Yaffe et al. 2009), whereas a history of severe hypoglycemic episodes is associated with a greater risk of dementia (Whitmer et al. 2009). Finally, pre-diabetes, impaired glucose regulation, and impaired insulin secretion have also been associated with dementia (Xu et al. 2007). The association of diabetes with dementia and AD is likely due to the convergent effects of multiple pathological processes that include cerebral macrovascular and microvascular injury, chronic hyperglycemia, insulin resistance, advanced glycation end products, oxidative stress, and inflammation (Craft 2009).

Cerebrovascular Lesions and Cardiovascular Disease

Systematic reviews of population-based studies reveal an approximately two- to four-fold increased risk of incident dementia associated with clinical stroke (post-stroke dementia) (Pendlebury and Rothwell 2009; Savva and Stephan 2010). It is conceivable that an association of clinical stroke with AD is rarely reported due to the fact that a history of stroke is part of the current criteria for excluding the diagnosis of AD. However, asymptomatic cerebrovascular lesions such as silent brain infarcts and white-matter lesions have been associated with an increased risk of dementia and AD (Vermeer et al. 2003; Troncoso et al. 2008), although the association with AD is likely to be due to the inclusion of mixed dementia cases. In addition, a case-control study found that spontaneous cerebral emboli were associated with an increased odds ratio of AD and VaD (Purandare et al. 2006). The Cardiovascular Health Study (CHS) found that cardiovascular disease was associated with an increased incidence of dementia, with the highest risk seen among people with peripheral arterial disease, suggesting that extensive peripheral atherosclerosis is a risk factor for dementia (Newman et al. 2005). Atrial fibrillation, heart failure, and severe atherosclerosis measured with ankle-to-brachial index are also associated with the increased risk of dementia and AD (Ott et al. 1997; Qiu et al. 2006; van Oijen et al. 2007; Laurin et al. 2007). Neuropathological data show that cerebrovascular lesions and AD pathologies often coexist in patients with dementia, suggesting that these lesions may be the results of coinciding processes converging to cause additive brain damage and promote clinical manifestation of the dementia syndrome.

Body Mass Index

A lifespan-dependent relationship between BMI and risk of the dementias has emerged in which a higher BMI in midlife is related to an elevated risk of dementia and AD later in life, whereas an accelerated decline in BMI during late life may anticipate the onset of dementia (Gustafson 2006). The CHS showed that obesity at midlife was related to a higher risk of late-life dementia, whereas BMI measured after age 65 years was inversely related to dementia risk (Fitzpatrick et al. 2009). The long-term follow-up studies found a gradual decline in BMI over the years preceding dementia onset (Stewart et al. 2005; Hassing et al. 2009), which is supported by several follow-up studies of older people that show an association of low BMI and decline in BMI with subsequent development of dementia and AD (Atti et al. 2008; Beydoun, Lhotsky, et al. 2008). A meta-analysis of cohort studies suggested an increased risk of dementia for being underweight (pooled relative risk [RR], 1.36; 95 percent confidence interval [CI], 1.07–1.73) and obesity (RR, 1.42; 95 percent CI, 0.93–2.18); the association of increased dementia risk with obesity was stronger in studies with a longer follow-up period (e.g., more than 10 years) and younger age at BMI measurement (Rosengren et al. 2005; Beydoun, Beydoun, and Wang 2008). Thus, while obesity in midlife is a risk factor for late-life dementia, late-life low BMI and weight loss can be interpreted as markers for the predrome of dementia. Overweight or obesity in midlife may increase dementia risk through its close association with hypertension, hypercholesterolemia, diabetes, and other vascular diseases.

High Serum Cholesterol

As with blood pressure and BMI, an age-dependent association with the risk of dementia is also suggested for serum cholesterol, such that high total cholesterol at midlife is more consistently associated with an increased risk of dementia diagnosed more than 20–30 years later, whereas no or an inverse association between total cholesterol and the risk of dementia is often reported in cohort studies of older people. Interestingly, such a pattern of association was confirmed with all-cause dementia and AD, but not with VaD, in a meta-analysis and a follow-up study of middle aged cohort (Anstey et al. 2008; Solomon et al. 2009). Long-term follow-up studies have shown that total cholesterol levels begin to decline more than a decade before the onset of dementia (Stewart et al. 2007). This implies that decreasing total cholesterol after middle age and a lower cholesterol level in late life may reflect ongoing disease processes and thus could be a marker for future development of dementia (Solomon et al. 2007).

Cross-sectional studies suggest a lower likelihood of dementia associated with the use of statins, but this could be due to different prescribing patterns by physicians for people with and without dementia, such that dementia patients were less likely to be prescribed with lipid-lowering drugs than nondemented people (Rodriguez et al. 2002). Several follow-up studies show no beneficial effect of statin therapy or only a modestly decreased risk of dementia (Qiu, Kivipelto, et al. 2009). Neuropathological studies also show inconsistent results whether use of statins is associated with a reduced burden of Alzheimer pathological markers and infarcts in the brain (Li et al. 2007; Arvanitakis, Schneider, et al. 2008). A systematic review of randomized controlled trials concludes that statins given in late life to individuals at risk of vascular disease have no effect in preventing dementia (McGuinness, Craig, et al. 2009).

Nutrients and Dietary Factors

Several follow-up studies have reported a decreased risk of AD and dementia associated with increasing dietary or supplementary intake of antioxidants (e.g., vitamins E and C) (Barberger-Gateau et al. 2007), although some negative results are also reported (Gray et al. 2008). Similarly, studies also showed mixed results on the association of serum vitamin B_{12} and folate with the risk of dementia and AD (Luchsinger and Mayeux 2004). The Cochrane review of eight randomized clinical trials concludes that supplementations of folic acid and vitamin B_{12} have no benefits on cognition in healthy or cognitively impaired older people, although they are effective in reducing serum homocysteine levels (Malouf and Evans 2008).

A higher adherence to "Mediterranean diet" (i.e., a dietary pattern with higher intake of fish, fruits, and vegetables rich in antioxidants) has been associated with a reduced risk of dementia independent of vascular factors and physical activity in some studies (Scarmeas et al. 2006, 2009), but not in the French Three-City Study (Féart et al. 2009). A diet rich in high polyunsaturated and fish-related fats is known to be associated with a lower risk of vascular disease; thus, it is plausible to extend the beneficial effects to dementia. In support of this hypothesis, a systematic review suggested that a high dietary intake of fish and omega-3 polyunsaturated fatty acids (PUFAs) was associated with a decreased risk of cognitive decline (Fotuhi et al. 2009). However, this review also found that only four out of eight observational studies suggested a reduced risk of dementia and AD associated with consumption of fish and PUFAs independent of multiple potential confounders, and in two studies the protective effect disappeared after controlling for confounders such as demographics and income. Furthermore, two recent studies added no additional evidence for a possible role of high consumption of fish and PUFAs in reducing the risk of dementia and AD (Kröger et al. 2009; Devore et al. 2009). Finally, randomized clinical trials have failed to show any beneficial role for the use of PUFAs in the treatment and secondary prevention of dementia among elderly people (Fotuhi et al. 2009).

High Serum Homocysteine

Elevated total homocysteine (tHcy) is associated with an increased risk of cardiac and cerebrovascular disease and thus may increase dementia risk. The follow-up study of the Framingham cohort of older residents reported a nearly double-increased risk of AD and dementia associated with increase of one standard deviation in tHcy levels (Seshadri et al. 2002). A meta-analysis of prospective cohort studies revealed that hyperhomocysteine was associated with a pooled RR of 2.5 (95 percent CI, 1.4–4.6) for AD (van Dam and van Gool 2009). Despite the association, the beneficial effect of reducing serum homocysteine levels by supplement-ing vitamin B_{12} and folate on cognitive function remains to be established. Neuroimaging study suggested that higher plasma tHcy levels are associ-ated with smaller brain volume and silent brain infarcts, even in healthy middle-aged adults, suggesting that both neurodegenerative and vascular mechanisms may underlie the association of tHcy with brain aging and dementia (Seshadri et al. 2008).

Inflammation

Inflammation is known to play a pivotal role in the pathogenesis of ath-erosclerosis. A higher level of serum C-reactive protein (CRP) in midlife was linked to an increased risk of AD and VaD, suggesting that inflam-matory markers may reflect both peripheral and cerebral vascular mech-anisms related to dementia, and the process can be a measurable long time before the dementia syndrome is manifested (Schmidt et al. 2002). Follow-up studies of older adults also showed an association between high levels of serum inflammatory markers (e.g., CRP and interleukin-1,6) and an increased incidence of dementia and AD (Engelhart et al. 2004; Tan et al. 2007). In addition, the systematic review of observational stud-ies confirms that long-term use of nonsteroidal anti-inflammatory drugs (NSAIDs) (e.g., more than 2 years) is associated with a decreased risk of AD and dementia (Etminan et al. 2003), which provides additional evi-dence supporting the involvement of inflammation in AD and dementia. Thus, it seems plausible to hypothesize that inflammatory mechanisms play a part in the neurodegenerative process. However, neuropathologi-cal studies found no evidence for an association between use of NSAIDs and the reduced burden of AD pathologies (Arvanitakis, Grodstein, et al. 2008). Furthermore, the clinical trial of celecoxib or naproxen in AD pre-vention failed to show any beneficial effect of these drugs against AD; instead, an increased risk of AD related to drug therapy was observed (Martin et al. 2008).

Smoking

Follow-up studies have frequently shown an increased risk of demen-tia and AD associated with cigarette smoking, although the association may vary by APOE ε4 allele status (Qiu, Kivipelto, et al. 2009; Alonso et al. 2009). Meta-analyses of follow-up studies indicate that current smok-ing, compared to never smoking, is associated with an increased risk for dementia, especially for AD, but the increased risk for VaD seems less evident (Anstey et al. 2007; Peters, Poulter, et al. 2008). Neuropathological data show that the number of neuritic plaques is increased with increasing amount of cigarette smoking (Tyas et al. 2003). Thus, in contrast to the protective effect initially suggested in earlier cross-sectional and case-control studies, prospective cohort studies have actually provided convincing evidence that cigarette smoking, even long-term secondhand smoking (Barnes et al. 2010), is a risk factor for dementia and AD. Smoking is known to cause damage to the vascular system, but it remains unclear whether and how smoking can lead to Alzheimer pathologies.

Alcohol Consumption

Alcohol abuse may cause "alcoholic" dementia. A population-based study found that heavier alcohol drinkers at middle age had more than a three-fold increased risk of developing dementia later in life, especially among the carriers of APOE ε4 allele (Anttila et al. 2004). By contrast, epidemiological studies often reported a reduced incidence of dementia and AD associated with light-to-moderate alcohol intake (e.g., 1–3 drinks per day) (Qiu, Kivipelto, et al. 2009), leading to the hypothesis that light-to-moderate alcohol consumption may protect against dementia and cognitive decline. Two systematic reviews of prospective studies showed that light-to-moderate alcohol drinkers had an approximately 30–40 percent reduced risk of AD and dementia (Peters, Peters, et al. 2008; Anstey et al. 2009). However, a neuroimaging study did not support any protective effect of moderate alcohol consumption on brain aging (Paul et al. 2008). Moreover, the apparent cognitive benefits of light-to-moderate alcohol intake could be due to potential biases that result from methodological limitations of the observational studies such as information bias, confounding of socioeconomic status and healthy lifestyles, and inconsistent approaches of alcohol assessments.

Clustering of Vascular Factors and Disorders

Vascular risk factors and related disorders often coexist among elderly people. Several studies have consistently shown that the risk of dementia increases with an increasing burden of vascular factors (Whitmer et al. 2005; Qiu, Xu, Winblad, et al. 2010). In addition, the risk indices at both middle age and late life provide a reasonable estimation for the probability of future development of dementia, in which a cluster of multiple cardiovascular risk factors plays a relevant role (Kivipelto et al. 2006; Barnes et al. 2009). Clinical observations have suggested that treatment of multiple vascular factors (e.g., high blood pressure, diabetes, and ath-erosclerotic disease) is associated with a slower cognitive decline in AD patients without cerebrovascular disease in a progressive gradient man-ner, that is, the more vascular factors that are treated, the smaller the decline in global cognitive function (Deschaintre et al. 2009). Finally, gene-environment interaction, such as interactions of APOE ε4 allele severe atherosclerosis and high blood pressure, may be important in determin-ing the risk of dementia (Hofman et al. 1997; Qiu, Winblad, et al. 2003).

The metabolic syndrome is a constellation of obesity, dyslipidemia, high blood pressure, and hyperglycemia. Follow-up studies found little evidence for the association between the metabolic syndrome in late life and the risk of dementia and AD (Muller et al. 2007; Raffaitin et al. 2009), although some components of the syndrome (e.g., diabetes) have been linked to the dementias. It is likely that, due to age-related metabolic changes, a cluster of late-life specific factors in the metabolic syndrome may not be superior to some of its individual components in defining the risk of dementia.

Psychosocial Factors

Evidence from epidemiological research has been accumulating that some psychosocial factors and healthy lifestyle may postpone the onset of dementia, possibly by enhancing cognitive reserve. These factors include early-life high education, adult-life rich social network and social engage-ment, mentally stimulating activity, and regular physical exercise.

High Educational Attainments

Numerous longitudinal studies have consistently shown that a higher educational achievement in early life is associated with a decreased inci-dence of dementia, and of AD in particular (De Ronchi et al. 1998; Qiu et al. 2001; Ngandu et al. 2007). A meta-analysis of cohort studies reported that the lowest education, compared with the highest, was associated with an approximately 60 percent increased risk of dementia and AD (Caama-no-Isorna et al. 2006). The reserve hypothesis has been proposed to inter-pret this association, such that education could enhance cognitive reserve, which provides compensatory mechanisms to cope with degenerative pathologies in the brain and therefore delay the onset of the dementia syndrome (Stern 2006; Fratiglioni and Wang 2007). In addition, high edu-cational achievement can be a surrogate or an indicator of high intelligent quotient, high socioeconomic status, better living environment in early life, and less occupational toxic exposures experienced over adulthood; all these conditions favor a protective effect against dementia (De Ronchi et al. 1998; Qiu et al. 2001).

Social Network and Social Engagement

A systematic review of longitudinal studies suggested that a poor social network or social disengagement in late life was associated with an elevated risk of dementia (Fratiglioni et al. 2004). The dementia risk was also increased in older people with social isolation or with less frequent or unsatisfactory contacts with relatives and friends (Fratiglioni, Wang, et al. 2000). Furthermore, late-life low social engagement and a decline in social engagement from middle age to late life could double the risk of dementia (Wang et al. 2002; Saczynski et al. 2006). Finally, being widowed from midlife onwards was associated with a substantially increased risk of dementia, suggesting that living with a partner might imply cognitive and social challenges that have a potential protective effect against the development of dementia later in life (Håkansson et al. 2009). It is hypothesized that a rich social network and a high level of social engagement reflect better social support, which leads to better access to resources and material goods (Fratiglioni et al. 2004). In addition, large social networks can also provide intellectual stimulations that affect cognitive function and various health outcomes through behavioral, psychological, and physiological pathways. Finally, in line with the cognitive reserve hypothesis, neuropathological data have shown that the size of social networks could modify the association between Alzheimer pathologies and cognitive function, such that cognitive function remains higher in individuals with a heavier burden of global neuropathologies if they also have larger social networks (Bennett et al. 2006).

Mentally Stimulating Activity

Mentally stimulating activities at leisure time, such as reading, playing board games and musical instruments, knitting, gardening, and dancing, have been associated with a reduced risk of developing AD and dementia (Verghese et al. 2003; Akbaraly et al. 2009). A few studies have shown that a greater complexity of work, particularly the complex work with data or people, could reduce the risk of dementia (Andel et al. 2005; Karp et al. 2009), especially for VaD (Kröger et al. 2008), suggesting that greater mental requirements during the working life also play a relevant role. Complex mental activity could enhance cognitive reserve and delay the onset of dementia. In addition, a neuroimaging study reported that a high level of complex mental activity across the lifespan was correlated with a reduced rate of hippocampal atrophy, which means that mental activity may also provide brain reserve (Valenzuela et al. 2008).

Physical Activity

Regular physical exercise was associated with a delayed onset of dementia among cognitively normal elderly (Fratiglioni et al. 2004). Even low intensity physical exercise such as walking may reduce the risk of dementia (Abbott et al. 2004; Larson et al. 2006). A study of Medicare beneficiaries in the United States showed that higher levels of physical activity were associated with a gradual reduction in dementia risk, suggesting a possible dose-response association (Scarmeas et al. 2009). A recent systematic review of prospective studies revealed that the highest physical activity, compared with the lowest, reduced the risk of dementia and AD by approximately 30–45 percent (Hamer and Chida 2009). Regular physical activity is likely to promote vascular and circulatory health by reducing blood pressure, serum lipids, BMI or obesity, and blood glucose. Because physical activity also contains components of social and cognitive activities, it may reduce the risk or postpone the onset of dementia also by providing cognitive reserve.

Miscellaneous

Hormone Replacement Therapy

Hormone replacement therapy in postmenopausal women has been frequently reported to be associated with a lower risk of AD and dementia in numerous observational studies (Zandi et al. 2002; Qiu, Kivipelto, et al. 2009). However, the large-scale clinical trial of the Women's Health Initiative Memory Study (WHI-MS) showed that estrogen therapy alone or in combination with progestin did not reduce the incidence of probable dementia and mild cognitive impairment (MCI); instead, the active treatment with estrogen or estrogen plus progestin was found to be associated with a two-fold increased risk for dementia and MCI (Shumaker et al. 2004). It has been argued that in the WHI-MS hormone replacement therapy was given 10 to 15 years after the menopause when the "window of critical time" for putative beneficial effects of estrogen therapy on cognition may have been missed; thus, use of hormone therapy at a younger age close to the time of menopause may reduce the risk of dementia later in life (Harman et al. 2005).

Occupational Exposures

Manual work involving goods production was associated with an increased risk of AD and dementia, suggesting the possible role of occupational exposure to toxics in the development of dementia (Qiu, Karp, et al. 2003). Occupational exposure to heavy metals such as aluminum and mercury is suggested to be a risk factor for AD; even high consumption of aluminum from drinking water is associated with an elevated risk of AD and dementia (Rondeau et al. 2009). However, this remains to be confirmed by further studies. In addition, occupational exposure to extremely low-frequency electromagnetic fields (ELF-EMFs) has been related to an increased risk of dementia and AD in a few follow-up studies (Feychting et al. 2003; Qiu, Fratiglioni, et al. 2004). The meta-analysis of epidemiological studies suggests an association of occupational ELF-EMF exposure with AD (Garcia et al. 2008). The biological plausibility linking high ELF-EMF exposure to Alzheimer pathologies has been previously described (Sobel and Davanipour 1996).

Other Factors

Traumatic brain injury has been extensively investigated as a possible risk factor for AD. The meta-analysis of case-control studies supported an association between a history of head injury and the increased risk of AD (Fleminger et al. 2003). In contrast, some longitudinal studies found that AD was not associated with head trauma or only associated with severe traumatic head injury (Himanen et al. 2006).

Several studies have reported an association of depression with subsequent development of dementia and AD. A meta-analysis of cohort studies yielded a pooled RR of 1.9 (95 percent CI, 1.6–2.3) for AD, and the sensitive analysis suggested that depression could be a risk factor, rather than a prodrome, for AD (Ownby et al. 2006). However, it remains debatable regarding whether depression is a preclinical symptom or a pure risk factor for dementia and AD (Amieva et al. 2008).

PREVENTION OF DEMENTIA

Identification of modifiable risk and protective factors for dementia provides potential for the primary prevention of the disease (Fratiglioni et al. 2008; Middleton and Yaffe 2009). Evidence from recent epidemiological research supports the notion that preventive strategies aiming at postponing the onset of dementia can be implemented in the general community.

Epidemiological Evidence for Intervention Toward Dementia: A Summary

Epidemiological evidence supporting the potential etiological role of modifiable risk and protective factors in dementia and AD is summarized in Table 1.1. Evidence is considered *strong* when several high-quality studies, especially with regard to randomized controlled trials, consistently report the same finding; *moderately strong* evidence is also from high-quality studies but with a limited number, or the quality of studies is moderately high (e.g., population-based prospective studies) but with numerous reports, and the finding is supported by systematic reviews and meta-analyses. Evidence from randomized placebo-controlled trials for primary intervention against dementia is currently limited for reasons such as: (1) most clinical trials have been conducted among older adults (e.g., 65 years or older) when traditional vascular risk factors are less important in dementia due to age-related pathophysiological changes (e.g., statin therapy); (2) dementia has been only considered a secondary endpoint in most clinical trials (e.g., antihypertensive therapy), in which clear benefits for primary endpoints (e.g., coronary heart disease and stroke) are shown usually in a short period of observation; and (3) intervention measures have been implemented in a period (e.g., 2–3 years) that is not sufficient long to show any efficacy.

At the moment, we can conclude that moderately strong evidence, mostly from prospective observational studies, supports the hypotheses that vascular and psychosocial factors over the lifespan are involved in the development and clinical manifestation of AD and dementia.

Intervention Strategies Against Dementia

Intervention Toward Vascular Factors and Related Disorders

Most vascular risk factors and related disorders are modifiable or treatable and can serve as targets in the development of primary preventative strategies against dementia. For example, antihypertensive therapy has been shown to reduce the risk of dementia in observational studies, and this finding was partly confirmed by clinical trials. Furthermore, studies have confirmed that obesity and diabetes can be prevented by changing dietary habits and lifestyles, and that health education may help someone quit smoking. Finally, preventing recurrent cerebrovascular disease and maintaining sufficient cerebral blood perfusion seems to be critical for postponing expression of the dementia syndrome in older people. Thus, controlling high blood pressure and obesity, especially from middle age,

Table 1.1
Summary of Epidemiological Evidence Supporting the Modifiable Etiological
Factors of Dementia and Alzheimer's Disease

Profile	Risk, protective, or precipitating factors	Epidemiological evidence
Vascular factors	*Midlife risk factors*: High blood pressure, diabetes, high body mass index (obesity or overweight), hyperlipidemia or high cholesterol, and smoking	Moderately strong
	Late-life risk factors: Very high and very low blood pressure, diabetes, atherosclerosis, heart disease, cerebral microvascular disease (e.g., white matter lesions and infarcts), plasma hyperhomocysteine, and smoking	Moderately strong
	Late-life protective factors: Use of antihypertensive medications, use of non-steroidal anti-inflammatory drugs, light-to-moderate alcohol consumption (*note*: the protective effect of alcohol intake may be due to information bias, residual confounding, etc.)	Moderately strong
	Late-life precipitating factors or markers: Weight loss, low blood pressure in very old or decline in blood pressure, and low cholesterol or decline in serum cholesterol	Limited
Psychosocial factors	*Protective factors (lifespan)*: High education, rich social network, mentally-stimulating activity, active social engagement, and regular physical activity	Moderately strong

and preventing diabetes and recurrent stroke could be the primary preventive measures against late-life dementia.

Intervention Toward Psychosocial Factors and Lifestyles

High educational achievements in early life can provide cognitive reserve that benefits the whole life in terms of cognitive health and delaying the onset of late-life dementia. Extensive social networks and active engagements in intellectually stimulating activities such as reading, doing crossword puzzles, and playing board games significantly lower the risk of dementia by providing cognitive reserve or by reducing psychosocial stress. Thus, it is likely that mentally and socially integrated lifestyles could postpone the onset of dementia. Regular physical exercise may reduce the risk of the dementias resulting from cerebral atherosclerosis. Leisure activities with all three components of physical, mental, and social activities may have the most beneficial effect on dementia prevention (Karp et al. 2006).

Taken together, the most promising strategy for the primary prevention of dementia may be to encourage people implementing multiple preventative measures throughout the life course, including high educational attainment in childhood and early adulthood, an active control of vascular factors (e.g., smoking) and disorders (e.g., hypertension and diabetes) over adulthood, and maintenance of mentally, physically, and socially active lifestyles during middle age and later in life.

CONCLUSIONS

Dementia is a major cause of functional dependence, institutionalization, and mortality among elderly people. As the population ages in the decades to come, dementia will reach an epidemic level, a scenario that poses a serious threat not only to public health but also to the social and economic development of the modern society. Epidemiological studies have shown that vascular risk factors in middle age and later in life significantly contribute to the development and progression of the dementia syndrome, whereas extensive social network and active engagement in social, physical, and mental activities may delay the onset of the dementing disorders. Hence, one of the promising strategies to deal with the tremendous challenge from the epidemic of dementia is to implement appropriate intervention measures from the life-course perspective, such as achieving high education in early life and engaging in mentally stimulating activity over the course of adulthood to enhance cognitive reserve, and maintaining vascular health by adopting a healthy lifestyle and optimally controlling vascular diseases to reduce the burden of vascular lesions in the brain. These preventive measures will enable people to maintain cognitive ability in late life, even though they may have developed a high load of Alzheimer pathologies in their brain.

REFERENCES

Abbott, R. D., L. R. White, G. W. Ross, K. H. Masaki, J. D. Curb, and H. Petrovitch. 2004. Walking and dementia in physically capable elderly men. *JAMA* 292 (12): 1447–1453.

Access Economics Pty Limited Report for Asia Pacific Members of Alzheimer's Disease International. 2006. Dementia in the Asia Pacific region: The epidemic is here. www.accesseconomics.com.au/publicationsreports/showreport.php?id=99) (accessed March 5, 2010).

Agüero-Torres, H., L. Fratiglioni, Z. Guo, M. Viitanen, and B. Winblad. 1999. Mortality from dementia in advanced age: A five-year follow-up study of incident dementia cases. *Journal of Clinical Epidemiology* 52 (8): 737–743.

Akbaraly, T. N., F. Portet, S. Fustinoni, J. F. Dartigues, S. Artero, O. Rouaud, J. Touchon, K. Ritchie, and C. Berr. 2009. Leisure activities and the risk of dementia in the elderly: Results from the Three-City Study. *Neurology* 73 (11): 854–861.

Alonso, A., T. H. Mosley, R. F. Gottesman, D. Catellier, A. R. Sharrett, and J. Coresh. 2009. Risk of dementia hospitalisation associated with cardiovascular risk factors in midlife and older age: The Atherosclerosis Risk in Communities (ARIC) study. *Journal of Neurology, Neurosurgery and Psychiatry* 80 (11): 1194–1201.

Amieva, H., M. Le Goff, X. Millet, J. M. Orgogozo, K. Peres, P. Barberger-Gateau, H. Jacqmin-Gadda, and J. F. Dartigues. 2008. Prodromal Alzheimer's disease: Successive emergence of the clinical symptoms. *Annals of Neurology* 64 (5): 492–498.

Andel, R., M. Crowe, N. L. Pedersen, J. Mortimer, E. Crimmins, B. Johansson, and M. Gatz. 2005. Complexity of work and risk of Alzheimer's disease: A population-based study of Swedish twins. *Journals of Gerontology: Series B Psychological Sciences and Social Sciences* 60 (5): P251–258.

Anstey, K. J., D. M. Lipnicki, and L. F. Low. 2008. Cholesterol as a risk factor for dementia and cognitive decline: A systematic review of prospective studies with meta-analysis. *American Journal of Geriatric Psychiatry* 16 (5): 343–354.

Anstey, K. J., H. A. Mack, and N. Cherbuin. 2009. Alcohol consumption as a risk factor for dementia and cognitive decline: Meta-analysis of prospective studies. *American Journal of Geriatric Psychiatry* 17 (7): 542–555.

Anstey, K. J., C. von Sanden, A. Salim, and R. O'Kearney. 2007. Smoking as a risk factor for dementia and cognitive decline: A meta-analysis of prospective studies. *American Journal of Epidemiology* 166 (4): 367–378.

Anttila, T., E. L. Helkala, M. Viitanen, I. Kareholt, L. Fratiglioni, B. Winblad, H. Soininen, J. Tuomilehto, A. Nissinen, and M. Kivipelto. 2004. Alcohol drinking in middle age and subsequent risk of mild cognitive impairment and dementia in old age: A prospective population based study. *British Medical Journal* 329 (7465): 539.

Arvanitakis, Z., F. Grodstein, J. L. Bienias, J. A. Schneider, R. S. Wilson, J. F. Kelly, D. A. Evans, and D. A. Bennett. 2008. Relation of NSAIDs to incident AD, change in cognitive function, and AD pathology. *Neurology* 70 (23): 2219–2225.

Arvanitakis, Z., J. A. Schneider, R. S. Wilson, J. L. Bienias, J. F. Kelly, D. A. Evans, and D. A. Bennett. 2008. Statins, incident Alzheimer disease, change in cognitive function, and neuropathology. *Neurology* 70 (19): 1795–1802.

Arvanitakis, Z., J. A. Schneider, R. S. Wilson, Y. Li, S. E. Arnold, Z. Wang, and D. A. Bennett. 2006. Diabetes is related to cerebral infarction but not to AD pathology in older persons. *Neurology* 67 (11): 1960–1965.

Atti, A. R., K. Palmer, S. Volpato, B. Winblad, D. De Ronchi, and L. Fratiglioni. 2008. Late-life body mass index and dementia incidence: Nine-year follow-up data from the Kungsholmen Project. *Journal of the American Geriatrics Society* 56 (1): 111–116.

Barberger-Gateau, P., C. Raffaitin, L. Letenneur, C. Berr, C. Tzourio, J. F. Dartigues, and A. Alperovitch. 2007. Dietary patterns and risk of dementia: The Three-City Cohort Study. *Neurology* 69 (20): 1921–1930.

Barnes, D. E., K. E. Covinsky, R. A. Whitmer, L. H. Kuller, O. L. Lopez, and K. Yaffe. 2009. Predicting risk of dementia in older adults: The late-life dementia risk index. *Neurology* 73 (3): 173–179.

Barnes, D. E., T. J. Haight, K. M. Mehta, M. C. Carlson, L. H. Kuller, and I. B. Tager. 2010. Secondhand smoke, vascular disease, and dementia incidence: Findings from the Cardiovascular Health Cognition Study. *American Journal of Epidemiology* 171 (3): 292–302.

Bennett, D. A., J. A. Schneider, Y. Tang, S. E. Arnold, and R. S. Wilson. 2006. The effect of social networks on the relation between Alzheimer's disease pathology and level of cognitive function in old people: A longitudinal cohort study. *Lancet Neurology* 5 (5): 406–412.

Bertram, L., M. B. McQueen, K. Mullin, D. Blacker, and R. E. Tanzi. 2007. Systematic meta-analyses of Alzheimer disease genetic association studies: The AlzGene database. *Nature Genetics* 39 (1): 17–23.

Beydoun, M. A., H. A. Beydoun, and Y. Wang. 2008. Obesity and central obesity as risk factors for incident dementia and its subtypes: A systematic review and meta-analysis. *Obesity Reviews* 9 (3): 204–218.

Beydoun, M. A., A. Lhotsky, Y. Wang, G. Dal Forno, Y. An, E. J. Metter, L. Ferrucci, R. O'Brien, and A. B. Zonderman. 2008. Association of adiposity status and changes in early to mid-adulthood with incidence of Alzheimer's disease. *American Journal of Epidemiology* 168 (10): 1179–1189.

Biessels, G. J., S. Staekenborg, E. Brunner, C. Brayne, and P. Scheltens. 2006. Risk of dementia in diabetes mellitus: A systematic review. *Lancet Neurology* 5 (1): 64–74.

Blennow, K., M. J. de Leon, and H. Zetterberg. 2006. Alzheimer's disease. *Lancet* 368 (9533): 387–403.

Brayne, C. 2006. Incidence of dementia in England and Wales: The MRC cognitive function and ageing study. *Alzheimer Disease and Associated Disorders* 20 (3): S47–S51.

Caamano-Isorna, F., M. Corral, A. Montes-Martinez, and B. Takkouche. 2006. Education and dementia: A meta-analytic study. *Neuroepidemiology* 26 (4): 226–232.

Canadian Study of Health and Aging Working Group. 2000. The incidence of dementia in Canada. *Neurology* 55 (1): 66–73.

Chiu, H. F. K., and M. Y. Zhang. 2000. Dementia research in China. *International Journal of Geriatric Psychiatry* 15 (10): 947–953.

Corrada, M. M., R. Brookmeyer, D. Berlau, A. Paganini-Hill, and C. H. Kawas. 2008. Prevalence of dementia after age 90—Results from the 90+Study. *Neurology* 71 (5): 337–343.

Craft, S. 2009. The role of metabolic disorders in Alzheimer disease and vascular dementia: Two roads converged. *Archives of Neurology* 66 (3): 300–305.

Cukierman-Yaffe, T., H. C. Gerstein, J. D. Williamson, R. M. Lazar, L. Lovato, M. E. Miller, L. H. Coker, et al. 2009. Relationship between baseline glycemic control and cognitive function in individuals with type 2 diabetes and other cardiovascular risk factors: The Action to Control Cardiovascular Risk in Diabetes-Memory in Diabetes (ACCORD-MIND) trial. *Diabetes Care* 32 (2): 221–226.

De Ronchi, D., L. Fratiglioni, P. Rucci, A. Paternico, S. Graziani, and E. Dalmonte. 1998. The effect of education on dementia occurrence in an Italian population with middle to high socioeconomic status. *Neurology* 50 (5): 1231–1238.

Deschaintre, Y., F. Richard, D. Leys, and F. Pasquier. 2009. Treatment of vascular risk factors is associated with slower decline in Alzheimer disease. *Neurology* 73 (9): 674–680.

Devore, E. E., F. Grodstein, F. J. van Rooij, A. Hofman, B. Rosner, M. J. Stampfer, J. C. Witteman, and M. M. Breteler. 2009. Dietary intake of fish and omega-3 fatty acids in relation to long-term dementia risk. *American Journal of Clinical Nutrition* 90 (1): 170–176.

Dong, M. J., B. Peng, X. T. Lin, J. Zhao, Y. R. Zhou, and R. H. Wang. 2007. The prevalence of dementia in the People's Republic of China: A systematic analysis of 1980–2004 studies. *Age and Ageing* 36 (6): 619–624.

Engelhart, M. J., M. I. Geerlings, J. Meijer, A. Kiliaan, A. Ruitenberg, J. C. van Swieten, T. Stijnen, A. Hofman, J. C. Witteman, and M. M. Breteler. 2004. Inflammatory proteins in plasma and the risk of dementia: The Rotterdam study. *Archives of Neurology* 61 (5): 668–672.

Etminan, M., S. Gill, and A. Samii. 2003. Effect of non-steroidal anti-inflammatory drugs on risk of Alzheimer's disease: Systematic review and meta-analysis of observational studies. *British Medical Journal* 327 (7407): 128.

Féart, C., C. Samieri, V. Rondeau, H. Amieva, F. Portet, J. F. Dartigues, N. Scarmeas, and P. Barberger-Gateau. 2009. Adherence to a Mediterranean diet, cognitive decline, and risk of dementia. *JAMA* 302 (6): 638–648.

Ferri, C. P., M. Prince, C. Brayne, H. Brodaty, L. Fratiglioni, M. Ganguli, K. Hall, et al. 2005. Global prevalence of dementia: A Delphi consensus study. *Lancet* 366 (9503): 2112–2117.

Feychting, M., F. Jonsson, N. L. Pedersen, and A. Ahlbom. 2003. Occupational magnetic field exposure and neurodegenerative disease. *Epidemiology* 14 (4): 413–419.

Fitzpatrick, A. L., L. H. Kuller, O. L. Lopez, P. Diehr, E. S. O'Meara, W. T. Longstreth Jr., and J. A. Luchsinger. 2009. Midlife and late-life obesity and the risk of dementia: The Cardiovascular Health Study. *Archives of Neurology* 66 (3): 336–342.

Fleminger, S., D. L. Oliver, S. Lovestone, S. Rabe-Hesketh, and A. Giora. 2003. Head injury as a risk factor for Alzheimer's disease: The evidence 10 years on; a partial replication. *Journal of Neurology, Neurosurgery and Psychiatry* 74 (7): 857–862.

Fotuhi, M., P. Mohassel, and K. Yaffe. 2009. Fish consumption, long-chain omega-3 fatty acids and risk of cognitive decline on Alzheimer disease: A complex association. *Nature Clinical Practice Neurology* 5 (3): 140–152.

Fratiglioni, L., L. J. Launer, K. Andersen, M. M. Breteler, J. R. Copeland, J. F. Dartigues, A. Lobo, J. Martinez-Lage, H. Soininen, and A. Hofman. 2000. Incidence of dementia and major subtypes in Europe: A collaborative study of population-based cohorts. *Neurology* 54 (11 Suppl 5): S10–S15.

Fratiglioni, L., S. Paillard-Borg, and B. Winblad. 2004. An active and socially integrated lifestyle in late life might protect against dementia. *Lancet Neurology* 3 (6): 343–353.

Fratiglioni, L., E. von Strauss, and C. Qiu. 2008. Epidemiology of the dementias of old age. In *The Oxford Textbook of Old Age Psychiatry*, ed. T. Dening, R. Jacoby, C. Oppenheimer, and A. Thomas, 391–406. London: Oxford University Press.

Fratiglioni, L., and H. X. Wang. 2007. Brain reserve hypothesis in dementia. *Journal of Alzheimer's Disease* 12 (1): 11–22.

Fratiglioni, L., H. X. Wang, K. Ericsson, M. Maytan, and B. Winblad. 2000. Influence of social network on occurrence of dementia: A community-based longitudinal study. *Lancet* 355 (9212): 1315–1319.

Ganguli, M., and E. G. Rodriguez. 1999. Reporting of dementia on death certificates: A community study. *Journal of American Geriatric Society* 47 (7): 842–849.

Garcia, A. M., A. Sisternas, and S. P. Hoyos. 2008. Occupational exposure to extremely low frequency electric and magnetic fields and Alzheimer disease: A meta-analysis. *International Journal of Epidemiology* 37 (2): 329–340.

Gatz, M., C. A. Reynolds, L. Fratiglioni, B. Johansson, J. A. Mortimer, S. Berg, A. Fiske, and N. L. Pedersen. 2006. Role of genes and environments for explaining Alzheimer disease. *Archives of General Psychiatry* 63 (2): 168–174.

Gray, S. L., M. L. Anderson, P. K. Crane, J. C. Breitner, W. McCormick, J. D. Bowen, L. Teri, and E. Larson. 2008. Antioxidant vitamin supplement use and risk of dementia or Alzheimer's disease in older adults. *Journal of American Geriatric Society* 56 (2): 291–295.

Green, R. C., L. A. Cupples, R. Go, K. S. Benke, T. Edeki, P. A. Griffith, M. Williams, et al. 2002. Risk of dementia among white and African American relatives of patients with Alzheimer disease. *JAMA* 287 (3): 329–336.

Gustafson, D. 2006. Adiposity indices and dementia. *Lancet Neurology* 5 (8): 713–720.

Haag, M. D., A. Hofman, P. J. Koudstaal, B. H. Stricker, and M. M. Breteler. 2009. Statins are associated with a reduced risk of Alzheimer disease regardless of lipophilicity: The Rotterdam Study. *Journal of Neurology, Neurosurgery and Psychiatry* 80 (1): 13–17.

Håkansson, K., S. Rovio, E. L. Helkala, A. R. Vilska, B. Winblad, H. Soininen, A. Nissinen, A. H. Mohammed, and M. Kivipelto. 2009. Association between mid-life marital status and cognitive function in later life: Population based cohort study. *British Medical Journal* 339: b2462.

Hamer, M., and Y. Chida. 2009. Physical activity and risk of neurodegenerative disease: A systematic review of prospective evidence. *Psychological Medicine* 39 (1): 3–11.

Harman, S. M., F. Naftolin, E. A. Brinton, and D. R. Judelson. 2005. Is the estrogen controversy over? Deconstructing the Women's Health Initiative Study: A critical evaluation of the evidence. *Annals of New York Academic Science* 1052: 43–56.

Hassing, L. B., A. K. Dahl, V. Thorvaldsson, S. Berg, M. Gatz, N. L. Pedersen, and B. Johansson. 2009. Overweight in midlife and risk of dementia: A 40-year follow-up study. *International Journal of Obesity (Lond)* 33 (8): 893–898.

Hayden, K. M., P. P. Zandi, N. A. West, J. T. Tschanz, M. C. Norton, C. Corcoran, J. C. S. Breitner, and K. A. Welsh-Bohmer. 2009. Effects of family history and apolipoprotein E ε4 status on cognitive decline in the absence of Alzheimer dementia: The Cache County Study. *Archives of Neurology* 66 (11): 1378–1383.

Hebert, L. E., P. A. Scherr, J. L. Bienias, D. A. Bennett, and D. A. Evans. 2003. Alzheimer disease in the US population: Prevalence estimates using the 2000 census. *Archives of Neurology* 60 (8): 1119–1122.

Helmer, C., P. Joly, L. Letenneur, D. Commenges, and J. F. Dartigues. 2001. Mortality with dementia: Results from a French prospective community-based cohort. *American Journal of Epidemiology* 154 (7): 642–648.

Helzner, E. P., N. Scarmeas, S. Cosentino, M. X. Tang, N. Schupf, and Y. Stern. 2008. Survival in Alzheimer disease: A multiethnic, population-based study of incident cases. *Neurology* 71 (19): 1489–1495.

Himanen, L., R. Portin, H. Isoniemi, H. Helenius, T. Kurki, and O. Tenovuo. 2006. Longitudinal cognitive changes in traumatic brain injury: A 30-year follow-up study. *Neurology* 66 (2): 187–192.

Hoffman, L. B., J. Schmeidler, G. T. Lesser, M. S. Beeri, D. P. Purohit, H. T. Grossman, and V. Haroutunian. 2009. Less Alzheimer disease neuropathology in medicated hypertensive than nonhypertensive persons. *Neurology* 72 (20): 1720–1726.

Hofman, A., A. Ott, M. M. Breteler, M. L. Bots, A. J. Slooter, F. van Harskamp, C. N. van Duijn, C. Van Broeckhoven, and D. E. Grobbee. 1997. Atherosclerosis, apolipoprotein E, and prevalence of dementia and Alzheimer's disease in the Rotterdam Study. *Lancet* 349 (9046): 151–154.

Huang, W., C. Qiu, E. von Strauss, B. Winblad, and L. Fratiglioni. 2004. APOE genotype, family history of dementia, and Alzheimer disease risk: A six-year follow-up study. *Archives of Neurology* 61 (12): 1930–1934.

Ikeda, M., K. Hokoishi, N. Maki, A. Nebu, N. Tachibana, K. Komori, K. Shigenobu, R. Fukuhara, and H. Tanabe. 2001. Increased prevalence of vascular dementia in Japan: A community-based epidemiological study. *Neurology* 57 (5): 839–844.

Jagger, C., K. Andersen, M. M. Breteler, J. R. Copeland, C. Helmer, M. Baldereschi, L. Fratiglioni, et al. 2000. Prognosis with dementia in Europe: A collaborative study of population-based cohorts. *Neurology* 54 (11 Suppl 5): S16–S20.

Jin, Y. P., M. Gatz, B. Johansson, and N. L. Pedersen. 2004. Sensitivity and specificity of dementia coding in two Swedish disease registries. *Neurology* 63 (4): 739–741.

Jorm, A. F., and D. Jolley. 1998. The incidence of dementia: A meta-analysis. *Neurology* 51 (3): 728–733.

Kalaria, R. N., G. E. Maestre, R. Arizaga, R. P. Friedland, D. Galasko, K. T. Hall, J. A. Luchsinger, et al. 2008. Alzheimer's disease and vascular dementia in developing countries: Prevalence, management, and risk factors. *Lancet Neurology* 7 (9): 812–826.

Karp, A., R. Andel, M. G. Parker, H. X. Wang, B. Winblad, and L. Fratiglioni. 2009. Mentally stimulating activities at work during midlife and dementia risk after age 75: Follow-up study from the Kungsholmen Project. *American Journal of Geriatric Psychiatry* 17 (3): 227–236.

Karp, A., S. Paillard-Borg, H. X. Wang, M. Silverstein, B. Winblad, and L. Fratiglioni. 2006. Mental, physical and social components in leisure activities equally contribute to decrease dementia risk. *Dementia and Geriatric Cognitive Disorders* 21 (2): 65–73.

Kawas, C., S. Gray, R. Brookmeyer, J. Fozard, and A. Zonderman. 2000. Age-specific incidence rates of Alzheimer's disease: The Baltimore Longitudinal Study of Aging. *Neurology* 54 (11): 2072–2077.

Kivipelto, M., T. Ngandu, T. Laatikainen, B. Winblad, H. Soininen, and J. Tuomilehto. 2006. Risk score for the prediction of dementia risk in 20 years among middle aged people: A longitudinal, population-based study. *Lancet Neurology* 5 (9): 735–741.

Kopf, D., and L. Frölich. 2009. Risk of incident Alzheimer's disease in diabetic patients: A systematic review of prospective trials. *Journal of Alzheimer's Disease* 16 (4): 677–685.

Korf, E. S., L. R. White, P. Scheltens, and L. J. Launer. 2004. Midlife blood pressure and the risk of hippocampal atrophy: The Honolulu-Asia Aging Study. *Hypertension* 44 (1): 29–34.

Kröger, E., R. Andel, J. Lindsay, Z. Benounissa, R. Verreault, and D. Laurin. 2008. Is complexity of work associated with risk of dementia? The Canadian Study of Health and Aging. *American Journal of Epidemiology* 167 (7): 820–830.

Kröger, E., R. Verreault, P. H. Carmichael, J. Lindsay, P. Julien, E. Dewailly, P. Ayotte, and D. Laurin. 2009. Omega-3 fatty acids and risk of dementia: The Canadian Study of Health and Aging. *American Journal of Clinical Nutrition* 90 (1): 184–192.

Kukull, W. A., R. Higdon, J. D. Bowen, W. C. McCormick, L. Teri, G. D. Schellenberg, G. van Belle, L. Jolley, and E. B. Larson. 2002. Dementia and Alzheimer disease incidence: A prospective cohort study. *Archives of Neurology* 59 (11): 1737–1746.

Larson, E. B., L. Wang, J. D. Bowen, W. C. McCormick, L. Teri, P. Crane, and W. Kukull. 2006. Exercise is associated with reduced risk for incident dementia among persons 65 years of age and older. *Annals of Internal Medicine* 144 (2): 73–81.

Launer, L. J., H. Petrovitch, G. W. Ross, W. Markesbery, and L. R. White. 2008. AD brain pathology: Vascular origins? Results from the HAAS autopsy study. *Neurobiology of Aging* 29 (10): 1587–1590.

Laurin, D., K. H. Masaki, L. R. White, and L. J. Launer. 2007. Ankle-to-brachial index and dementia: The Honolulu-Asia Aging Study. *Circulation* 116 (20): 2269–2274.

Li, G., E. B. Larson, J. A. Sonnen, J. B. Shofer, E. C. Petrie, A. Schantz, E. R. Peskind, M. A. Raskind, J. C. S. Breitner, and T. J. Montine. 2007. Statin therapy is associated with reduced neuropathologic changes of Alzheimer disease. *Neurology* 69 (9): 878–885.

Li, N. C., A. Lee, R. A. Whitmer, M. Kivipelto, E. Lawler, L. E. Kazis, and B. Wolozin. 2010. Use of angiotensin receptor blockers and risk of dementia in a predominantly male population: Prospective cohort analysis. *British Medical Journal* 340: b5465.

Llibre Rodriguez, J. J., C. P. Ferri, D. Acosta, M. Guerra, Y. G. Huang, K. S. Jacob, E. S. Krishnamoorthy, et al. 2008. Prevalence of dementia in Latin America, India, and China: A population-based cross-sectional survey. *Lancet* 372 (9637): 464–474.

Lobo, A., L. J. Launer, L. Fratiglioni, K. Andersen, A. Di Carlo, M. M. Breteler, J. R. Copeland, et al. 2000. Prevalence of dementia and major subtypes in Europe: A collaborative study of population-based cohorts. *Neurology* 54 (11 Suppl 5): S4–S9.

Lopes, M. A., S. R. Hototian, G. C. Reis, H. Elkis, and C. M. C. Bottino. 2007. Systematic review of dementia prevalence 1994 to 2000. *Dementia and Neuropsychologia* 1 (3): 230–240.

Lu, F. P., K. P. Lin, and H. K. Kuo. 2009. Diabetes and the risk of multi-system aging phenotypes: A systematic review and meta-analysis. *PLoS One* 4 (1): e4144.

Luchsinger, J. A., and R. Mayeux. 2004. Dietary factors and Alzheimer's disease. *Lancet Neurology* 3 (10): 579–587.

Malouf, R., and J. G. Evans. 2008. Folic acid with or without vitamin B12 for the prevention and treatment of healthy elderly and demented people. *Cochrane Database of Systematic Reviews* (4): CD004514.

Martin, B. K., C. Szekely, J. Brandt, S. Piantadosi, J. C. S. Breitner, S. Craft, D. Evans, R. Green, and M. Mullan. 2008. Cognitive function over time in the Alzheimer's disease anti-inflammatory prevention trial (ADAPT): Results of a randomized, controlled trial of naproxen and celecoxib. *Archives of Neurology* 65 (7): 896–905.

Matthews, F., and C. Brayne. 2005. The incidence of dementia in England and Wales: Findings from the five identical sites of the MRC CFA Study. *PLoS Medicine* 2 (8): e193.

McGuinness, B., D. Craig, R. Bullock, and P. Passmore. 2009. Statins for the prevention of dementia. *Cochrane Database of Systematic Reviews* (2): CD003160.

McGuinness, B., S. Todd, P. Passmore, and R. Bullock. 2009. Blood pressure lowering in patients without prior cerebrovascular disease for prevention of cognitive impairment and dementia. *Cochrane Database of Systematic Reviews* (4): CD004034.

Middleton, L. E., and K. Yaffe. 2009. Promising strategies for the prevention of dementia. *Archives of Neurology* 66 (10): 1210–1215.

Miech, R. A., J. C. Breitner, P. P. Zandi, A. S. Khachaturian, J. C. Anthony, and L. Mayer. 2002. Incidence of AD may decline in the early 90s for men, later for women: The Cache County Study. *Neurology* 58 (2): 209–218.

Mitchell, S. L., J. M. Teno, D. K. Kiely, M. L. Shaffer, R. N. Jones, H. G. Prigerson, L. Volicer, J. L. Givens, and M. B. Hamel. 2009. The clinical course of advanced dementia. *New England Journal of Medicine* 361 (16): 1529–1538.

Muller, M., M. X. Tang, N. Schupf, J. J. Manly, R. Mayeux, and J. A. Luchsinger. 2007. Metabolic syndrome and dementia risk in a multiethnic elderly cohort. *Dementia and Geriatric Cognitive Disorders* 24 (3): 185–192.

Mura, T., J. F. Dartigues, and C. Berr. 2010. How many dementia cases in France and Europe? Alternative projections and scenarios 2010–2050. *European Journal of Neurology* 17 (2): 252–259.

Newman, A. B., A. L. Fitzpatrick, O. Lopez, S. Jackson, C. Lyketsos, W. Jagust, D. Ives, S. T. Dekosky, and L. H. Kuller. 2005. Dementia and Alzheimer's disease incidence in relationship to cardiovascular disease in the Cardiovascular Health Study cohort. *Journal of the American Geriatrics Society* 53 (7): 1101–1117.

Ngandu, T., E. von Strauss, E. L. Helkala, B. Winblad, A. Nissinen, J. Tuomilehto, H. Soininen, and M. Kivipelto. 2007. Education and dementia: What lies behind the association? *Neurology* 69 (14): 1442–1450.

Nitrini, R., C. M. C. Bottino, C. Albala, N. S. C. Capunay, C. Ketzoian, J. J. L. Rodriguez, G. E. Maestre, A. T. A. Ramos-Cerqueira, and P. Caramelli. 2009. Prevalence of dementia in Latin America: A collaborative study of population-based cohorts. *International Psychogeriatrics* 21 (4): 622–630.

Ott, A., M. M. Breteler, M. C. de Bruyne, F. van Harskamp, D. E. Grobbee, and A. Hofman. 1997. Atrial fibrillation and dementia in a population-based study: The Rotterdam Study. *Stroke* 28 (2): 316–321.

Ownby, R. L., E. Crocco, A. Acevedo, V. John, and D. Loewenstein. 2006. Depression and risk for Alzheimer disease: Systematic review, meta-analysis, and metaregression analysis. *Archives of General Psychiatry* 63 (5): 530–538.

Paul, C. A., R. Au, L. Fredman, J. M. Massaro, S. Seshadri, C. DeCarli, and P. A. Wolf. 2008. Association of alcohol consumption with brain volume in the Framingham study. *Archives of Neurology* 65 (10): 1363–1367.

Peila, R., B. L. Rodriguez, and L. J. Launer. 2002. Type 2 diabetes, APOE gene, and the risk for dementia and related pathologies: The Honolulu-Asia Aging Study. *Diabetes* 51 (4): 1256–1262.

Peila, R., L. R. White, K. Masaki, H. Petrovitch, and L. J. Launer. 2006. Reducing the risk of dementia: Efficacy of long-term treatment of hypertension. *Stroke* 37 (5): 1165–1170.

Pendlebury, S. T., and P. M. Rothwell. 2009. Prevalence, incidence, and factors associated with pre-stroke and post-stroke dementia: A systematic review and meta-analysis. *Lancet Neurology* 8 (11): 1006–1018.

Peters, R., N. Beckett, F. Forette, J. Tuomilehto, R. Clarke, C. Ritchie, A. Waldman, et al. 2008. Incident dementia and blood pressure lowering in the Hypertension in the Very Elderly Trial cognitive function assessment (HYVET-COG): A double-blind, placebo controlled trial. *Lancet Neurology* 7 (8): 683–689.

Peters, R., J. Peters, J. Warner, N. Beckett, and C. Bulpitt. 2008. Alcohol, dementia and cognitive decline in the elderly: A systematic review. *Age and Ageing* 37 (5): 505–512.

Peters, R., R. Poulter, J. Warner, N. Beckett, L. Burch, and C. Bulpitt. 2008. Smoking, dementia and cognitive decline in the elderly: A systematic review. *BMC Geriatrics* 8: 36.

Purandare, N., A. Burns, K. J. Daly, J. Hardicre, J. Morris, G. Macfarlane, and C. McCollum. 2006. Cerebral emboli as a potential cause of Alzheimer's disease and vascular dementia: Case-control study. *British Medical Journal* 332 (7550): 1119–1122.

Qiu, C., L. Backman, B. Winblad, H. Agüero-Torres, and L. Fratiglioni. 2001. The influence of education on clinically diagnosed dementia incidence and mortality data from the Kungsholmen project. *Archives of Neurology* 58 (12): 2034–2039.

Qiu, C., L. Fratiglioni, A. Karp, B. Winblad, and T. Bellander. 2004. Occupational exposure to electromagnetic fields and risk of Alzheimer's disease. *Epidemiology* 15 (6): 687–694.

Qiu, C., A. Karp, E. von Strauss, B. Winblad, L. Fratiglioni, and T. Bellander. 2003. Lifetime principal occupation and risk of Alzheimer's disease in the Kungsholmen project. *American Journal of Industrial Medicine* 43 (2): 204–211.

Qiu, C., M. Kivipelto, H. Agüero-Torres, B. Winblad, and L. Fratiglioni. 2004. Risk and protective effects of the APOE gene towards Alzheimer's disease in the Kungsholmen project: Variation by age and sex. *Journal of Neurology, Neurosurgery and Psychiatry* 75 (6): 828–833.

Qiu, C., M. Kivipelto, and E. von Strauss. 2009. Epidemiology of Alzheimer's disease: occurrence, determinants, and strategies toward intervention. *Dialogues in Clinical Neuroscience* 11 (2): 111–128.

Qiu, C., B. Winblad, J. Fastbom, and L. Fratiglioni. 2003. Combined effects of APOE genotype, blood pressure, and antihypertensive drug use on incident AD. *Neurology* 61 (5): 655–660.

Qiu, C., B. Winblad, and L. Fratiglioni. 2005. The age-dependent relation of blood pressure to cognitive function and dementia. *Lancet Neurology* 4 (8): 487–499.

Qiu, C., B. Winblad, and L. Fratiglioni. 2009. Low diastolic pressure and risk of dementia in very old people: A longitudinal study. *Dementia and Geriatric Cognitive Disorders* 28 (3): 213–219.

Qiu, C., B. Winblad, A. Marengoni, I. Klarin, J. Fastbom, and L. Fratiglioni. 2006. Heart failure and risk of dementia and Alzheimer disease: A population-based cohort study. *Archives of Internal Medicine* 166 (9): 1003–1008.

Qiu, C., W. Xu, and L. Fratiglioni. 2010. Vascular and psychosocial factors for Alzheimer's disease: Epidemiological evidence toward intervention. *Journal of Alzheimer's Disease* 20 (3): 689–697.

Qiu, C., W. Xu, B. Winblad, and L. Fratiglioni. 2010. Vascular risk profiles for dementia and Alzheimer's disease in very old people: A population-based longitudinal study. *Journal of Alzheimer's Disease* 20 (1): 293–300.

Raffaitin, C., H. Gin, J. P. Empana, C. Helmer, C. Berr, C. Tzourio, F. Portet, J. F. Dartigues, A. Alperovitch, and P. Barberger-Gateau. 2009. Metabolic syndrome and risk for incident Alzheimer's disease or vascular dementia: The Three-City Study. *Diabetes Care* 32 (1): 169–174.

Rodriguez, E. G., H. H. Dodge, M. A. Birzescu, G. P. Stoehr, and M. Ganguli. 2002. Use of lipid-lowering drugs in older adults with and without dementia: A community-based epidemiological study. *Journal of the American Geriatrics Society* 50 (11): 1852–1856.

Rondeau, V., H. Jacqmin-Gadda, D. Commenges, C. Helmer, and J. F. Dartigues. 2009. Aluminum and silica in drinking water and the risk of Alzheimer's disease or cognitive decline: Findings from 15-year follow-up of the PAQUID cohort. *American Journal of Epidemiology* 169 (4): 489–496.

Rosengren, A., I. Skoog, D. Gustafson, and L. Wilhelmsen. 2005. Body mass index, other cardiovascular risk factors, and hospitalization for dementia. *Archives of Internal Medicine* 165 (3): 321–326.

Saczynski, J. S., L. A. Pfeifer, K. Masaki, E. S. Korf, D. Laurin, L. White, and L. J. Launer. 2006. The effect of social engagement on incident dementia: The Honolulu-Asia Aging Study. *American Journal of Epidemiology* 163 (5): 433–440.

Savva, G. M. and B. C. M. Stephan. 2010. Epidemiological studies of the effect of stroke on incident dementia: A systematic review. *Stroke* 41 (1): E41–E46.

Scarmeas, N., J. A. Luchsinger, N. Schupf, A. M. Brickman, S. Cosentino, M. X. Tang, and Y. Stern. 2009. Physical activity, diet, and risk of Alzheimer disease. *JAMA* 302 (6): 627–637.

Scarmeas, N., Y. Stern, R. Mayeux, and J. A. Luchsinger. 2006. Mediterranean diet, Alzheimer disease, and vascular mediation. *Archives of Neurology* 63 (12): 1709–1717.

Schmidt, R., H. Schmidt, J. D. Curb, K. Masaki, L. R. White, and L. J. Launer. 2002. Early inflammation and dementia: A 25-year follow-up of the Honolulu-Asia Aging Study. *Annals of Neurology* 52 (2): 168–174.

Schneider, J. A., Z. Arvanitakis, W. Bang, and D. A. Bennett. 2007. Mixed brain pathologies account for most dementia cases in community-dwelling older persons. *Neurology* 69 (24): 2197–2204.

Seshadri, S., A. Beiser, J. Selhub, P. F. Jacques, I. H. Rosenberg, R. B. D'Agostino, P. W. Wilson, and P. A. Wolf. 2002. Plasma homocysteine as a risk factor for dementia and Alzheimer's disease. *New England Journal of Medicine* 346 (7): 476–483.

Seshadri, S., and P. A. Wolf. 2007. Lifetime risk of stroke and dementia: Current concepts, and estimates from the Framingham Study. *Lancet Neurology* 6 (12): 1106–1114.

Seshadri, S., P. A. Wolf, A. S. Beiser, J. Selhub, R. Au, P. F. Jacques, M. Yoshita, I. H. Rosenberg, R. B. D'Agostino, and C. DeCarli. 2008. Association of plasma total homocysteine levels with subclinical brain injury. *Archives of Neurology* 65 (5): 642–649.

Shumaker, S. A., C. Legault, L. Kuller, S. R. Rapp, L. Thal, D. S. Lane, H. Fillit, et al. 2004. Conjugated equine estrogens and incidence of probable dementia and mild cognitive impairment in postmenopausal women: Women's Health Initiative Memory Study. *JAMA* 291 (24): 2947–2958.

Slooter, A. J., M. Cruts, S. Kalmijn, A. Hofman, M. M. Breteler, C. Van Broeckhoven, and C. M. van Duijn. 1998. Risk estimates of dementia by apolipoprotein E genotypes from a population-based incidence study: The Rotterdam Study. *Archives of Neurology* 55 (7): 964–968.

Sobel, E., and Z. Davanipour. 1996. Electromagnetic field exposure may cause increased production of amyloid beta and eventually lead to Alzheimer's disease. *Neurology* 47 (6): 1594–1600.

Solomon, A., I. Kareholt, T. Ngandu, B. Winblad, A. Nissinen, J. Tuomilehto, H. Soininen, and M. Kivipelto. 2007. Serum cholesterol changes after midlife and late-life cognition: Twenty-one-year follow-up study. *Neurology* 68 (10): 751–756.

Solomon, A., M. Kivipelto, B. Wolozin, J. F. Zhou, and R. A. Whitmer. 2009. Midlife serum cholesterol and increased risk of Alzheimer's and vascular dementia three decades later. *Dementia and Geriatric Cognitive Disorders* 28 (1): 75–80.

Sonnen, J. A., E. B. Larson, K. Brickell, P. K. Crane, R. Woltjer, T. J. Montine, and S. Craft. 2009. Different patterns of cerebral injury in dementia with or without diabetes. *Archives of Neurology* 66 (3): 315–322.

Stern, Y. 2006. Cognitive reserve and Alzheimer disease. *Alzheimer Disease and Associated Disorders* 20 (3 Suppl 2): S69–S74.

Stewart, R., K. Masaki, Q. L. Xue, R. Peila, H. Petrovitch, L. R. White, and L. J. Launer. 2005. A 32-year prospective study of change in body weight and incident dementia: The Honolulu-Asia Aging Study. *Archives of Neurology* 62 (1): 55–60.

Stewart, R., L. R. White, Q. L. Xue, and L. J. Launer. 2007. Twenty-six-year change in total cholesterol levels and incident dementia: The Honolulu-Asia Aging Study. *Archives of Neurology* 64 (1): 103–107.

Tan, Z. S., A. S. Beiser, R. S. Vasan, R. Roubenoff, C. A. Dinarello, T. B. Harris, E. J. Benjamin, et al. 2007. Inflammatory markers and the risk of Alzheimer disease: The Framingham study. *Neurology* 68 (22): 1902–1908.

Troncoso, J. C., A. B. Zonderman, S. M. Resnick, B. Crain, O. Pletnikova, and R. J. O'Brien. 2008. Effect of infarcts on dementia in the Baltimore Longitudinal Study of Aging. *Annals of Neurology* 64 (2): 168–176.

Tschanz, J. T., C. Corcoran, I. Skoog, A. S. Khachaturian, J. Herrick, K. M. Hayden, K. A. Welsh-Bohmer, et al. 2004. Dementia: The leading predictor of death in a defined elderly population: The Cache County Study. *Neurology* 62 (7): 1156–1162.

Tyas, S. L., L. R. White, H. Petrovitch, G. Webster Ross, D. J. Foley, H. K. Heimovitz, and L. J. Launer. 2003. Mid-life smoking and late-life dementia: The Honolulu-Asia Aging Study. *Neurobiology of Aging* 24 (4): 589–596.

Valenzuela, M. J., P. Sachdev, W. Wen, X. H. Chen, and H. Brodaty. 2008. Lifespan mental activity predicts diminished rate of hippocampal atrophy. *PLoS One* 3 (7): e2598.

van Dam, F., and W. A. van Gool. 2009. Hyperhomocysteinemia and Alzheimer's disease: A systematic review. *Archives of Gerontology and Geriatrics* 48 (3): 425–430.

van Oijen, M., F. J. de Jong, J. C. Witteman, A. Hofman, P. J. Koudstaal, and M. M. Breteler. 2007. Atherosclerosis and risk for dementia. *Annals of Neurology* 61 (5): 403–410.

Verghese, J., R. B. Lipton, M. J. Katz, C. B. Hall, C. A. Derby, G. Kuslansky, A. F. Ambrose, M. Sliwinski, and H. Buschke. 2003. Leisure activities and the risk of dementia in the elderly. *New England Journal of Medicine* 348 (25): 2508–2516.

Vermeer, S. E., N. D. Prins, T. den Heijer, A. Hofman, P. J. Koudstaal, and M. M. Breteler. 2003. Silent brain infarcts and the risk of dementia and cognitive decline. *New England Journal of Medicine* 348 (13): 1215–1222.

von Strauss, E., M. Viitanen, D. De Ronchi, B. Winblad, and L. Fratiglioni. 1999. Aging and the occurrence of dementia: Findings from a population-based cohort with a large sample of nonagenarians. *Archives of Neurology* 56 (5): 587–592.

Wang, H. X., A. Karp, B. Winblad, and L. Fratiglioni. 2002. Late-life engagement in social and leisure activities is associated with a decreased risk of dementia: A longitudinal study from the Kungsholmen project. *American Journal of Epidemiology* 155 (12): 1081–1887.

Whalley, L. J., F. D. Dick, and G. McNeill. 2006. A life-course approach to the aetiology of late-onset dementias. *Lancet Neurology* 5 (1): 87–96.

Whitmer, R. A., A. J. Karter, K. Yaffe, C. P. Quesenberry, and J. V. Selby. 2009. Hypo-glycemic episodes and risk of dementia in older patients with type 2 diabe-tes mellitus. *JAMA* 301 (15): 1565–1572.

Whitmer, R. A., S. Sidney, J. Selby, S. C. Johnston, and K. Yaffe. 2005. Midlife car-diovascular risk factors and risk of dementia in late life. *Neurology* 64 (2): 277–281.

Wolfson, C., D. B. Wolfson, M. Asgharian, C. E. M'Lan, T. Ostbye, K. Rockwood, and D. B. Hogan. 2001. A reevaluation of the duration of survival after the onset of dementia. *New England Journal of Medicine* 344 (15): 1111–1116.

Xie, J., C. Brayne, F. E. Matthews, and Council Med Res. 2008. Survival times in people with dementia: Analysis from population based cohort study with 14 year follow-up. *British Medical Journal* 336 (7638): 258–262.

Xu, W., C. Qiu, M. Gatz, N. L. Pedersen, B. Johansson, and L. Fratiglioni. 2009. Mid- and late-life diabetes in relation to the risk of dementia: A population-based twin study. *Diabetes* 58 (1): 71–77.

Xu, W., C. Qiu, B. Winblad, and L. Fratiglioni. 2007. The effect of borderline diabetes on the risk of dementia and Alzheimer's disease. *Diabetes* 56 (1): 211–216.

Zandi, P. P., M. C. Carlson, B. L. Plassman, K. A. Welsh-Bohmer, L. S. Mayer, D. C. Steffens, and J. C. Breitner. 2002. Hormone replacement therapy and incidence of Alzheimer disease in older women: The Cache County Study. *JAMA* 288 (17): 2123–2129.

Zhang, Z. X., G. E. Zahner, G. C. Roman, J. Liu, Z. Hong, Q. M. Qu, X. H. Liu, et al. 2005. Dementia subtypes in China: Prevalence in Beijing, Xian, Shanghai, and Chengdu. *Archives of Neurology* 62 (3): 447–453.

Chapter 2

Cost of Illness Studies and Neuropsychiatric Symptoms of Dementia

Wilm Quentin, Steffi G. Riedel-Heller, Melanie Luppa, Hanna Leicht, and Hans-Helmut König

Worldwide direct costs of dementia have been estimated to be US$156 billion (Wimo, Jonsson, and Winblad 2006), and annual costs of patients with neuropsychiatric symptoms of dementia have been found to amount to US$39,514 (Murman et al. 2002). Similar results of cost-of-illness (COI) studies of dementia are frequently reported in the scientific literature, policy discourses, and the media alike. They contribute to the impression that dementia is "very costly." And they make people worry that high costs per case combined with the projected increase in dementia prevalence in countries around the world will place a heavy burden on societies.

Of course, the main purpose of COI studies is not to make people worry. They are intended to provide estimates about the economic impact of diseases on different aspects of health systems and societies in order to assist policymakers in decisions of planning and financing (Bloom et al. 2001). However, unfortunately, methodological characteristics and estimated results of COI studies vary widely. Consequently, the usefulness of COI studies has come under debate because high variability puts into question the reliability of their results (Koopmanschap 1998).

This chapter aims to provide an overview to theory and practice of COI studies of dementia and uses the results of existing studies to outline the impact of neuropsychiatric symptoms of dementia on resource use and costs. It first reviews the theoretical health economics background of COI studies of dementia before exploring in more detail methodological characteristics of studies and sources of variation of their results. The following section then presents findings of a recent systematic literature review of COI studies of dementia by Quentin et al. (2010). Their findings demonstrate that results of COI-studies show consistent patterns while the exact size of costs varies greatly among studies. Drawing on the literature review and on results of existing COI studies analyzing the impact of neuropsychiatric symptoms of dementia, the subsequent section explores the likely role of neuropsychiatric symptoms of dementia in determining resource use and costs. Finally, the chapter summarizes the argument and concludes that neuropsychiatric symptoms of dementia are important determinants of costs of care. However, the exact size of costs depends on many factors that should be controlled through greater standardization of COI studies of dementia. Results of existing studies always need to be interpreted by considering the specific design, the setting, and other methodological characteristics outlined in this chapter.

BACKGROUND: HEALTH ECONOMICS AND DEMENTIA

COI studies of dementia are part of the health economics literature, which makes use of economic concepts in order to assess issues related to the allocation of resources to and within the health sector (Folland, Goodman, and Stano 2007). One concept essential for understanding the results of COI studies is the *opportunity costs* or *economic costs*. In all societies resources are scarce and decisions have to be taken between alternative uses of resources. If resources are committed to one alternative, society gives up the opportunity to enjoy the benefits of the other. Therefore, the opportunity cost of one item is what is given up in order to obtain it.

COI studies usually aim to estimate the opportunity costs of an illness, which are equal to the value of the forgone opportunity to use the resources used or lost due to the disease in another way. If there were no diseases at all, patients would be able to work, hospitals could be transformed into hotels, and doctors would have chosen to become bankers or painters. From a societal perspective, which is often adopted by economists in order to estimate the costs of dementia, the value of all resources that could have been employed in other ways to increase the welfare of society needs to be considered. As money is a medium to exchange and store value, the monetary value of the resources used or lost due to illness indicates what is given up as a result of the illness.

In order to estimate the opportunity costs of an illness, analysts usually proceed in two steps: First, they measure the quantity of resources consumed or lost due to illness (usually by following a sample of selected patients); and second, they attach monetary values (unit costs) to identified resources. In order to get an idea of the resources that are consumed, and of the determinants of resource consumption, it is useful to think about the normal course of the disease.

In progressive diseases like dementia, resource consumption is highly dependent on the stage of the disease. In early stages, demented patients are usually cared for in the community. They receive informal care and support in activities of daily living (ADLs) from mostly female caregivers (Harrow et al. 2004). As the disease progresses and functional ability deteriorates, patients become increasingly dependent on others. Caregivers sometimes have to cut down working hours in order to take care of their parents or relatives and may even incur excess healthcare costs themselves (Moore, Zhu, and Clipp 2001). At the same time, increasing dementia severity leads to augmenting demand for formal community support services. Eventually, many patients require institutional nursing-home care once the subjective caregiver burden becomes overwhelming (Yaffe et al. 2002). In addition, demented patients have been found to be high users of healthcare services (Hill et al. 2006; Bynum et al. 2004), even though the evidence in this field is not unambiguous (Kane and Atherly 2000). Attaching monetary values to all of the resources used (e.g., formal medical and informal care) and lost (lost productivity of patients and caregivers) and adding them up yields the opportunity cost of dementia. In theory, the methodology appears relatively straightforward. However, in practice, things are more complicated.

METHODOLOGICAL CHARACTERISTICS AND SOURCES OF VARIATION IN DEMENTIA COST-OF-ILLNESS STUDIES

COI studies vary widely in their methodological characteristics. They differ in their methods of sample selection and data collection and in the employed cost-estimation techniques. Methodological characteristics of COI studies are important since they determine what is measured and what is reported in their results. This section provides an overview to methodological differences between COI studies of dementia and highlights the impact that these differences can have on estimated results.

Differences in Sample Selection and Data Collection

Table 2.1 presents different approaches of COI studies to solving the methodological problems of sample selection and data collection. Since different approaches influence estimated results, they become important sources of variation between studies. The last column in Table 2.1 presents examples of characteristics of existing studies.

Sample Selection

As mentioned above, in most COI studies resource consumption for a sample of patients is measured. Important sources of variation between

Table 2.1
General Design Features and Sources of Variation between COI Studies of Dementia

Methodological Problem	Source of Variation	Characteristics of Studies (examples)
Sample selection	Identification of patients	Population screening
		Physician diagnosis
	Definition of dementia	Dementia (unspecified)
		Alzheimer's disease vs. vascular dementia, etc.
		Positive screening test (e.g., MMSE[a])
	Sample composition	Proportion of patients living in institutional care settings
		Proportion of patients in different stages of disease
		Proportion of patients with neuro-psychiatric symptoms of dementia
	Classification of patients into disease stages	Definition of severity (e.g., by MMSE, CDR[b])
		Number of stages
Data collection	Source of information	Questionnaire
		Analysis of medical claims data
	Study design	Retrospective
		Prospective
	Time period	1 month
		4 years

[a] MMSE = Mini Mental State Examination
[b] CDR = Clinical Dementia Rating Scale

studies arise from different methods of identifying patients, different definitions of dementia, the resulting divergence in the composition of samples, and from differences in the methods used to classify patients into different stages of disease.

The method for *identification of patients*, for example, whether an entire population is screened or whether patients are recruited from general practitioners or specialists, influences the sample composition: Studies using population screenings in order to identify patients are more likely to include a larger number of patients in earlier stages of the disease than studies recruiting patients from specialist practices. The resulting differences between samples (e.g., higher numbers of patients living in institutional-care settings) are bound to influence estimated costs.

Similarly, the study *definition of dementia* can influence sample composition. In cases where an unspecified dementia diagnosis is sufficient for study inclusion, the sample may include varying proportions of patients with specific types of dementia. For example, the proportion of patients with vascular dementia (VaD) included in a study of "dementia patients" could be higher than one would expect in the general population. Consequently, resource consumption of "demented patients" would be overestimated as VaD patients have been found to have higher costs in earlier stages of dementia than patients with Alzheimer's disease (AD) (Wimo and Winblad 2003).

Furthermore, studies analyzing stage dependency of costs can differ in their approach to the *classification of patients into different stages of severity*. On the one hand, they can apply different measures of severity. Some use the Mini Mental State Examination (MMSE) in order to assess the cognitive state of their sampled patients and classify patients accordingly. Other studies use measures of functional disability such as dependency in activities of daily living or instrumental activities of daily living in order to classify patients. On the other hand, researchers can classify patients into different numbers of stages of severity. Of course, depending on the way patients are classified into different stages of disease, reported cost estimates for mild, moderate, and severe dementia vary considerably.

Data Collection

Concerning data collection, studies can use various sources of information, can collect data retrospectively or prospectively, and may cover different periods of time. The method of data collection is likely to influence the accuracy of measurement. The most accurate estimates of resource consumption are likely to result from prospective studies relying on multiple sources of information and covering long periods of time.

However, *sources of information* used in existing studies vary widely. They include interviews with patients, caregivers, and physicians either by phone or in person as well as administered or mailed questionnaires. Established questionnaires for data collection are the Resource Utilisation in Dementia (RUD) Instrument (Wimo et al. 2000) and the Client Service Receipt Inventory (Beecham and Knapp 1992). In addition, patient records or registries and medical claims databases of different payers are used for identifying costs of formal care.

The *study design* determines whether data is collected retrospectively or prospectively, or whether both methods of data collection are used. Prospective studies have the advantage that they allow greater standardization of data collection, for example, by providing diaries to patients and caregivers in order to facilitate recording of resource consumption. In addition, they make it possible to follow patients over the course of the disease, which is an advantage as it allows estimating incidence costs of dementia (see below).

Furthermore, studies differ in the *time periods* covered by data collection. Some studies collect data on resource use for only one month (e.g., Langa et al. 2001). Other studies track patients over a time period of up to four years (Zhu et al. 2008). Shorter time periods, are in general, more likely to produce biased estimates as the impact of extraordinary events or seasonal variation has a stronger influence than if data are collected over a longer time period. On the other hand, if patients, caregivers, or physicians have to recall resource consumption over a longer time period, it is more likely that important elements are omitted. Many studies, therefore, use several data-collection points over a long period of time in order to increase the robustness of their estimates.

Cost-Estimation Technique

The problem of high variation between COI studies of dementia is further compounded by differences in cost estimation techniques employed by different studies. Table 2.2 shows methodological problems in estimating costs of dementia that can be solved in different ways. COI studies adopt different approaches to the definition of costs, the measurement of resource use, and the valuation of resources. The last column in Table 2.2 presents examples of characteristics of existing studies.

Defining Costs of Dementia

The *perspective* of a study is important as it determines which cost categories have to be considered as a cost of a disease (Drummond et al.

Table 2.2
**Cost-Estimation Technique and Sources of Variation between COI
Studies of Dementia**

Methodological Problem	Source of Variation	Characteristics of Studies (examples)
Defining costs of dementia	Perspective	Society
		Specific payers
		Families
	Inclusion of cost categories	Formal medical care
		Formal non-medical care
		Informal care
		Indirect costs
	Prevalence vs. incidence costs	Prevalence cost study
		Incidence cost study
	Objectives	Estimation of total costs of demented patients
		Estimation of net costs of dementia
Measurement of resource use	Costing approach	Bottom-up approach
		Top-down approach
	Measurement of informal care	Including all time spent with the patients
		Including only time spent providing assistance with ADL[a] and IADL[b]
Valuation of used resource	Valuation of formal care	Use of national cost schedules
		Use of prices
		Use of cost study
	Valuation of informal care	Replacement cost approach
		Opportunity cost approach

[a]Activities of daily living.
[b]Instrumental activities of daily living.

2005). For example, from a societal perspective, lost earnings of patients and informal caregiving time are important costs of dementia. However, from other perspectives, for example, from the perspective of Medicare, they are completely irrelevant. A study adopting a Medicare perspective would be concerned exclusively with estimating the financial costs of those resources that are covered under Medicare.

Theoretically, the number of *included cost categories* should follow logically from the adopted perspective. A study adopting a societal perspective should include all of the following cost categories: inpatient care (IP), outpatient care (OP) (e.g., ambulatory care, hospital outpatient, emergency room, general practitioner), drugs (nootropics and others), nonmedical care (physiotherapy, nursing home care, domestic care, home help, day care, home health visits, and so on), informal care (e.g. support by family members), and indirect costs (lost productivity). However, the number of included cost categories varies considerably between studies and it is not always consistent with the stated perspective.

The definition of the costs of dementia also determines whether *prevalence* or *incidence costs* are estimated. Most COI studies of dementia estimate prevalence costs, meaning that they are concerned with costs of demented patients during a specific year. Prevalence cost studies are less difficult to perform than incidence cost studies as they only look at the costs of patients during a specific year. Incidence cost studies follow patients over the course of the disease and usually aim to estimate costs from onset of the disease until death. They are more difficult since they require prospective analysis of patients over an extended period of time. However, the generated information is very useful as it can be more easily incorporated into economic evaluations of different interventions (Koopmanschap 1998).

Furthermore, depending on the *objectives* of the study, COI studies of dementia may aim to estimate either total costs or net costs of the disease. Total-cost studies of dementia aim to estimate total costs of all care received by their sampled patients. Consequently, their results include all costs associated with the entire variety of pathologies that frequently occur in elderly populations (e.g., cardiovascular disease or cancer). Net-cost studies try to account for the fact that not all costs incurred by demented patients are actually caused by dementia (Langa et al. 2001). The ideal COI study estimating net costs of dementia would be able to appropriately identify all costs due to dementia and omit all costs attributable to other reasons (Akobundu et al. 2006). Different approaches to estimating net costs of dementia exist. However, it remains difficult to exactly identify the costs specifically due to a disease (Lee, Meyer, and Clouse 2001).

Measurement of Resource Use

Different *costing approaches* exist that allow estimating costs of a disease. Costs can be estimated either by using a bottom-up approach or a top-down approach. Most COI studies of dementia use a bottom-up approach. They measure resource use by looking at individual services and aggregating resources until total resource use of patients has been estimated. Then monetary values are assigned. The bottom-up approach can proceed even further up and estimate national costs by multiplying estimated costs per patient with prevalence data for the number of patients in the country. Conversely, the top-down approach starts from highly aggregated data, for example, national registries and national accounts, and proceeds downwards. In the process, average resource use of patients is estimated by disaggregating total costs into smaller units and allocating them to specific diseases. The top-down approach has the advantage that it can be used to produce comparable cost estimates across different diseases (Koopmanschap 1998), facilitating comparative analyses of burden of disease. However, top-down studies are usually less detailed than bottom-up studies and do not generate information about informal care and indirect costs.

Since *informal care* is an important cost category in COI studies of dementia, differences in measurement and valuation of informal care can have a particularly large impact on estimated results. When *measuring* the time requirements for informal care, some studies look at all time spent with the patient, others only include time spent providing ADL and instrumental activities of daily living (IADL) assistance, while still others include informal care only up to a maximum of 16 hours per day in order to allow for at least 8 hours of sleep of caregivers. Depending on the chosen method, total estimated hours of informal caregiving time differ between studies.

Valuation of Resource Use

The valuation of consumed resources can have a large impact on estimated costs. It ultimately determines the monetary value of the resources that are consumed and lost due to illness. Often studies use secondary sources of information like national cost schedules in order to attach monetary values to measured resources. In other cases, market prices of used resources are determined. However, only few studies explicitly describe the assigned values. Therefore, it is often difficult to assess the appropriateness of chosen values.

The *valuation of informal care* is even more complicated as no market prices are available that could be used as unit costs. In theory, several solutions to this problem exist (McDaid 2001). Most dementia COI studies use either the opportunity cost approach or the replacement cost approach. The opportunity cost approach tries to estimate costs of forgone opportunities by asking caregivers about how they would make use of their time if they were not engaged in the provision of informal care. Depending on their answers, caregiving time is then valued either at the market wage rate, at a rate for the contribution to household production or the rate for leisure time. The alternative replacement cost approach assigns monetary values to caregiver time according to what it would cost to replace informal caregiving activities with formal care. If the alternative approaches result in different monetary values per hour of informal caregiving time, they can have a considerable impact on estimated costs of informal care.

A SYSTEMATIC LITERATURE REVIEW OF COST-OF-ILLNESS STUDIES OF DEMENTIA

The previous section has illustrated the high degree of variability among COI studies of dementia that results from differences in sample selection, data collection, and cost-estimation technique. A recent systematic literature review by Quentin et al. (2010) provides an overview to methods and results of COI studies of dementia focusing on stage dependency of costs. Their findings document the high degree of variability described in the previous section. Yet, by summarizing costs for different stages of disease, their results demonstrate that estimates of existing studies show consistent patterns of increasing costs from mild over moderate to severe dementia. This section presents methods, results, and limitations of their literature review.

Review Methods

Quentin et al. (2010) performed a systematic literature search in Medline (Pubmed), Cochrane Library, and NHS Economic Evaluations Database (NHSEED) between May and July 2008. They searched for COI studies of dementia from Europe and North America, restricting their search to studies that appeared after 1996 since earlier studies had been included in two prior literature reviews (Wimo, Ljunggren, and Winblad 1997; Ernst and Hay 1997). Twenty-eight studies were selected that fulfilled the following criteria: The primary objective of the study was the estimation of costs of dementia; the study had a sample size greater than 20; it included at least the cost categories of formal nonmedical care or informal care; and the main outcome of the study was reported as average costs per patient and time period presented separately for different stages of disease.

Studies were divided into two groups: (1) total-cost studies assessing total costs of demented individuals, and (2) net-cost studies, which tried to discern net costs of dementia (costs specifically caused by dementia). Within these groups, subgroups were formed according to the care setting of patients included in the study. Furthermore, reported costs of different cost categories (e.g., inpatient care, outpatient care, nursing home care, family caregiving) were aggregated to the categories of formal care and informal care. When the original studies presented cost estimates for more than three stages of disease (mild, moderate, severe), presented results were assigned to the appropriate stages of dementia on the basis of reported MMSE scores (mild: ≥18, moderate: 10–17, severe: ≤9) or the original studies' definitions. When studies presented costs for only two stages of disease, the lower estimate was classified as mild dementia and the higher estimate as severe dementia unless specified otherwise by the original studies' authors. All cost estimates were converted into 2006 USD purchasing power parities (PPP) (OECD 2008).

Review Results

Study Characteristics

Table 2.3 summarizes characteristics of the 28 included studies. Their region of origin was evenly distributed between Europe (n = 14) and North America (n = 14). Among European studies, most studies were from Scandinavia and the United Kingdom, while eastern and southern Europe, with the exception of Spain, were not represented in the sample. Concerning the dementia type, 21 studies looked at costs of patients with AD, of which six studies also included patients with VaD or other dementias. Two studies aimed to identify differences between costs of AD patients and VaD patients (Andersen et al. 1999; Wimo and Winblad 2003). Three studies looked at patients with "cognitive impairment," and four studies did not specify the type of dementia. Even within the same diagnosis, definitions of dementia varied. Seventeen studies required a formal dementia diagnosis based on established criteria (e.g., National Institute of Neurological and Communicative Disorders and Stroke and the Alzheimer's Disease and Related Disorders Association; NINCDS-ADRDA). Seven studies required a positive screening test (e.g., MMSE) or did not specify their definition of dementia. Most studies relied on interviews to collect information on resource use by patients during a certain time period prior to the interview. Concerning patient sample characteristics, the median sample size was 337 patients, reported mean age was mostly in the late seventies, and most samples were predominantly female.

Concerning cost-estimation methods, studies differed widely. Sixteen studies analyzed costs from a societal perspective, four from the perspective of specific payers, and four from the perspective of families. Most studies included several cost categories of formal care. Nineteen

Table 2.3
Characteristics of Included COI Studies of Dementia (N = 28)

Characteristic	
Region: N (%)	
United States	11 (39%)
Canada	3 (11%)
Europe	14 (50%)
Sample Size	
Median (range)	337 (50 – 8.736)
Mean	880
Included Diagnoses: N (%)	
(Multiple diagnoses possible)	
Alzheimer's disease	21 (75%)
Vascular dementia	6 (21%)
Other dementias	4 (14%)
Dementia (unspecified)	4 (14%)
Cognitive impairment	3 (11%)
Diagnostic Criteria: N (%)	
Formal diagnoses (e.g. according to NINCDS-ADRDA[a])	17 (61%)
Physician diagnosis (unspecified)	4 (14%)
Other (e.g., MMSE) / not described	7 (25%)
Method for Data Collection / Data source: N (%)	
(Multiple methods possible)	
Interview	21 (75%)
Questionnaire	4 (14%)
Patient records	3 (11%)
Medical claims	3 (11%)
Not described	1 (4%)
Adopted Perspective: N (%)	
(Multiple perspectives possible)	
Society	16 (57%)
Payers	5 (18%)
Families	4 (14%)
Not described	4 (14%)
Included Cost Categories: N (%)	
(Multiple categories possible)	
Formal nonmedical care	23 (82%)
Ambulatory care	
Inpatient care	20 (71%)
Informal care	19 (68%)
Drugs	19 (68%)
Study Objectives	
Total costs	19 (68%)
Net costs	4 (14%)
Both	5 (18%)

Table 2.3 (*Continued*)

Funding Source	
Pharmaceutical companies	16 (57%)
Public funds	6 (21%)
Other (e.g. Alzheimer's Association)/not described	6 (21%)

Source: Adapted from König et al., Stadienspezifische Kosten der Demenz: Ergebnisse eines systematischen Literaturuberblicks, in *Versonrgungsforschung fur
demenziell erkrankte Menschen*, ed. Dibelius and Maier, with permission.
[a]National Institute of Neurological and Communicative Disorders and Stroke–
Alzheimer's Disease and Related Disorders Association.

studies estimated cost of informal care. In addition, studies pursued different objectives: 19 studies looked at total costs of demented patients while
9 others tried to estimate net costs of dementia or looked at both total
and net costs of dementia. When looking at the sources of funding, most
studies included financial contributions from pharmaceutical companies
but several studies were financed exclusively through public funds. More
information on the methods for valuation of informal care is provided in
the original review article (Quentin et al. 2010).

Estimated Costs

Table 2.4 summarizes results of analyzed studies. It presents estimated
costs from total-cost studies and net-cost studies separately for patients
living in different care settings, and it further differentiates between costs
for formal and informal care. The table shows the range of estimated average costs from analyzed studies and the median of their results. At first
sight, the large range of estimated costs in each field might appear confus-
ing. However, after close examination, consistent patterns of increasing
costs from mild over moderate to severe dementia emerge.

In most total-cost studies, costs more than double from mild to severe
dementia. For example, Table 2.4 shows that the range of average total costs
estimated by different studies for community-dwelling patients in the mild
stage of dementia was between US$7,124 and $56,192, whereas average
total costs reported for patients in the severe stage were between $8,544 and
$115,450. Accordingly, the median of estimated results reported in different
studies increased from about $18,000 to about $36,000. In net-cost studies, the
increase of costs was even more pronounced: The median of estimated costs
for community-dwelling patients increased from about $18,000 to about
$63,000. However, in general, costs estimated in net-cost studies tended to
be smaller than costs estimated in comparable total-cost studies.

Table 2.4

Results of Included COI Studies of Dementia by Study Objectives, Level of Severity, Care Setting, and Cost Category

		Estimated Costs per Year in USD-PPP (2006)		
		Number of studies Range of costs [Median]		
Care Setting	Cost Category	Mild Dementia	Moderate Dementia	Severe Dementia
Total Cost Studies (24 studies)				
Community-dwelling patients	Formal care costs	n = 9 1,268–14,388 [6,341]	n = 6 5,234–32,283 [9,837]	n = 9 4,255–36,428 [13,649]
	Informal care costs	n = 8 783–41,677 [14,212]	n = 6 615–54,544 [15,937]	n = 8 1,225–78,504 [36,354]
	Total costs	n = 7 7,124–56,192 [18,041]	n = 7 5,849–87,057 [25,331]	n = 8 8,544–115,450 [36,354]
Mixed group of patients	Formal care costs	n = 13 2,255–29,127 [10,261]	n = 11 7,592–34,897 [21,537]	n = 13 11,764–56,118 [29,549]
	Informal care costs	n = 6 3,932–13,039 [5,841]	n = 5 4,050–9,001 [7,496]	n = 6 2,392–14,261 [8,071]
	Total costs	n = 8 3,992–35,338 [12,340]	n = 7 16,462–34,264 [25,492]	n = 8 21,977–74,555 [38,204]
Institutional-ized patients	Formal care cost	n = 2 21,990–42,319 [31,640]	n = 2 28,665–44,941 [36.803]	n = 2 35,518–48,162 [41,840]
	Informal care costs	n = 2 1,028–1,875 [1,452]	n = 2 790–3,576 [2,183]	n = 2 834–2,306 [1,570]
	Total costs	n = 2 23,865–42,319 [33,092]	n = 2 32,240–45,731 [38,986]	n = 2 37,825–48,994 [43,410]

Table 2.4 (*Continued*)

Net Cost Studies (9 Studies)				
Community-dwelling patients	Formal care costs	n = 7 1,007–11,143 [3,330]	n = 7 166–28,996 [7,208]	n = 7 986–33,285 [9,816]
	Informal care costs	n = 8 197–41,677 [5,647]	n = 8 29–54,544 [12,042]	n = 8 639–78,504 [33,103]
	Total costs	n = 7 1,470–52,947 [18,388]	n = 7 195–83,770 [28,767]	n = 7 2,890–112,307 [62,916]
Mixed group of patients[a]	Formal care costs	n = 3 2,553–11,720 [8,373]	n = 2 13,433–18,567 [16,000]	n = 3 4,595–27,359 [26,052]

Source: Adapted from König et al., Stadienspezifische Kosten der Demenz: Ergebnisse eines systematischen Literaturuberblicks, in *Versonrgungsforschung fur demenziell erkrankte Menschen*, ed. Dibelius and Maier, with permission.
Note: USD-PPP = US$–purchasing power parities.
[a]Studies only report costs of formal care.

Furthermore, the patterns of increasing costs and the proportion of formal and informal care differ between care settings. In mild dementia, total-cost studies of patients living in institutional-care settings found higher costs (about US$33,000) than total-cost studies of community-dwelling patients (about $18,000). In contrast, in severe dementia, estimated costs of patients living in different care settings were similar. In studies analyzing samples of community-dwelling patients, costs increased mostly for informal care and accounted for about two-thirds of costs in the severe stage. In studies including community-dwelling and institutionalized patients (mixed group), costs for formal care increased more strongly from mild to severe dementia, which could be attributed to increasing proportions of institutionalized patients from mild to severe dementia in this group of studies. In studies of institutionalized patients, the proportion of informal-care costs remained relatively small across all stages of dementia.

Limitations

Reported results vary considerably even within the presented subgroups of studies and within the cost categories of formal and informal care. On the one hand, these variations are related to limitations of the original studies. For example, some studies excluded certain cost categories or excluded patients with severe comorbidities; other studies used extremely high values for the valuation of informal care.

On the other hand, variations are related to limitations of the review method, which had to ignore certain differences between studies in order to be able to compare their results. The review formed subgroups according to the care setting of patients and aggregated various cost categories into the categories of formal and informal care. However, studies differed considerably within subgroups. The samples of patients analyzed in the original studies varied greatly: Some studies included "dementia patients"; others recruited only AD patients. Studies used various methods to classify patients into different stages of disease; and informal-care costs were estimated through very different approaches.

These limitations need to be considered when drawing on the results of the review by Quentin et al. (2010). However, despite all methodological differences between studies and variation of results, the patterns of increasing costs are clear enough to allow drawing conclusions for the effect of neuropsychiatric symptoms on costs of dementia.

COST-OF-ILLNESS OF DEMENTIA: THE ROLE OF NEUROPSYCHIATRIC SYMPTOMS

Two findings of the presented literature review are particularly important for a discussion about the role of neuropsychiatric symptoms (NPS) in determining resource use and costs of dementia: First, the review shows that informal care accounts for an important part of total resources used and constitutes the majority of costs of dementia care in community-dwelling patients; second, it indicates that costs of institutionalization are considerable already in early stages of dementia. The implications of these findings for costs of NPS can be explored by looking at existing studies of the importance of NPS in determining caregiver burden and nursing home placement. In addition, some studies exist that have specifically looked at the effect of NPS on cost-of-illness of dementia.

Caregiver Burden and Determinants of Nursing Home Placement: The Role of Neuropsychiatric Symptoms

Multiple studies have assessed the role of neuropsychiatric symptoms in determining caregiver burden and nursing home placement. Almost 30 years ago, Greene et al. (1982) found behavioral problems to be important determinants of caregiver burden. More recently, these findings were confirmed by studies that looked at the specific type of neuropsychiatric symptom with the highest impact on caregiver burden as measured by standardized interviews of caregivers. For example, Craig et al. (2005) have found sleep disturbance, aggression/agitation, and depression/dysphoria to be particularly distressing to caregivers. Another stream of research has looked at the time spent by caregivers on dealing with NPS of dementia. Beeri et al. (2002) found that caregivers spent about one-third of their time with managing behavioral and psychiatric symptoms. And Murman et al. (2002) found that patients with NPS required 3.5 hours more of caregiving per day than patients without these symptoms.

Nursing home placement is the result of a complex set of interacting variables, including caregiver, patient, social, and cultural variables (Yaffe et al. 2002). However, high caregiver burden and presence of NPS of dementia are two particularly important factors influencing the likeliness of patients to be admitted to nursing homes. Even when controlling for other factors, Yaffe et al. (2002) found caregiver burden and age over 75 years to be the most important determinants of nursing home placement. Phillips and Diwan (2003) estimated that patients with NPS enter nursing homes nearly two years earlier than those without.

These findings combined with the results of the literature review by Quentin et al. (2010) suggest that NPS are important determinants of costs of care for demented patients. Informal-care costs account for the majority of costs in community-dwelling patients and NPS are important determinants of caregiver burden. Consequently, total costs of care related to NPS of dementia can be expected to be considerable. In addition, neuropsychiatric symptoms of dementia contribute to increasing costs by leading to earlier nursing home placement. Since costs of nursing home placement are important even in the early stages of disease, the impact on total costs is likely to be important.

COI Studies Focusing on Neuropsychiatric Symptoms of Dementia

A small number of studies have looked specifically at the contribution of neuropsychiatric symptoms of dementia on costs of dementia care. Table 2.5 provides an overview to the characteristics of two of these studies, which compared groups of patients with different levels of neuropsychiatric symptoms of dementia. Both studies are from North America and estimated total costs of dementia care of a sample of patients which they divided into two groups: one group with a low score on the neuropsychiatric inventory (NPI) and one group with a high NPI score. Herrmann

Table 2.5
**Characteristics of COI Studies Focusing on Neuropsychiatric
Symptoms of Dementia**

Author (year)	Herrmann et al. 2006	Murman et al. 2002
General study characteristics		
Country	Canada	USA
Dementia type	Dementia (AD/VaD/other)	Alzheimer's disease
Method for data collection	Mailed questionnaire	Interview
Sample characteristics		
Size	500	128
Mean age	76.3	76.2
% receiving long-term care (patients with low/high NPI)	0%	(12%/27%)
Funding source	Industry	National Institute on Aging
Perspective	Society	n/d (Society)
Objectives	Total cost study	Total cost study
Included cost categories		
Inpatient care	+	+
Outpatient care	+	+
Drugs	+	+
Nonmedical	+	+
Informal	+	+
Indirect	+	-
Valuation of informal care		
Unit cost value (in 2006 US$-PPP)	98.01/day	5.82/hr, 9.02/hr, 10.68/hr (low, mid-range, high estimate)

Note: AD = Alzheimer's disease; n/d = not described; NPI = neuropsychiatric inventory; VaD = vascular dementia.

et al. (2006) studied patients living in the community, whereas Murman et al. (2002) included a certain number of patients receiving long term care. Both included a wide range of formal and informal care costs. In addition, Herrmann et al. (2006) included indirect costs by estimating the opportunity costs of the time that patients were prevented from performing their regular activities.

Table 2.6 presents the results of the two COI studies focusing on neuropsychiatric symptoms of dementia. It is important to note that the studies estimated costs for disparate groups of patients. Herrmann et al. (2006)

Table 2.6

Results of COI Studies Focusing on Neuropsychiatric Symptoms of Dementia

Author (year)	Mean annual costs per patient (in 2006 USD-PPP)							
	Patients with low NPI				Patients with high NPI			
	Definition of Group	Formal	Informal	Total	Definition of Group	Formal	Informal	Total
Herrmann et al. 2006	NPI = 0	2,479	2,098	7,091	NPI >0	4,255	4,877	16,119
Murman et al. 2002	NPI <13	10,074	13,039	23,113	NPI ≥13	20,485	14,261	44,993

Note: NPI = neuropsychiatric inventory.

defined their "low NPI group" as patients with no neuropsychiatric symptoms, whereas the "low NPI group" of Murman et al. (2002) included all patients with an NPI score less than 13. Both studies found that costs of patients in the high NPI group were about twice as high as costs in the low NPI group. However, the size of costs varied considerably, which is not particularly surprising as the assessed groups of patients were very different.

Both studies also used regression analyses in order to determine the effect of a one-point increase in NPI score on total costs of dementia care. Herrmann et al. (2006) estimated that costs would increase by US$346 for every one-point increase in NPI, while Murman et al. (2002) estimated the effect to lie somewhere between US$281 and $466 depending on the valuation of informal care (all in 2006 US$-PPP). The estimated effect of neuropsychiatric symptoms of dementia on costs, therefore, appears to be similar. However, it has to be considered that the estimate of Herrmann et al. (2006) includes indirect costs (the value of the time that patients were prevented from performing their regular activities), which they found to be considerable, whereas Murman et al. (2002) did not include this cost category. Presumably, further differences existed in the measurement and valuation of informal care, which are, however, difficult to evaluate.

CONCLUSION

This chapter has described the theoretical background and methodological characteristics of COI studies of dementia. It has highlighted the importance of considering methodological differences between studies when interpreting their results. Different approaches to sample selection, data collection, definition of costs, and measurement and valuation of resources determine the size of estimated costs in COI studies of dementia. Users of results of COI studies should be careful with generalizing results of COI studies since they are always specific to the study setting, the sample of patients, and the cost-estimation techniques. However, if these methodological characteristics are considered, estimated results can be useful for determining the impact of dementia on specific aspects of health systems and societies.

The literature review by Quentin et al. (2010) demonstrated that costs increase from mild over moderate to severe dementia and that costs differ by care setting and depend on whether total or net costs of dementia are estimated. Informal-care costs were confirmed to account for the majority of costs in community-dwelling patients and costs of patients living in institutional-care settings were important already in the early stages of disease. Since neuropsychiatric symptoms of dementia are an important determinant of caregiver burden and nursing home placement, their impact on costs of dementia is considerable. Existing studies have found that costs of patients with neuropsychiatric symptoms of dementia are much higher than costs of patients without these symptoms. However, again, methodological differences between studies complicate comparisons of their results.

An international consensus statement exists that defines how to measure benefits in dementia treatment trials (Katona et al. 2007), and reference cases have been developed for the presentation of cost-effectiveness results (NICE 2008). A similar international consensus on a dementia-specific reference case for conducting COI studies of dementia and presenting their results could improve quality of studies, facilitate comparisons, and increase certainty that results are reliable and transferable to other settings.

ACKNOWLEDGMENT: This publication is part of the German Research Network on Dementia (KND) and the German Research Network on Degenerative Dementia (KNDD) and was funded by the German Federal Ministry of Education and Research (grants KND: 01GI0102, 01GI0420, 01GI0422, 01GI0423, 01GI0429, 01GI0431, 01GI0433, 01GI0434; grants KNDD: O1GI0710, 01GI0711, 01GI0712, 01GI0713, 01GI0714, 01GI0715, 01GI0716).

REFERENCES

Akobundu, E., J. Ju, L. Blatt, and C. D. Mullins. 2006. Cost-of-illness studies: A review of current methods. *Pharmacoeconomics* 24 (9): 869–890.

Andersen, C. K., J. Sogaard, E. Hansen, A. Kragh-Sorensen, L. Hastrup, J. Andersen, K. Andersen, A. Lolk, H. Nielsen, and P. Kragh-Sorensen. 1999. The cost of dementia in Denmark: The Odense Study. *Dement Geriatr Cogn Disord* 10 (4): 295–304.

Beecham, J., and M. Knapp. 1992. Costing psychiatric interventions. In *Measuring Mental Health Needs*, ed. G. Thornicroft, C. R. Brewin, and J. K. Wing, 179–190. London: Gaskell.

Beeri, M. S., P. Werner, M. Davidson, and S. Noy. 2002. The cost of behavioral and psychological symptoms of dementia (BPSD) in community dwelling Alzheimer's disease patients. *Int J Geriatr Psychiatry* 17 (5): 403–408.

Bloom, B. S., D. J. Bruno, D. Y. Maman, and R. Jayadevappa. 2001. Usefulness of US cost-of-illness studies in healthcare decision making. *Pharmacoeconomics* 19 (2): 207–213.

Bynum, J. P., P. V. Rabins, W. Weller, M. Niefeld, G. F. Anderson, and A. W. Wu. 2004. The relationship between a dementia diagnosis, chronic illness, Medicare expenditures, and hospital use. *J Am Geriatr Soc* 52 (2): 187–194.

Craig, D., A. Mirakhur, D. J. Hart, S. P. McIlroy, and A. P. Passmore. 2005. A cross-sectional study of neuropsychiatric symptoms in 435 patients with Alzheimer's disease. *Am J Geriatr Psychiatry* 13 (6): 460–468.

Drummond, M. F., M. J, Sculpher, G, W. Torrance, B. J. O'Brien, and G. L. Stoddart. 2005. Cost analysis. In *Methods for the Economic Evaluation of Health Care Programmes*, 3rd ed., 49–102. New York: Oxford University Press.

Ernst, R. L., and J. W. Hay. 1997. Economic research on Alzheimer disease: A review of the literature. *Alzheimer Dis Assoc Disord* 11 (Suppl 6): 135–145.

Folland, S., A, C. Goodman, and M. Stano. 2007. Introduction. In *The Economics of Health and Health Care*, 5th ed., 1–19. Upper Saddle River, NJ: Pearson Prentice-Hall.

Greene, J. G., R. Smith, M. Gardiner, and G. C. Timbury. 1982. Measuring behavioural disturbance of elderly demented patients in the community and its effects on relatives: A factor analytic study. *Age Ageing* 11 (2): 121–126.

Harrow, B. S., D. F. Mahoney, A. B. Mendelsohn, M. G. Ory, D. W. Coon, S. H. Belle, and L. O. Nichols. 2004. Variation in cost of informal caregiving and formal-service use for people with Alzheimer's disease. *Am J Alzheimers Dis Other Demen* 19 (5): 299–308.

Herrmann, N., K. L. Lanctot, R. Sambrook, N. Lesnikova, R. Hebert, P. McCracken, A. Robillard, and E. Nguyen. 2006. The contribution of neuropsychiatric symptoms to the cost of dementia care. *Int J Geriatr Psychiatry* 21 (10): 972–976.

Hill, J., H. Fillit, S. K. Thomas, and S. Chang. 2006. Functional impairment, healthcare costs and the prevalence of institutionalisation in patients with Alzheimer's disease and other dementias. *Pharmacoeconomics* 24 (3): 265–280.

Kane, R. L., and A. Atherly. 2000. Medicare expenditures associated with Alzheimer disease. *Alzheimer Dis Assoc Disord* 14 (4): 187–195.

Katona, C., G. Livingston, C. Cooper, D. Ames, H. Brodaty, and E. Chiu. 2007. International Psychogeriatric Association consensus statement on defining and measuring treatment benefits in dementia. *Int Psychogeriatr* 19 (3): 345–354.

Koopmanschap, M. A. 1998. Cost-of-illness studies. Useful for health policy? *Pharmacoeconomics* 14 (2): 143–148.

Langa, K. M., M. E. Chernew, M. U. Kabeto, A. R. Herzog, M. B. Ofstedal, R. J. Willis, R. B. Wallace, L. M. Mucha, W. L. Straus, and A. M. Fendrick. 2001. National estimates of the quantity and cost of informal caregiving for the elderly with dementia. *J Gen Intern Med* 16 (11): 770–778.

Lee, D. W., J. W. Meyer, and J. Clouse. 2001. Implications of controlling for comorbid conditions in cost-of-illness estimates: A case study of osteoarthritis from a managed care system perspective. *Value Health* 4 (4): 329–334.

McDaid, D. 2001. Estimating the costs of informal care for people with Alzheimer's disease: Methodological and practical challenges. *Int J Geriatr Psychiatry* 16 (4): 400–405.

Moore, M. J., C. W. Zhu, and E. C. Clipp. 2001. Informal costs of dementia care: Estimates from the National Longitudinal Caregiver Study. *J Gerontol B Psychol Sci Soc Sci* 56 (4): S219–228.

Murman, D. L., Q. Chen, M. C. Powell, S. B. Kuo, C. J. Bradley, and C. C. Colenda. 2002. The incremental direct costs associated with behavioral symptoms in AD. *Neurology* 59 (11): 1721–1729.

NICE. 2008. *Guide to the methods of technology appraisal*. London: National Institute for Health and Clinical Excellence (NICE).

OECD. 2008. *Health Data 2008: Statistics and Indicators for 30 Countries*. Organisation for Economic Co-operation and Development (OECD).

Phillips, V. L., and S. Diwan. 2003. The incremental effect of dementia-related problem behaviors on the time to nursing home placement in poor, frail, demented older people. *J Am Geriatr Soc* 51 (2): 188–193.

Quentin, W., S. G. Riedel-Heller, M. Luppa, A. Rudolph, and H. H. Konig. 2010. Cost-of-illness studies of dementia: A systematic review focusing on stage dependency of costs. *Acta Psychiatr Scand* 121 (4): 243–259.

Wimo, A., L. Jonsson, and B. Winblad. 2006. An estimate of the worldwide prevalence and direct costs of dementia in 2003. *Dement Geriatr Cogn Disord* 21 (3): 175–181.

Wimo, A., G. Ljunggren, and B. Winblad. 1997. Costs of dementia and dementia care: A review. *Int J Geriatr Psychiatry* 12 (8): 841–856.

Wimo, A., G. Nordberg, W. Jansson, and M. Grafstrom. 2000. Assessment of informal services to demented people with the RUD instrument. *Int J Geriatr Psychiatry* 15 (10): 969–971.

Wimo, A., and B. Winblad. 2003. Societal burden and economics of vascular dementia: Preliminary results from a Swedish-population-based study. *Int Psychogeriatr* 15 (Suppl 1): 251–256.

Yaffe, K., P. Fox, R. Newcomer, L. Sands, K. Lindquist, K. Dane, and K. E. Covinsky. 2002. Patient and caregiver characteristics and nursing home placement in patients with dementia. *JAMA* 287 (16): 2090–2097.

Zhu, C. W., R. Torgan, N. Scarmeas, M. Albert, J. Brandt, D. Blacker, M. Sano, and Y. Stern. 2008. Home health and informal care utilization and costs over time in Alzheimer's disease. *Home Health Care Serv Q* 27 (1): 1–20.

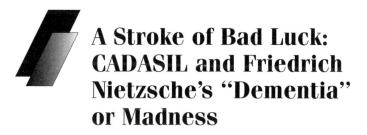

Chapter 3

A Stroke of Bad Luck: CADASIL and Friedrich Nietzsche's "Dementia" or Madness

Paul M. Butler

Philosophy is its own time raised to the level of thought.
G. W. F. Hegel (1821/1991)

The early eighteenth-century Prussian philosopher Georg Wilhelm Friedrich Hegel envisaged history as a dynamic, dialectic system—an ineluctable process of unfolding epochs. *Reason*, seen as the highest form of human cognition, is forever ensconced within these historical movements. Regardless of the absolute veridicality of Hegel's thought, he proposes an interesting way to think about reason and history (Hegel 1837/1997). Logical analysis is restricted to comprehending its object using the tools available within a given stage of history. Likewise, science and the art of medicine are bound by the limits of historically constrained reason. This is well illustrated by pondering the vastly different ways human reason has apprehended natural reality across time (i.e., from the Ptolemaic epicyles to Steven Hawking's arrow of time or Aelius Galen's circulatory model to William Harvey's heart-pump model).

Medical diagnoses will always only be as accurate as the categories that contain them. Take, for instance, the history of stroke and the diagnosis of "softening of the brain" in the early 1800s. In 1814 Jean Andre Rochoux maintained that apoplexy or *ramollissement* (softening) of the brain was exclusively the result of hemorrhagic bleeding. No other categories or ways of thinking about brain lesions existed at this time in medical history. It was not until 1823, when Leon Rostan proposed that ossification of the arteries was associated with parenchymous brain lesions that the concept of brain softening was divided into hemorrhagic and occlusive-based lesions (Paciaroni and Bogousslavsky 2009).

And so it is today in clinical neurology; our reason is trapped in history. Of course, multitudinous diagnostic categories now exist as tools for the practicing physician compared to just 100 years ago, but pathologic etiologies yet to be discovered still hover beyond our conceptual grasp. What was seen as "softening of the brain" in 1810 and diagnosed as an embolic stroke due to atrial fibrillation in 2010 will be phrased in a molecular cardiac basis (an undiscovered channelopathy?) in the future.

With this line of thought in mind, I introduce here a potential diagnosis unknown to physicians of the late nineteenth century to explain the dementia of Friedrich Nietzsche. When Nietzsche was brought to Dr. Otto Binswanger's clinic in Jena, Switzerland, in January 1889, the diagnostic category most fitting to explain his sudden onset of bizarre ideas, grandiosity, dementia, and apparent Argyll-Robertson pupils was *paresis paralytica* (tertiary syphilis) (Volz 1990). This diagnosis was very reasonable at that time in medical history because dementia presenting in a middle-aged adult male was nearly always due to syphilitic infection. So what physicians saw in 1889 as syphilitic *paresis* is ascertained, at least in my estimation, as genetically testable CADASIL (cerebral autosomal dominant arteriopathy with subcortical infarcts and leukoencephalopathy) with dementia and perhaps, in the indeterminate future, *reason* will diagnostically supplant our present-day diagnosis with a new category, such as Type II CADASIL, endophenotype 10b with features of epigenetic modulation (for want of a better imaginary example).

OVERVIEW OF NIETZSCHE'S CASE PRESENTATION

> For my life's terrible and almost unremitting martyrdom makes me thirst for the end, and there have been some signs which allow me to hope that the stroke which will liberate me is not too distant.
>
>   Nietzsche (1880/1996)

I conducted a comprehensive review of Nietzsche's medical records and over 500 letters written by Nietzsche (see Nietzsche 1971, 1985, 1996; Frenzel 1967; Volz 1990). Translations from primary sources reveal that he suffered from shifting headaches beginning in adolescence. Further, this evidence clearly demonstrates that Nietzsche was specifically tormented by migraine with aura and with motor symptoms giving him an IHS classification of (familial, vide infra) hemiplegic migraine: IHS1.2.4 (International Headache Society 2004). Nietzsche's headaches emerged during his mid-twenties, peaked in his thirties, and attenuated in his forties. They were trigger-sensitive to weather, travel, and dietary habits and exhibited prolonged duration, photosensitivity, emesis, gastrointestinal pain, and fatigue. Medical records and correspondence demonstrate these headache attacks occurred for many hours, often causing tonic eye cramps and reversible paralysis of the right oculomotor muscles. His right eyelid would droop and his gaze would move into the right lower temporal quadrant. Dizziness, disturbance of speech, temporary loss of consciousness, facial hemi-paralysis, and feelings of numbness accompanied the headaches. Nietzsche described a "flickering in front of the eye" and "numerous danger signals" prior to the onset of these attacks (Volz 1990).

Nietzsche's correspondence also suggests mood disorder. He entertained thoughts of death, experiencing profound depression during the 1870s and early 1880s with an emergent hypomania in the early to mid-1880s. There is a sudden progression to fulminant mania by the time of his mental collapse at the end of 1888. Nietzsche's intense depression alternated with euphoric moods. He wrote letters, within the same month to the same individual, stating that he "hungered for the end" believing that "the cerebral *coup de grace* is close enough at hand." Just days later he wrote, "My joyous thirst for knowledge brings me to heights where I can triumph over all torment and despair. On the whole I'm happier than ever before in my life." In an explosion of 10 days of racing thoughts and flights of ideas during the winter of 1882, Nietzsche produced book 1 of *Thus Spake Zarathustra*. Just months later, he wrote book 2 over another 10-day stretch of prolonged creativity. For a relatively isolated individual, Nietzsche exhibited pressured speech and loose concatenations of thought in a written form known clinically as hypergraphia.

A progressive and predominately right-sided retinal inflammation was noted throughout his life in medical records, in addition to a rapidly developing myopia and eventual blindness. Several physicians commented on this "mysterious inflammatory mechanism" that caused "light granulations" and "retinitis pigmentosa." In 1884 Nietzsche reported a sudden change in vision not connected with headache that likely reflected a stroke-induced Charles Bonnet syndrome. He described "blots, veils, and darkening" in his visual fields as an "opacification." With his eyes closed Nietzsche experienced hallucinations filled with fantastic colorful flowers that flowed and changed in brilliant displays of movement. A sudden change in Nietzsche's mental status occurred during the final week of 1888.

He sent off cryptic letters signed "The Anti-Christ" and "The Man on the Cross." This was followed by multiple nonresolving ischemic-like attacks ultimately causing subcortical dementia initially presenting as a pseudo-bulbar palsy, gait disturbance, and emotional lability. Nietzsche developed a labile affect, tearful outbursts and inappropriate laughter, dysfunction in cranial nerves IX-XII—Binswanger noted tongue deviation to the right and spasmodic left shoulder jerking—in addition to left body upper motor neuron dysfunction evidenced by left ankle clonus and an exaggerated patellar reflex. Under full-time familial care, Nietzsche slowly became bed-ridden and demented, and died in 1900 after suffering several strokes.

NIETZSCHE'S CASE DETAILS

Family History

Because of Nietzsche's fame, his family medical history is partly known. Nietzsche was born in 1844 to an already sick father, Karl Ludwig Nietzsche. In brief, Nietzsche's melancholic father also experienced intense headaches from adolescence until death at age 35. Beginning in his thirties, he dealt with increasingly labile mood, epileptic-like fits, and multiple strokes leading to facial hemi-paralysis, blindness, and eventual dementia and death. Autopsy revealed a "softening of the brain" affecting 25% of brain tissue. Additionally, records state that Karl's father, Friedrich August Ludwig Nietzsche, suffered from similar symptoms. So three successive paternal generations, Friedrich August, Karl Ludwig, and Friedrich Nietzsche, suffered from similar symptoms and untimely deaths.

Nietzsche's Health from 1844 to 1888

Ocular Disturbances

Nietzsche struggled with his vision throughout life and saw many eye doctors. An ophthalmologist, Dr. Vater, diagnosed Nietzsche with myopia in early childhood.

Dr. Schelbach examined Nietzsche's vision at age five and noted congenital differences in Nietzsche's pupils (anisocoria). The right pupil was abnormally shaped, significantly larger than the left, and reacted slowly to light. Dr. Schelbach's records note the young Nietzsche's mother, Franziska, also had an uneven right pupil slow to react to light.

Even though the right eye was congenitally worse, Nietzsche still needed eye correction for both eyes. His vision deteriorated from early childhood at varying rates until eventual blindness occurred before death. In 1873 Dr. Schiesse again noted the right pupillary shape disparity in addition to small pigment granulations on the retina of both sides. He diagnosed "retinitis pigmentosa" in both eyes and "strabismus convergens" in the right eye. In 1877 Dr. Kruger also noticed an inflammatory process present in both retinas that seemed radically changed from previous years. He diagnosed this inflammation as "chorio-retinitis centralis." He further observed retinal exudates that were spreading toward the macula of both eyes.

In January 1884 Nietzsche reported a sudden change in vision not connected with headache. He experienced "blots, veils, and darkening" in his visual fields, which he described in one word as "opacification." Resa Schirnhofer, a friend of Nietzsche, visited him in 1884 during this abrupt change in vision, and later wrote that he saw fantastic colors after closing his eyes—colorful flowers that flowed and changed in brilliant displays of movement. Hallucinations result from many potential causes, such as schizophrenia, temporary psychosis, and Parkinson's disease, but the relationship between vision loss and hallucinatory experiences in Nietzsche suggests Charles Bonnet syndrome (CBS). CBS is characterized by vivid, elaborate, and recurrent visual hallucinations in the absence of external stimuli in individuals with preserved intellectual functioning. Associated with anomalies at any juncture of the visual system, the condition can be episodic, periodic, or chronic. Macular degeneration and stroke-induced lesion in the visual system accounts for approximately 75–85% of CBS cases.

Headaches

As early as 11 years old, Nietzsche missed school due to headaches and eye pain. His letters suggest that he began to suffer from increasingly frequent and intense headache attacks throughout his 20s and 30s. Sometime between 1870 and 1871 he began to suffer from migrainous attacks. The situation became progressively worse over the next decade.

He complains in a letter to his colleague and friend Carl von Gersdorff, who Nietzsche had befriended at Schulpforta, "I've been through a very bad time, and there may be an even worse one to come. My stomach could no longer be tamed, even with an absurdly strict diet. Chronic headaches of the fiercest sort, which lasted for days. Vomiting on an empty stomach, for hours on end. In short the machine seemed to want to disintegrate, and I won't deny having wished several times that it would do just that. Great fatigue, difficulty getting about, hypersensitivity to light . . ." (Nietzsche 1971). Writing to Dr. Otto Eiser in January of 1880 he asserts, "And yet!—constant pain, a feeling much like seasickness several hours each day, a semi-paralysis which makes speaking difficult and, for a change of pace, furious seizures (the last involved three days and nights of vomiting; I lusted for death)" (Nietzsche 1971).

Nietzsche registered several important somatic complaints that are consistent with a diagnosis of migraine with aura (MA). His MA attacks involved fully reversible homonymous visual symptoms, unilateral sensory loss, and dysphasic speech. His headaches were prolonged and accompanied by photosensitivity, emesis, gastrointestinal pain, and fatigue. Medical evidence suggests that individuals more susceptible to triggers are likely to have headaches with a longer history of duration, more premonitory symptoms, throbbing, pressure, stabbing, nausea, photophobia, rhinorrhea, tearing of eyes, and higher headache frequency. These individuals are likely to choose rest during headaches and suffer from anxiety, depression, mood swings, and general pain. Nietzsche's MA attacks match well with this picture. His MAs lessened in the 1880s but returned suddenly in the summer 1888.

Mood Disorders

Nietzsche's correspondence also supports a diagnosis of major depression during the 1870s and early 1880s with an emergent hypomania in the early to mid-1880s. Just prior to the expression of subcortical dementia at the end of 1888 and beginning of 1889, Nietzsche's behavior shifted from hypomanic to manic and was accompanied by a psychotic break from reality. In the early 1880s, Nietzsche reached the nadir of his depression. His writings were not being acknowledged for their brilliance, plans of love and marriage with the young Russian Lou Salomé ended abruptly, and he distanced himself from his mother and sister. In August of 1883 he wrote, "I am now working like a man who is 'putting his house in order before departing.'" Nietzsche's intense depression began to alternate with a mood of euphoria.

Beginning in the 1870s, Nietzsche's struggle with melancholic moods and suicidal ideation became apparent to his closest friends and colleagues. In 1877 Nietzsche writes to Malwida von Meysenbug, a close friend he met through his prior friendship with Richard Wagner, "on the ship I had only the blackest thoughts, my only doubts about suicide concerned where the sea might be deepest, so that one would not be immediately fished out again and have to pay a debt of gratitude to one's rescuers in a terrible mass of gold—sometimes such a feeling of emptiness comes over me that I want to scream" (Nietzsche 1996).

In March 1883 he writes, "My dear friend—I've lost interest in everything. Deep down, an unyielding black melancholy. And weariness too. Most of the time I'm in bed. I've suffered too much and sacrificed too much; I feel so incomplete, so inexpressibly conscious of having bungled and botched my whole creative life. It's all hopeless. I won't do anything worthwhile again. Why do anything anymore!" (Nietzsche 1971).

Just a year later he writes an ecstatic letter to Peter Gast asserting,

> Thoughts have emerged on my horizon the likes of which I've never seen—I won't even hint at what they are, but shall maintain my own unshakeable calm. I suppose now I'll have to live a few years longer! Ah, my friend, I sometimes think that I lead a highly dangerous life, since I'm one of those machines that can burst apart. The intensity of my feelings makes me shudder and laugh. Several times I have been unable to leave my room, for the ridiculous reason that my eyes were inflamed. Why? Because I'd cried too much on my wanderings the day before. Not sentimental tears, mind you, but tears of joy, to the accompaniment of which I sang and talked nonsense, filled with a new vision far superior to that of other men. (Nietzsche, 1971)

In an explosion of ten days of racing thoughts and flight of ideas during the winter of 1882, Nietzsche produced Book One of *Thus Spake Zarathustra*. Just months later, he wrote Book Two over another ten-day stretch of prolonged creativity (Nietzsche 1971). While the evidence from his letters first suggests a diagnosis of major depression, as time elapsed his depressive episodes gave rise to cycling moods consistent with bipolar. For a relatively isolated individual, the pressured speech and loose concatenations of thought were expressed in written form, known as hypergraphia.

Nietzsche's Health from 1888 to 1900

In late December 1888 Nietzsche experienced a profound change in mental status. In early January 1889 he allegedly collapsed while in public. Nietzsche was brought to Dr. Ludwig Wille's psychiatric clinic near the Alsatian border for three days. He was an unruly patient, bursting into song or scream at any moment and demonstrating constant motor agitation. His gait was stumbling and not steady, and he seemed stiff at times. Next, Nietzsche was moved to Basel, where the patient records state, "Pupillary disparity, right larger than left, reaction sluggish. Convergent strabismus-acute myopia. Tongue heavily furred, no deviation, no tremor! Facial nerve almost normal; right nasolabial fold slightly contracted. Exaggerated patellar reflex; plantar reflexes normal" (Volz 1990).

Within a few days Nietzsche was moved to a clinic in Jena that was managed by a well-known physician, Dr. Otto Binswanger (who first described Binswanger's disease, coined by Alois Alzheimer). Both Wille and Binswanger diagnosed Nietzsche with *paralytica progressiva* due to syphilis. With this assessment, both doctors assumed Nietzsche only had two years to live. Dr. Binswanger's medical notes on Nietzsche give,

> Pupils right wide, left rather narrower, left contracted with slight irregularity, all reactions normal on left, on right only reaction to convergence, consensual reactions only on left . . . symmetrical smile, tongue non-tremulous with deviations to right . . . Romberg negative . . . screws left shoulder up spasmodically when walking . . . slight ankle clonus on left . . . head percussion not sensitive, facial nerves sensitive.

After several weeks, Nietzsche seemed to improve with no further deterioration. His mother surreptitiously removed him from the clinic to bring him home to care for him full-time. By 1893 he was completely bedridden and retained no memories of his life as a writer. During 1898 and 1899, Nietzsche suffered at least two more strokes that left him unable to speak or walk. On August 24, 1900, Nietzsche died either from another stroke or a pneumonia-like infection. Nietzsche was buried alongside his father's grave next to the parsonage in Röcken, Germany.

DIAGNOSIS AND DISCUSSION

Table 3.1 displays a historical list of diagnoses in the literature posited to explain Nietzsche's condition. Following the emergence of new diagnostic categories since 1889, novel diagnostic possibilities now exist to explain Nietzsche's constellation of symptoms. Nietzsche's persistent medical issues are explainable with one unifying, genetically testable diagnosis: cerebral autosomal dominant arteriopathy with subcortical infarcts and leukoencephalopathy (CADASIL). The diagnosis of CADASIL explains Friedrich's, Karl Ludwig's, and Friedrich August Nietzsche's condition. In this section I present our diagnosis and consider competing ideas.

CADASIL is likely the cause of Nietzsche's illness. It takes all of his relevant findings into account: retinal abnormalities, migraine with aura, mood disorders, early onset history of stroke-like episodes, pseudobulbar palsy, dementia, and three generations of paternal family history. A positive genetic test of Nietzsche's DNA for a *NOTCH3* gene mutation would be diagnostic.

Table 3.1
List of Previous Diagnostic Attempts to Explain Nietzsche's Illness

Diagnosis	Source
Paresis paralytica (neurosyphilis)	Binswanger 1889; Mobius 1902; Lange-Eichbaum 1930
Slow-growing benign brain tumor	Hildebrandt 1926
Bipolar disease and multi-infarct dementia	Cybulska 2000
Schizophrenia	Schain 2001
Meningioma of right optic nerve	Sax 2003
Frontotemporal dementia (FTD)	Orth and Trimble 2006
Meningioma of right medial sphenoid wing	Owen, Schaller, and Binder 2007
Cerebral autosomal dominant arteriopathy with subcortical infarcts and leukoencephalopathy (CADASIL)	Butler (this chapter), Hemelsoet, Hemelsoet, and Devreese 2008

CADASIL is a genetic mutation in the *NOTCH3* protein on chromosome 19p13.2-p13.1. This autosomal dominant condition leads to microangiopathy of the brain. The presentation of CADASIL is variable even among family members. CADASIL is suspected when stroke-like episodes occur before the age of 60, accompanied by MA, executive dysfunction, or behavioral abnormalities.

TIAs (transient ischemic attacks) occur in 85% of symptomatic individuals with the average age of onset at 46 (range 19–67 years). Ischemic episodes are recurrent, leading to severe disability usually including gait disturbance, urinary incontinence, and pseudobulbar palsy. Eighty-five percent of patients develop cognitive dysfunction and eventual dementia. These symptoms fit Nietzsche's disease progression. He presented with gait disturbance and pseudobulbar palsy in 1889, slowly progressing over the course of years to a demented, bedridden, and paralyzed state.

Migraine occurs in about 40% of CADASIL patients with the first attack occurring at a mean age of 26 years. Of the CADASIL patients with migraine 90% have MA. In some families with CADASIL, MA is the most prominent symptom. Again, Nietzsche's presentation clinically matches. His correspondences evince the development of MA by his mid- to late 20s.

Approximately 30% of individuals with CADASIL develop psychiatric disturbances, with depression, bipolar, and personality changes being most common. Undoubtedly Nietzsche struggled with major depression and mood swings that suggest bipolar disorder. Full-blown mania with delusions of grandeur afflicted him by the end of 1888.

Epilepsy is less common (~10% of CADASIL patients) and tends to develop in middle age. Although Nietzsche mentioned having a seizure in a letter cited earlier from January 1880, it is hard to interpret exactly what Nietzsche meant by his limited use of that term. However, seizures clearly afflicted Nietzsche's father. Most likely, Karl's episodes of loss of consciousness were either seizure-induced or TIA-induced syncope. Both seizure and TIAs are common in CADASIL, so differentiating between them is unimportant for diagnosis in this case. Nietzsche's family history supports the finding that CADASIL's clinical manifestations are variable even among relatives.

Most recently, retinal abnormalities have been linked to CADASIL. Retinal vascular abnormalities, inflammation, and vision loss have all been implicated. Nietzsche's right-sided retinal exudates, vision loss, and alleged eye movement abnormalities were likely expressions of CADASIL. Recent research findings suggest that CADASIL can lead to diminished optic nerve fiber layers, retinal vasculopathies, retinal inflammation, visual field loss, eye movement abnormalities, and visual-spatial defects.

By reasonable assumption, Nietzsche has a positive family history. His father suffered from numerous stroke-like episodes before the age of 60, struggled with depression, and developed pseudobulbar affect and potential palsy. There is evidence of seizures, hemi-facial paralysis, dysarthria, cognitive decline, dementia, and eventual death from stroke. CADASIL explains this array of seemingly disparate symptoms. Although less is known about him, Karl's father was afflicted by a similar array of symptoms. This pattern fits the autosomal dominance inheritance pattern of CADASIL. Genetics studies have traced original mutations back to the 1600s in some Northern European communities. It is therefore reasonable to assume the existence of CADASIL mutations in Nietzsche's patrilineage based on historical, demographic, and founder effect studies.

CADASIL as cause for Nietzsche's illness is testable. Because the common *NOTCH3* mutations are well established and currently tested for genetically, it is possible to obtain nuclear DNA from Nietzsche, amplify the gene of interest via polymerase chain reaction techniques, and test for CADASIL with 90% sensitivity. The author is actively pursuing this research goal. DNA can be extracted from minute salivary samples sealed in time between envelope folds or stamps adhered by Nietzsche during his lifetime. Theoretically, preserved DNA samples from envelopes sealed by Nietzsche's saliva could be amplified in the region of the *NOTCH3* gene and tested for CADASIL. This would provide incontrovertible evidence for this diagnosis.

Concurrent to the preparation of this publication, an independent research effort by Hemelsoet, Hemelsoet, and Devreese (2008) also suggests CADASIL as a potential diagnosis for Nietzsche. Herein, we extend the confidence in the diagnosis of CADASIL by including evidence for three successive generations of disease, Nietzsche's history of migraine *with* aura, psychiatric disturbance, fits, and retinal abnormalities. Without evidence to extend the paternal history of disease to three generations, CADASIL becomes less likely. With a two-generation model, the recessive form of CADASIL, known as CARASIL (Maeda's syndrome), must remain on the differential diagnosis in addition to other more common nongenetic sources of multi-infarct dementia, such as Binswanger's disease (ironic to Nietzsche's case) or cerebrovascular disease. Our evidence of three successive paternal generations with similar symptomology greatly increases confidence in the diagnosis of CADASIL (Volz 1990). Further, I suggest clear evidence that Nietzsche suffered from migraine with aura and not migraine without aura as argued by Hemelsoet et al. Migraine with aura and *not* migraine without aura is clinical evidence of CADASIL (Oberstein, Boon, and Dichgins 2006.) Further, we explain Nietzsche's retinal abnormalities as a manifestation of CADASIL pathology (Parisi et al. 2007; Robinson 2001; Warner 2004). His blindness and subsequent Charles Bonnet syndrome also fit with our diagnosis.

The neurosyphilis hypothesis has repeatedly been questioned even at the time of Nietzsche's diagnosis. Sax (2003) summarized the key weaknesses in the syphilis hypothesis: the lack of documentation of syphilitic infection, Nietzsche's prolonged life after his 1889 collapse, the laterality of his symptoms, lack of tremulous tongue, and the extended history of his headaches. Also, the alleged Argyll-Robertson pupils noted in Nietzsche's medical notes from Binswanger were due to congenital anisocoria, which was a condition unknown to the physicians at the Jena clinic.

Owen, Schaller, and Binder (2007) suggest that Nietzsche had a slow-growing medial sphenoid meningioma. This is plausible because intracranial mass lesions can cause lateral visual symptoms, headaches, cranial nerve dysfunction, psychiatric disturbances, and dementia. Several ideas argue against a brain mass as cause for all of Nietzsche's illnesses. There is a significant female-to-male predominance in medial sphenoid meningiomas, headaches are rare and tend to be dull and brief, tumors typically emerge in the sixth and seventh decades of life, and common predisposing factors include family history, focal trauma, and radiation exposure—none of which apply to Nietzsche (Demchuk and Forsyth 1997; Zachariah 2008).

Cybulska (2000) suggests Nietzsche suffered from bipolar disorder followed by multi-infarct dementia. Cybulska's diagnosis lacks definitive testability and cannot explain the retinal findings, family history, and cranial nerve findings. Likewise, several other diagnostic possibilities, such as schizophrenia, frontotemporal dementia (FTD), and mitochondrial myopathy–encephalopathy–lactic acidosis–stroke syndrome (MELAS) fail to make sense of the paternal family history and Nietzsche's seemingly disparate illnesses. MELAS is worth consideration because its heterogeneous manifestations potentially explain Nietzsche's retinal disturbances, headaches, vomiting, psychiatric disturbance, and stroke-like episodes. However, Nietzsche did not have a maternal history indicative of MELAS. With the exception of congenital anisocoria, records suggest Franziska was healthy throughout her life; she died from cancer at the age of 71, her mother lived to 82, and her daughter (Elisabeth, Nietzsche's sister) lived to 89.

CONCLUSION

Nietzsche has a positive three-generation family history—his father suffered from numerous stroke-like episodes before the age of 60, struggled with depression, and developed pseudobulbar affect and potential palsy. There is evidence of seizures, hemi-facial paralysis, dysarthria, cognitive decline, dementia, and eventual death from stroke ("softening of the brain"). CADASIL explains this array of seemingly disparate symptoms. Although less is known, Karl's father was afflicted by a similar array of symptoms. This pattern fits the autosomal dominant inheritance pattern of CADASIL (Rufa et al. 2007). Genetics studies have traced original mutations back to the 1600s in some Northern European communities. It is therefore reasonable to assume the existence of CADASIL mutations in Nietzsche's patrilineage based on historical, demographic, and founder effect studies (Mykkanen et al. 2004).

CADASIL as cause for Nietzsche's illness is testable. Because the common *NOTCH3* mutations are well established, it is possible to obtain Nietzsche's nuclear DNA from historical samples, amplify the region of interest (19p13.1–19p13.2) via PCR techniques, and test for CADASIL. The author is actively pursuing this research goal: DNA can be extracted from minute salivary samples sealed in time between envelope folds or stamps adhered by Nietzsche during his lifetime.

The best analytical tools at the time of Binswanger's diagnosis pointed to syphilitic paresis of the insane. Present-day reason leads us to believe Nietzsche (and his paternal lineage) suffered from a rare genetic mutation in the *NOTCH3* gene. Neurologists of the future will likely comprehend the diagnostic complexities with conceptual categories yet-to-be revealed.

POSTSCRIPT: THE INFLUENCE OF CADASIL ON NIETZSCHE'S LIFE AND THOUGHT

This research is important for understanding Nietzsche's biography, and potentially for the interpretation of his life's work. If Nietzsche was indeed afflicted by CADASIL, understanding the course and pathophysiology of this condition gives reason to Nietzsche's extreme suffering with one unifying diagnosis. Only Nietzsche fully comprehended the depth of his suffering, how powerfully it shaped his life and thought.

To illustrate the effect CADASIL had on Nietzsche's life and thought, I will first consider Nietzsche's supposed stylistic preference for pithy and profound statements in the form of aphorisms. Due to CADASIL-induced retinopathy, migraines with aura, and epileptic fits, Nietzsche's vision continually degraded with temporary blindness occurring during some of his worst attacks. These attacks occurred from several hours to days. His struggle intensified throughout the 1870s until he was forced to resign his professorship in 1879. During these fits, friends or family would care for him, reading aloud to him or recording his dictations as Nietzsche lay still in a dimly lit room. Elisabeth, Nietzsche's sister, recalled him saying he would have been a bookworm if it were not for his fits, migrainous attacks, and ill health (Volz 1990). Nietzsche was often allowed brief windows of time to collect his own thoughts without the invasion of ill health. This likely shaped his stylistic preference in part—driving him to master the form of aphorism. Nietzsche filled countless notebooks with aphoristic insights from early adulthood until the full development of subcortical dementia in 1889. These aphoristic notes were the basis for many of his publications, such as *Beyond Good and Evil*, *The Antichrist*, and *Genealogy of Morals*. In *The Antichrist*, Nietzsche writes, "it is my ambition to say in ten sentences what everyone else says in a book." Nietzsche became a dedicated master of the aphorism, in part because of the impact of CADASIL during his productive life.

After resigning from professorship at the University of Basel in 1879, Nietzsche spent the 10 years prior to his collapse moving seasonally from Northern Italy, Austria, France, Germany, and Switzerland. Nietzsche's personal library contained books on weather patterns, which he likely consulted, as he sought the perfect climate to attenuate the various triggers to his intense migraine attacks. Nietzsche accompanied this itinerant lifestyle with an ascetic diet—he refrained from consuming tea, alcohol, and tobacco, for instance. These behaviors were built around Nietzsche's trial-and-error approach to control all of the factors that triggered his CADASIL-associated attacks, and led to a largely isolated life, which Nietzsche intermittently filled with periods of brilliant literary productivity. One of Nietzsche's colleagues, Paul Deussen, commented on Nietzsche's eccentric behavior and lifestyle (due to negotiating his illnesses) after visiting the demented Nietzsche in the April 1889, writing,

> No one can say to what extent the seeds of insanity were already present as a disposition in this highly talented mind. But if Nietzsche had not diligently separated himself from human society, in which he occupied such an honorable position, if he had kept his position, established a family, and allowed the fruits of his mind to mature slowly, instead of pursuing his thoughts in solitude with ascetic over-exertion of his energies on tiring walks during the day and at night compelling elusive sleep by stronger and stronger narcotics— who knows whether he might not still be living with us in full health and be able to offer us, instead of the torso of his posthumous works, the perfected divine image of an eccentric but highly noteworthy worldview. (Deussen 1890/1922)

The pain Nietzsche endured due to CADASIL strongly shaped him as a thinker, an artist, and a philosopher. From a young age Nietzsche demonstrated musical talent. He composed pieces and played improvisational piano with considerable skill. One of the titles of his compositions from 1861 arranged when he was only 17 years old was entitled *Schmerz ist der Grundton der Natur* or translated "Pain is the elemental tone of Nature." Lou Salomé, an alleged romantic and intellectual interest of Nietzsche's, later wrote that he was "a sadomasochist toward himself" attempting to find some contorted version of pleasure in the psychic and physiologic pain he was forced to endure (Volz 1990).

In 1879 following the completion of *The Wanderer and His Shadow*, Nietzsche wrote in a letter, "The completed *Wanderer* is to me something almost unbelievable . . . the entire "humanity" with the 2 supplements is from a time of the most bitter and continual pains—and yet seems to me to be a thing full of health. This is my triumph."

Nietzsche firmly believed that "everything deep loves a mask." Nietzsche continually layered meanings into his writings that interleaved his own personal experiences within depth psychological insight, aesthetics, and philosophical conjecture. Nietzsche's CADASIL-induced Charles Bonnet Syndrome experience echoes in his section of the *Logic of the Dream*. In *Human, All Too Human*, he wrote, "If we close our eyes, the brain produces a host of light-impressions and colours" and likely in reference to his life's pain he later wrote in *Twilight of the Idols*, "*increscunt animi, virescit volnere virtus*" ("the spirit grows, strength is restored by wounding") (Nietzsche 2003, 2006).

Summarizing the profound physical suffering and mental anguish he endured, Nietzsche proffered,

> in combating my sick conditions I always instinctively chose the *right* means. . . . I took myself in hand, I myself made myself healthy again. . . . I made out of my will to health, to *life*, my philosophy. . . . For pay heed to this: it was in the years of my lowest vitality that I *ceased* to be a pessimist: the instinct for self-recovery *forbade* me to a philosophy of indigence and discouragement. (Nietzsche 1989)

Nietzsche wrote those words just months before the onset of his subcortical dementia. Four years earlier he asserted in *Beyond Good and Evil* (1955): "I have come to realize what every great philosophy up to now has been: the personal confession of its originator, a type of involuntary and unaware memoir." Still earlier, in an unpublished notebook from 1873, he wrote, "For what purpose humanity is there should not even concern us: why you are there, that you should ask yourself: and if you have no ready answer, then set for yourself goals, high and noble goals, and perish in pursuit of them! I know of no better life purpose than to perish in attempting the great and the impossible" (Nietzsche 2009).

As many opinions exist as the number of profound thinkers who have attempted to interpret Nietzsche's philosophical teaching (e.g., Heidegger 1961/1984; Lampert 1993; Rosen 1995). If Nietzsche did in fact suffer from CADASIL, this does not adjudicate among the many laudable attempts to delineate Nietzsche's philosophical thought. I merely suggest that the pathophysiology of CADASIL profoundly shaped the person of Nietzsche, his life events, thought, and philosophy. Nietzsche built many of his philosophical teachings, such as *will to power*, *eternal return of the same*, and the idea of the *übermensch*, around his personal experience with physical and mental pain. Nietzsche proffered,

> A philosopher who has traversed many kinds of health, and keeps traversing them, has passed through an equal number of philosophies; he simply cannot keep from transposing his states every time into the most spiritual form and distance: this art of transfiguration is philosophy. (Nietzsche 1974)

ACKNOWLEDGMENT: Special thanks go to Dorothe Poggel, PhD for help with translation of original German medical records. Also, I thank Peter

Bergethon, MD for help contributing commentary and constructive criticism for the manuscript. Special thanks also go to Patrick McNamara, PhD and Benjamin Wolozin, PhD, MD for early support of this project.

REFERENCES

Cybulska, E. M. 2000. The madness of Nietzsche: A misdiagnosis of the millennium? *Journal of Hospital Medicine* 61 (8): 571–575.

Demchuk, A., and P. Forsyth. 1997. Headache in the cancer patient. In *Handbook of Clinical Neurology,* ed. P. K. Vinken, G. W. Bruyn, and C. J. Vecht, 25 (69): Neuro-Oncology, pt. 3, 241–266.

Deussen, Paul. 1890/1922. Erinnerungen an Friedrich Nietzsche. Leipzig: Brockhaus. As cited in *Conversations with Nietzsche: A Life in the Words of His Contemporaries,* ed. Sander L. Gilman, trans. David J. Parent. New York: Oxford University Press.

Frenzel, Ivan. 1967. *Friedrich Nietzsche: An Illustrated Biography.* New York: Pegasus.

Hegel, Georg Wilhelm Friedrich. 1821/1991. *Elements of the Philosophy of Right.* Edited by Allen W. Wood, translated by H. B. Nisbet. Cambridge: Cambridge University Press.

Hegel, Georg Wilhelm Friedrich. 1837/1997. *Reason in History.* Translated by Robert S. Hartman. Upper Saddle River, NJ: Prentice-Hall.

Heidegger, Martin. 1961/1984. *Nietzsche: Volumes 1 and 2, The Will to Power as Art* and *The Eternal Recurrence of the Same.* Translated by David Farrell Krell. San Francisco: HarperCollins.

Hemelsoet, D., K. Hemelsoet, and D. Devreese. 2008. The neurological illness of Friedrich Nietzsche. *Acta Neurologica Belgica* 108: 9–16.

Hildebrandt, K. 1926. *Gesundheit und krankheit in Nietzsches leben und werk.* Berlin: Karger.

International Headache Society, Headache Classification Subcommittee. 2004. The international classification of headache disorders. *Cephalalgia,* 24.

Koszka, C. 2009. Friedrich Nietzsche (1844–1900): A classical case of mitochondrial encephalomyopathy with lactic acidosis and stroke-like episodes (MELAS) syndrome? *Journal of Medical Biography* 17: 161–164.

Lampert, L. 1993. *Nietzsche and Modern Times: A Study of Bacon, Descartes, and Nietzsche.* New Haven, CT: Yale University Press.

Lange-Eichbaum, W. 1930. Nietzsche als psychiatrisches problem. *Deutsche Medizinische Wochenschrift,* 1538.

Mobius, P. J. 1902. *Ueber das pathologische bei Nietzsche.* Wiesbaden: J. F. Bergmann.

Mykkanen, K., M. L. Savontaus, V. Juvonen, et al. 2004. Detection of the founder affect in Finnish CADASIL families. *Journal of European Human Genetics* 12: 813–819.

Nietzsche, Friedrich. 1955. *Beyond Good and Evil.* Translated by Marianne Cowan. Chicago: Henry Regnary.

Nietzsche, Friedrich. 1971. *Nietzsche: A Self-portrait from His Letters.* Edited and translated by Peter Fuss and Henry Shapiro. Cambridge: Harvard University Press.

Nietzsche, Friedrich. 1974. *The Gay Science: With a Prelude in Rhymes and an Appendix of Songs.* Translated by Walter Kaufmann. New York: Vintage Books.

Nietzsche, Friedrich. 1985. *Selected Letters: Nietzsche.* Translated by A. N. Ludovici and edited by O. Levy. London: Soho Book Company.

Nietzsche, Friedrich. 1989. *On the Genealogy of Morals and Ecce Homo.* Translated by Walter Kaufmann and R. J. Hollingdale. New York: Vintage Books.

Nietzsche, Friedrich. 1996. *Selected Letters of Friedrich Nietzsche.* Edited and translated by Christopher Middleton. Chicago: Hackett Publishing.

Nietzsche, Friedrich. 2003. *Twilight of the Idols and the Antichrist.* Translated by R. J. Hollingdale. New York: Penguin Books.

Nietzsche, Friedrich. 2006. *Human, All Too Human: A Book for Free Spirits.* Translated by R. J. Hollingdale. New York: Cambridge University Press.

Nietzsche, Friedrich. 2009. *Writings from the Early Notebooks.* Edited by Raymond Geuss and Alexander Nehamas. New York: Cambridge University Press.

Oberstein, S. L., E. Boon, and M. Dichgans. 2006. CADASIL: Cerebral autosomal dominant arteriopathy with subcortical infarcts and leukoencephalopathy. http://www.nih.gov/genetics/CADASIL (accessed November 1, 2009).

Orth, M., and M. R. Trimble. 2006. Friedrich Nietzsche's mental illness—general paralysis of the insane vs. frontotemporal dementia. *Acta Psychiatrica Scandanavia,* 439–445.

Owen, C., C. Schaller, and D. K. Binder. 2007. The madness of Dionysus: A neurosurgical perspective on Friedrich Nietzsche. *Journal of Neurosurgery Online* 61 (3): 626–632.

Paciaroni, M., and J. Bogousslavsky. 2009. How did stroke become of interest to neurologists? *Neurology* 73: 724–728.

Parisi, V., F. Pierelli, G. Coppola, et al. 2007. Reduction of optic nerve fiber layer thickness in CADASIL. *European Journal of Neurology* 14 (6): 627–631.

Robinson, W. 2001. Retinal findings in cerebral autosomal dominant arteriopathy with subcortical infarcts and leukoencephalopathy (CADASIL). *Survey of Ophtalmology* 45 (5): 445–448.

Rosen, S. 2004. *The Mask of Enlightenment: Nietzsche's Zarathustra.* New Haven, CT: Yale University Press.

Rufa, A., F. Guideri, M. Acampa, et al. 2007. Cardiac autonomic nervous system and risk of arrhythmias in cerebral autosomal dominant arteriopathy with subcortical infarcts and leukoencephalopathy (CADASIL). *Stroke* 38: 276–280.

Sax, L. 2003. What was the cause of Nietzsche's dementia? *Journal of Medical Biography* 11: 47–54.

Schain, R. 2001. *The Legend of Nietzsche's Syphilis.* Westport, CT: Greenwood.

Volz, P. 1990. *Nietzsche im labyrinth seiner krankeit: Eine medizininische-biographische untersuchung.* Würburg: Königshausen and Neumann.

Vukicevic, M., and K. Fitzmaurice. 2008. Butterflies and black lacy patterns: The prevalence and characteristics of Charles Bonnet hallucinations in an Australian population. *Journal of Clinical and Experimental Ophthalmology* 36: 659–665.

Warner, J. 2004. Vasculopathies affecting the eye. *Journal of Neuro-Ophthalmology* 24: 164–169.

Zachariah, S. 2008. Meningioma, sphenoid wing. http://www.emedicine.com (accessed March 1, 2008).

Chapter 4

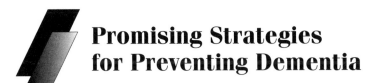 **Promising Strategies
for Preventing Dementia**

Laura E. Middleton

Age is the greatest risk factor for dementia, with the prevalence of dementia nearly doubling with every five years of age. The oldest-old, which
generally refers to people 85 years of age and older, are the fastest growing demographic in the United States. Increasing longevity over the com-
ing decades is expected to cause a dramatic increase in the prevalence of
dementia. The resources required to care for people with dementia will
rise along with the prevalence.

Healthcare systems are largely unprepared for the expected rise in
prevalence and for the complex care many people with dementia require.
People with severe dementia depend on caregivers or medical staff to
complete basic activities of daily living such as eating, bathing, and toilet-
ing. Co-morbid illnesses are common in people with dementia and require
concurrent treatment; however, pharmaceutical treatments can exacerbate
cognitive impairment, especially if multiple medications are taken concurrently. Outside of health care, significant demands are placed on the
caregivers of people with dementia, often spouses. Caregivers frequently
have lost productivity and increased absenteeism (Alzheimer's Association 2008). Furthermore, caregivers are at increased risk for adverse health
outcomes such as depressive and anxiety disorders (Schulz and Martire
2004).

Dementia does not appear to be an inevitable part of aging. Some
people do not develop dementia despite extreme old age and even in the
presence of neuropathic features normally associated with dementia. As a

result, increasing attention is been paid to identifying successful prevention strategies.

It is important to note that prevention may not be "all or none." Prevention may translate into less severe symptoms or delayed onset of disease.
However, if the onset of Alzheimer's disease (the most common form of
dementia) can be delayed by five years, the expected prevalence would
decrease by 1 million cases after 10 years and more than 4 million cases
after 50 years in the United States (Brookmeyer, Gray, and Kawas 1998).

Current pharmaceutical treatment for dementia can only modestly
improve symptoms and cannot cure or prevent dementia. As a result,
prevention of dementia through identification and modification of risk
factors is critical. Researchers have identified many risk and protective
factors through observational studies. Clinical trials confirming the relationship are often still preliminary. In this chapter, we will discuss some
of the most promising strategies for the prevention of dementia, including
cognitive activity, physical activity, social engagement, diet, and vascular
risk-factor control.

PREVENTION STRATEGIES

Cognitive Activity

People who engage in higher levels of cognitive activity appear to have
lower risk of dementia than those who participate in less. Aside from age,
education is arguably the most established risk factor for dementia. People
who are more educated have lower rates of Alzheimer's disease and all-
cause dementia than those with less education (Stern 2009). High levels of
education are also associated with slower cognitive decline during normal
aging (Albert et al. 1995; Colsher and Wallace 1991; Snowdon, Ostwald,
and Kane 1989).

Interestingly, people who are more highly educated may have faster
cognitive decline after the onset of Alzheimer's disease than those who
are less educated, though not all studies agree (Fritsch et al. 2002; Stern
2009). Some researchers suggest that this occurs because people with more
education can withstand greater neuropathic load before they show symptoms of Alzheimer's disease. There is some evidence to support this theory. One study reported that people who were more educated had greater
neuropathic loads before presenting symptoms of dementia compared to
those who were less educated (Bennett et al. 2003). This ability to withstand neuropathic load is referred to as "cognitive reserve"; occupational
attainment and leisure activity are also thought to contribute to cognitive
reserve (Stern 2009).

Research has emerged to suggest that cognitive activity, more generally, is also associated with reduced risk of cognitive decline and dementia (Stern 2009). Several prospective observational studies indicate that people who engage in mentally stimulating activities—such as learning, reading, or playing games—at younger ages (Carlson, Helms, et al. 2008) or older ages (Fratiglioni and Wang 2007) are less likely to develop dementia compared to those people who do not engage in these activities.

Moreover, interventional trials have demonstrated that cognitive training can improve cognitive performance in older adults regardless of baseline cognitive status (normal cognition; mild cognitive impairment, MCI; or dementia). In the ACTIVE trial, a large clinical trial of 2802 elderly people, training in memory, reasoning, and speed of processing were associated with improvements in cognitive performance equivalent to a 7- to 14-year reduction of normal aging effects (Ball et al. 2002). However, the benefits of cognitive training in this study and others appeared to be specific to the domain trained. Cognitive training does not appear to generalize across domains or improve daily functioning (Acevedo and Loewenstein 2007; Ball et al. 2002). Furthermore, there is some evidence to suggest that older people with memory impairment may be less able to make gains from memory training than those without impairment (Unverzagt et al. 2007). However, people with memory impairment appear to be equally able to make gains in reasoning and reaction time with training.

Although the role of cognitive training in people with dementia is unclear, cognitive activity appears to be a promising strategy to improve cognition in old age—and may thereby prevent or reduce the risk of dementia. However, because interventions to date show little benefit to daily function, future trials should investigate whether adapted multi-domain interventions, designed to mimic daily life, might be effective in improving global cognition and daily functioning. Simple interventions that include mental activities such as playing games or learning a new skill, which are associated with reduced rates of dementia and cognitive decline in observational studies (Wilson et al. 2002), might be effective in interventions. Trials should also investigate whether cognitive interventions might prevent the onset of dementia by including a long follow-up period.

Physical Activity

The evidence for physical activity as a potentially protective factor against the risk of dementia has expanded greatly over the last decade. Studies using a variety of ages, definitions of exercise, and countries have concluded that people who are more physically active have a lower risk of dementia. Specifically, physically active people may have a lower incidence of Alzheimer's disease and vascular dementia, though the association is more consistent for the former (Ravaglia et al. 2008; Rockwood and Middleton 2007).

The positive relationship between physical activity and the risk of dementia seems to hold true for physical activity both at older and younger ages. Most observational studies have examined physical activity in older populations (at least 65 years) and have had only a short follow-up time (approximately 5 years). Nearly all conclude that people who are physically active at older ages have 10–45% less risk of dementia at follow up than those who are inactive (Rockwood and Middleton 2007).

A number of studies have investigated the association between mid-life physical activity and late life cognitive impairment. People who are more physically active at mid-life seem to have a lower incidence of both Alzheimer's disease and all-cause dementia in late life, especially if the physical activity is performed during leisure time (Rockwood and Middleton 2007; Rovio et al. 2005, 2007). People who are active at mid-life also have lower risk of MCI in late life than those who are inactive (Geda et al. 2010).

Few studies have examined the relationship between physical activity in early life and cognition in old age. However, it appears that people who are physically active in early life also have better cognition in old age. Two studies indicated that people who were active in early life (teens to 30s) had better information processing speed and slower memory decline in later life (Dik et al. 2003; Richards, Hardy, and Wadsworth 2003). In another study, people who were physically active at teen age had lower risk of cognitive impairment in late life. Interestingly, physical activity status at teen age was more strongly related to reduced likelihood of cognitive impairment in late life than physical activity status at age 30, age 50, or in late life in this study (Middleton et al. 2010). It is reasonable to suggest that a longer duration of exercise is better than shorter, even though the benefits of exercise can be realized at any point in the life span. Age should not be a contra-indication to taking up an exercise program, other things being equal.

Significantly, physical activity is associated with augmented rates of stable or improved cognition and reduced rates of cognitive decline in people of all cognitive abilities (Lytle et al. 2004; Middleton et al. 2009; Weuve et al. 2004). Regardless of cognitive status, those people who are physically active seem to have better cognitive function and slower cognitive decline than those who are sedentary. However, it is unclear from observational studies whether physical activity improves cognition, delays impairment, or whether, in some cases, it prevents cognitive impairment entirely.

Interventional studies have confirmed that even short periods of exercise training can improve cognitive performance. A meta-analysis concluded that people who were not previously physically active showed improvements in cognitive functioning after exercising for as little as four months (Angevaren et al. 2008). Exercise interventions may also reduce the rate of cognitive decline in people with cognitive impairment (Lautenschlager et al. 2008). Executive function appears to be the cognitive domain most benefited by exercise (Colcombe and Kramer 2003).

The mechanisms by which physical activity affects cognition are likely complex and multifactorial. People who exercise have higher levels of brain-derived neurotrophic factors, which are implicated in neuroplasticity and neurological repair. Physical activity also reduces vascular risk; vascular risk factors are, as discussed later, associated not only with increased risk of vascular dementia but also of Alzheimer's disease. In addition, rats with high levels of voluntary physical activity also have less β-amyloid plaque formation, a hallmark of Alzheimer's disease (Dishman et al. 2006; Ott et al. 1999).

Despite the promising results from controlled trials to date, the trials of exercise interventions in relation to cognition have generally been low to moderate in both size and quality (Angevaren et al. 2008). Larger trials are needed to definitively determine the role of physical activity in the maintenance of cognitive performance and the prevention of dementia in old age. Such trials are underway. For example, the Lifestyle Interventions and Independence for Elders (LIFE) Study will begin in 2010 and will randomize 1600 people to either exercise or control groups and will follow them for an average of 2.7 years. The LIFE Study includes cognitive function as a secondary outcome. While we wait for results from ongoing trials, however, physical activity can be carefully recommended—if not for cognitive impairment, then for other health outcomes strongly linked to physical activity such as cardiovascular disease and some types of cancer (Warburton, Nicol, and Bredin 2006).

Social Engagement

Higher social engagement, measured in a variety of manners, appears to be associated with reduced risk of dementia. People who have an extensive social network have lower likelihood of dementia than those with few social connections (Seidler et al. 2003). Participation in socially engaging leisure activities—such as visits with friends and relatives, going to movies, clubs, centers, and church/synagogues, and volunteering—is also associated with reduced risk of dementia (Fratiglioni and Wang 2007).

Some suggest that social activity may increase cognitive reserve, similar to cognitive activity, so that people who are socially active can maintain cognitive performance even with neuropathic features normally associated with dementia (Fratiglioni and Wang 2007). Indeed, one study indicated that people with broader social networks had better cognitive performance, especially for memory, at a given neuropathic load (Bennett et al. 2006). However, the direction of this relationship is less clear. It may be that people who are able to maintain cognitive performance despite neuropathic feature normally associated with dementia are also more able to maintain social networks. The results of one study suggest as much. In this study, the relationship between low social engagement and high risk of dementia was restricted to those subjects who experienced a decline in social engagement from mid-life to late life (Saczynski et al. 2006). This suggests that low social engagement may be an early symptom of cognitive impairment rather than a risk factor.

There are no controlled trials that examined social engagement on its own in relation to dementia risk or cognitive outcomes. As a result, the importance of social engagement in a successful prevention strategy is still unclear. However, a volunteering intervention that was designed to include social, cognitive, and physical components showed a trend towards improved cognition in the intervention group compared to a control group. The volunteering intervention appeared to be most beneficial to those with baseline cognitive impairment (Carlson, Saczynski, et al. 2008).

Further studies are needed to determine whether social interventions might curb cognitive decline. However, the interactions between social activity, cognitive activity, and physical activity are difficult to disengage (Figure 4.1). One study concluded that each component is equally important in the protection against dementia (Karp et al. 2006). As a result, interventions that include cognitive, social, and physical components might be the best strategy to reduce the risk of cognitive impairment; research should further investigate this possibility. A larger, controlled trial should be instigated to evaluate whether multidomain interventions (cognitive, physical, and social) might be able to improve cognitive outcomes in those at risk for dementia.

Diet

Many risk factors for dementia (hypertension, diabetes, and obesity) and pathologic features (inflammation) associated with dementia can be modified by diet. Thus, it is reasonable to suggest that the risk of dementia

Figure 4.1

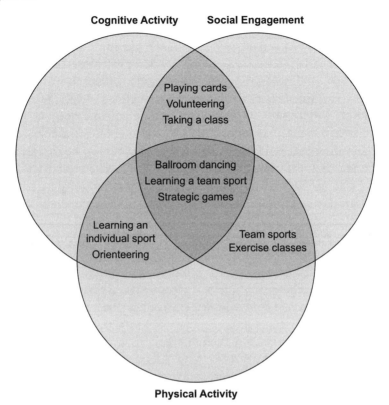

The cognitive, social, and physical components of leisure activity may evenly contribute to the prevention of dementia. Many leisure activities have all three types (cognitive, social, and physical) of stimulation.

itself could be modified by diet. Results from several observational studies support this hypothesis.

In most studies, adherence to a Mediterranean diet is associated with lower likelihood of Alzheimer's disease and all-cause dementia, as is greater consumption of fruit and vegetables, which is characteristic of a Mediterranean diet (Barberger-Gateau et al. 2007; Feart et al. 2009; Scarmeas et al. 2006). Adherence to a Mediterranean diet may also slow cognitive decline (Feart et al. 2009). Other studies found that people who consume high amounts of fish have lower dementia risk and slower cognitive decline (Barberger-Gateau et al. 2002; Kalmijn et al. 1997; Morris et al. 2003; van Gelder et al. 2007).

The reason for the association between fish, fruit, and vegetable intake and dementia risk has not been definitely identified but may be related to anti-oxidative, anti-inflammatory, or metabolic effects. On a component level, some attribute the relationship between Mediterranean diet and cognition to antioxidants and/or polyunsaturated fatty acids—consumption of each is associated with reduced risk of dementia and improved cognition in observational studies (Gillette Guyonnet et al. 2007). However, it may be that overall diet is more important than any one component.

The interest in antioxidants in relation to dementia risk stemmed from the observation that oxidative stress may contribute to neuropathic features associated with Alzheimer's disease. This observation led to the hypothesis that a high dietary intake of antioxidants might slow cognitive decline and lower the risk of dementia. Indeed, in some studies, people with higher intake of vitamin E and C (both antioxidants) through diet or supplements have slower cognitive decline and a lower risk of Alzheimer's disease. However, the relationship has not been consistent. Other large, prospective observational studies found no association between vitamin intake and dementia risk (Gillette Guyonnet et al. 2007). Furthermore, randomized controlled trial evidence has, at best, been inconsistent, with most studies finding no relationship between vitamin E supplementation and cognitive performance (Gillette Guyonnet et al. 2007; Isaac, Quinn, and Tabet 2008; Kang et al. 2006; Yaffe, Clemons, et al. 2004). This suggests that the association between antioxidants and cognitive impairment in observational studies may be due to uncontrolled confounding or other biases, rather than causation. Alternatively, vitamin supplementation may only be beneficial for those who are vitamin deficient.

Studies regarding consumption of long-chain omega-3 fatty acids, one type of essential polyunsaturated fatty acid common in many types of fish, have been similarly inconclusive (Fotuhi, Mohassel, and Yaffe 2009; van de Rest et al. 2008). Despite associations in observational studies, randomized controlled trials have not found a consistent association between omega-3 fatty acid supplementation and cognitive outcomes (Fotuhi, Mohassel, and Yaffe 2009). Omega-3 fatty acid supplementation also had no effect on memory and attention in cognitively healthy elderly people (van de Rest et al. 2008). However, most studies have been limited by a short follow up period.

The relationship between diet and dementia is likely confounded by numerous variables such as education, physical activity, vascular disease, and socioeconomic status. This may explain the inconsistent results of observational and controlled trials. Alternatively, it may be that one supplement is not sufficient to improve cognition or prevent dementia but that overall diet and lack of deficiencies is more important in optimizing cognitive outcomes. Interventions should examine the effect of supplementation on cognition in people who are deficient versus sufficient. Furthermore, an intervention focused on comprehensive dietary education and modification may have more of an effect than individual supplements. However, given that adherence to a Mediterranean diet is associated with reduced risk of mortality and cardiovascular disease (Sofi et al. 2008), people who adopt healthy diets are likely to have positive health outcomes regardless of the effect on cognitive functioning.

Increasing attention has recently been paid to vitamin D as a means to prevent dementia. Although evidence is very preliminary and generally cross-sectional, some studies suggest that higher serum 25-hydroxyvitamin D may be associated with better global cognition (Annweiler et al. 2009). Vitamin D is also associated with a number of risk factors for dementia including diabetes, cerebrovascular disease, and depression (Grant 2009). Future prospective observational and controlled trials should examine vitamin D intake in relation to cognition, particularly in people deficient in Vitamin D as is common in institutionalized elderly people.

Vascular Risk-Factor Reduction

Although Alzheimer's disease and vascular dementia have traditionally been viewed as distinct disorders, it is now generally agreed that the two rarely occur in isolation. Both types of dementia share many risk factors and pathologic features with atherosclerosis (Launer 2002). Even mild cerebrovascular disease appears to increase the risk of cognitive impairment for any level of Alzheimer's disease pathology (Snowdon et al. 1997). Thus, control of vascular risk factors might reduce the likelihood or severity of dementia, regardless of type.

Traditional cardiovascular risk factors such as hypertension, dyslipidemia, and diabetes appear to increase the risk of developing dementia in old age (Table 4.1). Hypertension is arguably the most studied vascular risk factors in relation to cognition, with inconsistent results. People with hypertension in mid-life had increased likelihood of dementia in late life in a number of observational studies (Launer et al. 2000; Qiu, Winblad, and Fratiglioni 2005). However, the relationship between late life hypertension and cognitive impairment is less clear. Both high systolic blood pressure and low systolic blood pressure in late life have been associated with augmented risk for dementia (Qiu, Winblad, and Fratiglioni 2005; Wu et al. 2003). Another study found no association between late life blood pressure and the incidence of dementia (Johnson et al. 2008). The reason for

Table 4.1
Summary of Evidence Regarding Vascular Risk Factors for Dementia

Risk Factor	Observational Studies	Trials
Hypertension	• Mid-life hypertension is associated with increased risk of dementia in late life. The association between late-life hypertension and dementia is less consistent. • People with hypertension who take antihypertensive medications have reduced risk of dementia compared to those who do not in most studies.	• Antihypertensives have not consistently reduced the risk of dementia/ cognitive impairment among people with hypertension. However, cognitive outcomes have generally been secondary and studies may be underpowered
Diabetes	• In most studies, people with diabetes in mid- or late life have higher risk of MCI and dementia. • Diabetics have faster cognitive decline in normal aging. • Diabetics may have slower cognitive decline after dementia onset, possibly due to onset with less severe neuropathic features.	• In a trial with no control group, diabetics showed improved cognition with glycemic management.
Dyslipidemia	• People with high levels of low-density lipoproteins have increased risk of cognitive impairment and vascular dementia in late life. • Statin therapy does not appear to reduce the risk of cognitive impairment among those with dyslipidemia.	• Two large, randomized-controlled trials suggested that statins do not improve cognitive outcomes.

Table 4.1 (*Continued*)

Obesity	• Obesity at mid-life is associated with higher risk of dementia in late life.	—
	• In late life, very high BMI or very low BMI may be associated with increased likelihood of dementia, possibly because obesity is a risk factor for dementia but weight loss may be an early symptom of the disease.	
Metabolic Syndrome	• People with metabolic syndrome have increased risk of cognitive impairment and cognitive decline in late life.	—
	• The effects of each vascular risk factor may be additive.	

these inconsistent results is unknown but it may reflect that hypertension is a risk factor for dementia but that hypotension is an early symptom of the disease.

If hypertension in mid-life is a risk factor for dementia, then it follows that antihypertensives have the potential to reduce the risk of dementia in people with hypertension. In observational studies, this appears to be the case. In a number of studies, people with hypertension who took antihypertensives had a lower risk of dementia than those who do not (Korf et al. 2004; Skoog 2009; Skoog et al. 2005). However, the results from controlled trials have been less consistent (Fillit et al. 2008; Peters et al. 2008; Prince et al. 1996). The largest study, the Hypertension in the Very Elderly Trial (HYVET), was not entirely conclusive but favored treatment of hypertension to improve cognitive outcomes when the results were combined into a meta-analysis with previous studies. However, most trials—including HYVET—were designed to examine other primary outcomes (Peters et al. 2008; Prince et al. 1996). The trials did not include detailed cognitive

measures and may not have been sufficiently powered to detect a relationship between antihypertensives and cognitive outcomes.

There is general accord that people with diabetes in late life have higher
risk of dementia and MCI compared to those who do not (Luchsinger,
Reitz, et al. 2007; Ott et al. 1999; Yaffe, Blackwell, et al. 2004), though some
studies show no association between the two (Luchsinger and Gustafson
2009). Similarly, mid-life diabetes is associated with augmented risk of
dementia in some but not all studies. The relationship with diabetes seems
to be stronger and more consistent for vascular dementia and vascular
cognitive impairment than for Alzheimer's disease and amnestic MCI
(Hassing et al. 2002; Luchsinger and Gustafson 2009; MacKnight et al.
2002; Whitmer 2007).

Counterintuitively, studies report that people who are treated for
diabetes have a greater likelihood of dementia than those who are not
(Luchsinger et al. 2001; Ott et al. 1999); however, this relationship is likely
confounded by severity, where people who receive treatment have more
severe diabetes than those who are not treated. Diabetics with hypoglycemic episodes, a complication of uncontrolled diabetes, also have a higher
risk of dementia (Whitmer et al. 2009).

Diabetes is also associated with faster cognitive decline in normal aging
(Gregg et al. 2000). In contrast, diabetics have slower cognitive decline
after Alzheimer's disease onset (Sanz et al. 2009). The slower decline after
Alzheimer's disease onset may occur because diabetics have less severe
Alzheimer's disease neuropathic features at onset. Indeed, there is evidence to suggest that people with dementia who have type 2 diabetes
have fewer plaques and neurofibrillary tangles than people with dementia only, indicating that people with diabetes may have more severe
symptoms of cognitive impairment for a given level of neuropathology
(Beeri et al. 2005).

Results from one controlled trial suggested that glycemic control by
medical management improved cognitive outcomes in type 2 diabetics;
however the trial was not placebo controlled (Ryan et al. 2006). Consequently, the results are very preliminary. The Action to Control Cardiovascular Risk in Diabetes Memory in Diabetes Study (ACCORD-MIND)
examined whether intense glycemic control improved cognitive outcomes
relative to standard care in type 2 diabetics who are 60 years or older
(Williamson et al. 2007). At baseline, those with better insulin control as
measured by A1C had better cognitive performance on a number of tests
(Cukierman-Yaffe et al. 2009). Although the longitudinal cognitive results
have not yet been released, the main ACCORD study was terminated
early due to an excess of deaths in the intense glycemic control group

relative to the standard control group (Hoogwerf 2008). It is unlikely that any potential cognitive benefits could justify the excess deaths associated with intense glycemic control.

Other vascular risk factors are also associated with increased likelihood of cognitive impairment, though evidence is more limited. Dyslipidemia is associated with enhanced risk of cognitive impairment in old age. People with high levels of low-density lipoproteins in late life have increased risk of cognitive impairment and dementia with stroke (Moroney et al. 1999; Yaffe et al. 2002). A number of observational trials have examined whether statin therapy is associated with reduced risk of cognitive impairment in people with dyslipidemia but the results are not convincing. Most cross-sectional studies found a link between statin use and lower likelihood of dementia but longitudinal studies did not (Rockwood 2006). Furthermore, two large, randomized controlled trials concluded that statin therapy did not improve cognitive outcomes (Heart Protection Study Collaborative Group 2002; Trompet et al. 2009). Consequently, current evidence suggests that statin therapy may not have a role in dementia prevention.

Obesity at mid-life, as measured using body mass index (BMI) or waist circumference, is also associated with higher likelihood of dementia in late life (Gustafson et al. 2003; Whitmer et al. 2005). However, the relationship is less consistent in later-life. In people 76 years and older, the relationship between BMI and dementia may resemble a U-shaped curve, where those with very high or low BMI have increased risk of dementia. (Luchsinger, Patel, et al. 2007) It is possible that high body fat is a risk factor for dementia while weight loss is a symptom of dementia pathology prior to diagnosis.

A cluster of three or more vascular risk factors (hypertension, hyperglycemia, abdominal obesity, and/or low high-density lipoprotein) is referred to as the metabolic syndrome. Not surprisingly, people with the metabolic syndrome also have augmented risk of cognitive impairment and cognitive decline in a number of studies (Komulainen et al. 2007; Vanhanen et al. 2006; Yaffe et al. 2007). One study suggested that the effects of each vascular risk factor were approximately additive (Yaffe 2007). Interestingly, another study found that metabolic syndrome was associated with slower cognitive decline in the oldest old (van den Berg et al. 2007). Why this is so is unclear but may reflect differential survival in this age group.

The mechanisms linking vascular risk factors to cognitive impairment are likely multifactorial. Since it is more common to have multiple vascular risk factors than just one, it is difficult to establish mechanistic links between individual vascular risk factors and dementia. The direct relationship between hypertension, cerebrovascular disease (in its most severe case, stroke), and subsequent dementia is well established. Cerebrovascular disease may also be the mechanistic pathway linking obesity, diabetes, and dyslipidemia with cognitive impairment. The degenerative changes in the cerebrovascular vessels may also cause dysfunction of both the endothelium and blood-brain barrier, causing the endothelial cells to produce an excess of free radicals and subsequent oxidative stress. This may result in increased blood-brain barrier permeability to proteins, leading to β-amyloid accumulation (Duron and Hanon 2008).

There is also a growing body of work that suggests a direct link between insulin and Alzheimer's disease pathology. Specifically, *in vitro* studies indicate that insulin causes a significant increase in extracellular β-amyloid levels (Luchsinger and Gustafson 2009). Consequently, people with insulin resistance, such as type II diabetics, or those with precursor hyperinsulemia, may have increases in β-amyloid levels caused by elevated insulin levels.

In addition, adipose tissue secretes both metabolic and inflammatory factors (Launer et al. 1995). Specifically, the secretion of inflammatory adipocytokines may be involved in neurodegenerative pathways. It is unclear, however, whether adipose tissue is directly linked to cognitive impairment or whether the adipose tissue is a marker of insulin resistance and hyperinsulinemia (Launer et al. 1995). Another mechanistic pathway may be cholesterol, which is a key regulator of neuronal function thought to contribute to regulation of β-amyloid plaque deposition in the brain (Fillit et al. 2008).

There are several areas that still need to be studied with regards to vascular risk management and cognition. Lifestyle management of vascular risk factors should be examined in relation to cognition in people with high vascular risk. In addition, a large, randomized controlled trial of medical management for glycemic control in diabetics is needed to definitely determine whether standard glycemic control improves cognitive outcomes; however, given the cardiovascular benefits of standard glycemic control, a randomized controlled trial to examine the cognitive benefits is unlikely to occur.

Despite the inconsistent or missing results regarding vascular risk management (Table 4.1), it is relatively agreed that people with vascular risk factors are also at augmented risk for dementia compared to those without vascular risk factors. As a result, clinicians treating people with vascular risk factors should be aware of and screen for symptoms of cognitive impairment. Preventative strategies—which may include lifestyle management and medications targeting dementia pathologic features—may be efficacious in reducing the likelihood of dementia in this high-risk group.

Figure 4.2

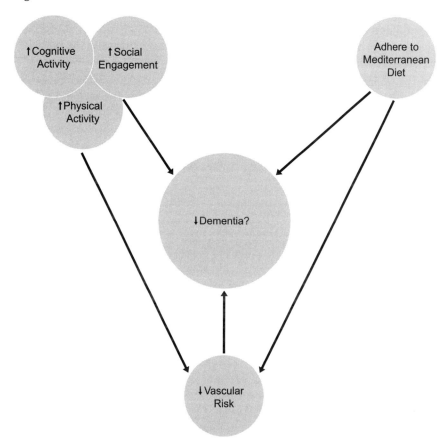

Interaction between promising strategies for the prevention of dementia.

CONCLUSION

Understanding how behavioral and biological factors might alter the risk of dementia is crucial to the prevention of the disease. Observational studies have identified factors including cognitive activity, physical activity, social activity, vascular risk factors, and diet that could be important both in identifying people at risk for dementia and for interventional strategies to reduce the risk. Though preliminary interventional studies have been less conclusive, future trials should continue to examine the impact of risk-factor modification on cognitive outcomes. Given that the risk factors are largely correlated—people who are more active generally have a better diet and lower vascular risk, it may be that living a healthy, engaged life is the best way to prevent dementia and that any one single factor is insufficient to prevent the disease (Figure 4.2). Future trials should continue to examine the implication of risk factor modification and, in particular, how we might combine interventions for optimal results. In the most optimistic view, dementia could be delayed or even prevented by these interventions. At worst, people will improve their overall health and enjoy a more cognitively and socially engaging life.

ACKNOWLEDGMENT: Dr. Middleton is supported in part by a Canadian Institutes of Health Research Fellowship.

REFERENCES

Acevedo, A., and D. A. Loewenstein. 2007. Nonpharmacological cognitive interventions in aging and dementia. *J Geriatr Psychiatry Neurol* 20 (4): 239–249.

Albert, M. S., K. Jones, C. R. Savage, L. Berkman, T. Seeman, D. Blazer, and J. W. Rowe. 1995. Predictors of cognitive change in older persons: MacArthur studies of successful aging. *Psychol Aging* 10 (4): 578–589.

Alzheimer's Association. 2008. *Alzheimer's disease facts and figures 2008*. http:// www.alz.org/national/documents/report_alzfactsfigures2008.pdf (accessed March 24, 2008).

Angevaren, M., G. Aufdemkampe, H. J. Verhaar, A. Aleman, and L. Vanhees. 2008. Physical activity and enhanced fitness to improve cognitive function in older people without known cognitive impairment. *Cochrane Database Syst Rev* (3): CD005381.

Annweiler, C., G. Allali, P. Allain, S. Bridenbaugh, A. M. Schott, R. W. Kressig, and O. Beauchet. 2009. Vitamin D and cognitive performance in adults: A systematic review. *Eur J Neurol* 16 (10): 1083–1089.

Ball, K., D. B. Berch, K. F. Helmers, J. B. Jobe, M. D. Leveck, M. Marsiske, J. N. Morris, et al. 2002. Effects of cognitive training interventions with older adults: A randomized controlled trial. *JAMA* 288 (18): 2271–2281.

Barberger-Gateau, P., L. Letenneur, V. Deschamps, K. Peres, J. F. Dartigues, and S. Renaud. 2002. Fish, meat, and risk of dementia: Cohort study. *BMJ* 325 (7370): 932–933.

Barberger-Gateau, P., C. Raffaitin, L. Letenneur, C. Berr, C. Tzourio, J. F. Dartigues, and A. Alperovitch. 2007. Dietary patterns and risk of dementia: The Three-City cohort study. *Neurology* 69 (20): 1921–1930.

Beeri, M. S., J. M. Silverman, K. L. Davis, D. Marin, H. Z. Grossman, J. Schmeidler, D. P. Purohit, et al. 2005. Type 2 diabetes is negatively associated with Alzheimer's disease neuropathology. *J Gerontol A Biol Sci Med Sci* 60 (4): 471–475.

Bennett, D. A., J. A. Schneider, Z. Arvanitakis, J. F. Kelly, N. T. Aggarwal, R. C. Shah, and R. S. Wilson. 2006. Neuropathology of older persons without cognitive impairment from two community-based studies. *Neurology* 66 (12): 1837–1844.

Bennett, D. A., R. S. Wilson, J. A. Schneider, D. A. Evans, C. F. Mendes de Leon, S. E. Arnold, L. L. Barnes, and J. L. Bienias. 2003. Education modifies the relation of AD pathology to level of cognitive function in older persons. *Neurology* 60 (12): 1909–1915.

Brookmeyer, R., S. Gray, and C. Kawas. 1998. Projections of Alzheimer's disease in the United States and the public health impact of delaying disease onset. *Am J Public Health* 88 (9): 1337–1342.

Carlson, M. C., M. J. Helms, D. C. Steffens, J. R. Burke, G. G. Potter, and B. L. Plassman. 2008. Midlife activity predicts risk of dementia in older male twin pairs. *Alzheimers Dement* 4 (5): 324–331.

Carlson, M. C., J. S. Saczynski, G. W. Rebok, T. Seeman, T. A. Glass, S. McGill, J. Tielsch, K. D. Frick, J. Hill, and L. P. Fried. 2008. Exploring the effects of an "everyday" activity program on executive function and memory in older adults: Experience Corps. *Gerontologist* 48 (6): 793–801.

Colcombe, S., and A. F. Kramer. 2003. Fitness effects on the cognitive function of older adults: A meta-analytic study. *Psychol Sci* 14 (2): 125–130.

Colsher, P. L., and R. B. Wallace. 1991. Longitudinal application of cognitive function measures in a defined population of community-dwelling elders. *Ann Epidemiol* 1 (3): 215–230.

Cukierman-Yaffe, T., H. C. Gerstein, J. D. Williamson, R. M. Lazar, L. Lovato, M. E. Miller, L. H. Coker, et al. 2009. Relationship between baseline glycemic control and cognitive function in individuals with type 2 diabetes and other cardiovascular risk factors: The action to control cardiovascular risk in diabetes-memory in diabetes (ACCORD-MIND) trial. *Diabetes Care* 32 (2): 221–226.

Dik, M., D. J. Deeg, M. Visser, and C. Jonker. 2003. Early life physical activity and cognition at old age. *J Clin Exp Neuropsychol* 25 (5): 643–653.

Dishman, R. K., H. R. Berthoud, F. W. Booth, C. W. Cotman, V. R. Edgerton, M. R. Fleshner, S. C. Gandevia, et al. 2006. Neurobiology of exercise. *Obesity (Silver Spring)* 14 (3): 345–356.

Duron, E., and O. Hanon. 2008. Vascular risk factors, cognitive decline, and dementia. *Vasc Health Risk Manag* 4 (2): 363–381.

Feart, C., C. Samieri, V. Rondeau, H. Amieva, F. Portet, J. F. Dartigues, N. Scarmeas, and P. Barberger-Gateau. 2009. Adherence to a Mediterranean diet, cognitive decline, and risk of dementia. *JAMA* 302 (6): 638–648.

Fillit, H., D. T. Nash, T. Rundek, and A. Zuckerman. 2008. Cardiovascular risk factors and dementia. *Am J Geriatr Pharmacother* 6 (2): 100–118.

Fotuhi, M., P. Mohassel, and K. Yaffe. 2009. Fish consumption, long-chain omega-3 fatty acids and risk of cognitive decline or Alzheimer disease: A complex association. *Nat Clin Pract Neurol* 5 (3): 140–152.

Fratiglioni, L., and H. X. Wang. 2007. Brain reserve hypothesis in dementia. *J Alzheimers Dis* 12 (1): 11–22.

Fritsch, T., M. J. McClendon, K. A. Smyth, and P. K. Ogrocki. 2002. Effects of educational attainment and occupational status on cognitive and functional decline in persons with Alzheimer-type dementia. *Int Psychogeriatr* 14 (4): 347–363.

Geda, Y. E., R. O. Roberts, D. S. Knopman, T. J. Christianson, V. S. Pankratz, R. J. Ivnik, B. F. Boeve, E. G. Tangalos, R. C. Petersen, and W. A. Rocca. 2010. Physical exercise, aging, and mild cognitive impairment: A population-based study. *Arch Neurol* 67 (1): 80–86.

Gillette Guyonnet, S., G. Abellan Van Kan, S. Andrieu, P. Barberger-Gateau, C. Berr, M. Bonnefoy, J. F. Dartigues, et al. 2007. IANA task force on nutrition and cognitive decline with aging. *J Nutr Health Aging* 11 (2): 132–152.

Grant, W. B. 2009. Does vitamin D reduce the risk of dementia? *J Alzheimers Dis* 17 (1): 151–159.

Gregg, E. W., K. Yaffe, J. A. Cauley, D. B. Rolka, T. L. Blackwell, K. M. Narayan, and S. R. Cummings. 2000. Is diabetes associated with cognitive impairment and cognitive decline among older women? Study of Osteoporotic Fractures Research Group. *Arch Intern Med* 160 (2): 174–180.

Gustafson, D., E. Rothenberg, K. Blennow, B. Steen, and I. Skoog. 2003. An 18-year follow-up of overweight and risk of Alzheimer disease. *Arch Intern Med* 163 (13): 1524–1528.

Hassing, L. B., B. Johansson, S. E. Nilsson, S. Berg, N. L. Pedersen, M. Gatz, and G. McClearn. 2002. Diabetes mellitus is a risk factor for vascular dementia, but not for Alzheimer's disease: A population-based study of the oldest old. *Int Psychogeriatr* 14 (3): 239–248.

Heart Protection Study Collaborative Group. 2002. MRC/BHF Heart Protection Study of cholesterol lowering with simvastatin in 20,536 high-risk individuals: A randomised placebo-controlled trial. *Lancet* 360 (9326): 7–22.

Hoogwerf, B. J. 2008. Does intensive therapy of type 2 diabetes help or harm? Seeking accord on ACCORD. *Cleve Clin J Med* 75 (10): 729–737.

Isaac, M. G., R. Quinn, and N. Tabet. 2008. Vitamin E for Alzheimer's disease and mild cognitive impairment. *Cochrane Database Syst Rev* (3): CD002854.

Johnson, K. C., K. L. Margolis, M. A. Espeland, C. C. Colenda, H. Fillit, J. E. Manson, K. H. Masaki, et al. 2008. A prospective study of the effect of hypertension and baseline blood pressure on cognitive decline and dementia in postmenopausal women: The Women's Health Initiative Memory Study. *J Am Geriatr Soc* 56 (8): 1449–1458.

Kalmijn, S., L. J. Launer, A. Ott, J. C. Witteman, A. Hofman, and M. M. Breteler. 1997. Dietary fat intake and the risk of incident dementia in the Rotterdam Study. *Ann Neurol* 42 (5): 776–782.

Kang, J. H., N. Cook, J. Manson, J. E. Buring, and F. Grodstein. 2006. A randomized trial of vitamin E supplementation and cognitive function in women. *Arch Intern Med* 166 (22): 2462–2468.

Karp, A., S. Paillard-Borg, H. X. Wang, M. Silverstein, B. Winblad, and L. Fratiglioni. 2006. Mental, physical, and social components in leisure activities equally contribute to decrease dementia risk. *Dement Geriatr Cogn Disord* 21 (2): 65–73.

Komulainen, P., T. A. Lakka, M. Kivipelto, M. Hassinen, E. L. Helkala, I. Haapala, A. Nissinen, and R. Rauramaa. 2007. Metabolic syndrome and cognitive function: A population-based follow-up study in elderly women. *Dement Geriatr Cogn Disord* 23 (1): 29–34.

Korf, E. S., L. R. White, P. Scheltens, and L. J. Launer. 2004. Midlife blood pressure and the risk of hippocampal atrophy: The Honolulu-Asia Aging Study. *Hypertension* 44 (1): 29–34.

Launer, L. J. 2002. Demonstrating the case that AD is a vascular disease: Epidemiologic evidence. *Ageing Res Rev* 1 (1): 61–77.

Launer, L. J., K. Masaki, H. Petrovitch, D. Foley, and R. J. Havlik. 1995. The association between midlife blood pressure levels and late life cognitive function: The Honolulu-Asia Aging Study. *JAMA* 274 (23): 1846–1851.

Launer, L. J., G. W. Ross, H. Petrovitch, K. Masaki, D. Foley, L. R. White, and R. J. Havlik. 2000. Midlife blood pressure and dementia: The Honolulu-Asia aging study. *Neurobiol Aging* 21 (1): 49–55.

Lautenschlager, N. T., K. L. Cox, L. Flicker, J. K. Foster, F. M. van Bockxmeer, J. Xiao, K. R. Greenop, and O. P. Almeida. 2008. Effect of physical activity on cognitive function in older adults at risk for Alzheimer disease: A randomized trial. *JAMA* 300 (9): 1027–1037.

Luchsinger, J. A., and D. R. Gustafson. 2009. Adiposity, type 2 diabetes, and Alzheimer's disease. *J Alzheimers Dis* 16 (4): 693–704.

Luchsinger, J. A., B. Patel, M. X. Tang, N. Schupf, and R. Mayeux. 2007. Measures of adiposity and dementia risk in elderly persons. *Arch Neurol* 64 (3): 392–398.

Luchsinger, J. A., C. Reitz, B. Patel, M. X. Tang, J. J. Manly, and R. Mayeux. 2007. Relation of diabetes to mild cognitive impairment. *Arch Neurol* 64 (4): 570–575.

Luchsinger, J. A., M. X. Tang, Y. Stern, S. Shea, and R. Mayeux. 2001. Diabetes mellitus and risk of Alzheimer's disease and dementia with stroke in a multiethnic cohort. *Am J Epidemiol* 154 (7): 635–641.

Lytle, M. E., J. Vander Bilt, R. S. Pandav, H. H. Dodge, and M. Ganguli. 2004. Exercise level and cognitive decline: The MoVIES project. *Alzheimer Dis Assoc Disord* 18 (2): 57–64.

MacKnight, C., K. Rockwood, E. Awalt, and I. McDowell. 2002. Diabetes mellitus and the risk of dementia, Alzheimer's disease and vascular cognitive impairment in the Canadian Study of Health and Aging. *Dement Geriatr Cogn Disord* 14 (2): 77–83.

Middleton, L. E., D. E. Barnes, L. Y. Lui, and K. Yaffe. 2010. Physical activity over the life course and its association with cognitive performance and impairment in old age. *J Am Geriatr Soc* 58 (7): 1322–1326.

Middleton, L. E., A. Mitnitski, N. Fallah, S. A. Kirkland, K. Rockwood. 2009. Changes in cognition and mortality in relation to exercise in late life: A population based study. *PLoS One* 3 (9): e3124.

Moroney, J. T., M. X. Tang, L. Berglund, S. Small, C. Merchant, K. Bell, Y. Stern, and R. Mayeux. 1999. Low-density lipoprotein cholesterol and the risk of dementia with stroke. *JAMA* 282 (3): 254–260.

Morris, M. C., D. A. Evans, J. L. Bienias, C. C. Tangney, D. A. Bennett, R. S. Wilson, N. Aggarwal, and J. Schneider. 2003. Consumption of fish and n-3 fatty acids and risk of incident Alzheimer disease. *Arch Neurol* 60 (7): 940–946.

Ott, A., R. P. Stolk, F. van Harskamp, H. A. Pols, A. Hofman, and M. M. Breteler. 1999. Diabetes mellitus and the risk of dementia: The Rotterdam Study. *Neurology* 53 (9): 1937–1942.

Peters, R., N. Beckett, F. Forette, J. Tuomilehto, R. Clarke, C. Ritchie, A. Waldman, et al. 2008. Incident dementia and blood pressure lowering in the Hypertension in the Very Elderly Trial Cognitive function assessment (HYVET-COG): A double-blind, placebo controlled trial. *Lancet Neurol* 7 (8): 683–689.

Prince, M. J., A. S. Bird, R. A. Blizard, and A. H. Mann. 1996. Is the cognitive function of older patients affected by antihypertensive treatment? Results from 54 months of the Medical Research Council's trial of hypertension in older adults. *BMJ* 312 (7034): 801–805.

Qiu, C., B. Winblad, and L. Fratiglioni. 2005. The age-dependent relation of blood pressure to cognitive function and dementia. *Lancet Neurol* 4 (8): 487–499.

Ravaglia, G., P. Forti, A. Lucicesare, N. Pisacane, E. Rietti, M. Bianchin, and E. Dalmonte. 2008. Physical activity and dementia risk in the elderly: findings from a prospective Italian study. *Neurology* 70 (19 Pt 2): 1786–1794.

Richards, M., R. Hardy, and M. E. Wadsworth. 2003. Does active leisure protect cognition? Evidence from a national birth cohort. *Soc Sci Med* 56 (4): 785–792.

Rockwood, K. 2006. Epidemiological and clinical trials evidence about a preventive role for statins in Alzheimer's disease. *Acta Neurol Scand Suppl* 185: 71–77.

Rockwood, K., and L. Middleton. 2007. Physical activity and the maintenance of cognitive function. *Alzheimers Dement* 3 (2 Suppl): S38–44.

Rovio, S., I. Kareholt, E. L. Helkala, M. Viitanen, B. Winblad, J. Tuomilehto, H. Soininen, A. Nissinen, and M. Kivipelto. 2005. Leisure-time physical activity at midlife and the risk of dementia and Alzheimer's disease. *Lancet Neurol* 4 (11): 705–711.

Rovio, S., I. Kareholt, M. Viitanen, B. Winblad, J. Tuomilehto, H. Soininen, A. Nissinen, and M. Kivipelto. 2007. Work-related physical activity and the risk of dementia and Alzheimer's disease. *Int J Geriatr Psychiatry* 22 (9): 874–882.

Ryan, C. M., M. I. Freed, J. A. Rood, A. R. Cobitz, B. R. Waterhouse, and M. W. Strachan. 2006. Improving metabolic control leads to better working memory in adults with type 2 diabetes. *Diabetes Care* 29 (2): 345–351.

Saczynski, J. S., L. A. Pfeifer, K. Masaki, E. S. Korf, D. Laurin, L. White, and L. J. Launer. 2006. The effect of social engagement on incident dementia: The Honolulu-Asia aging study. *Am J Epidemiol* 163 (5): 433–440.

Sanz, C., S. Andrieu, A. Sinclair, H. Hanaire, and B. Vellas. 2009. Diabetes is associated with a slower rate of cognitive decline in Alzheimer disease. *Neurology* 73 (17): 1359–1366.

Scarmeas, N., Y. Stern, R. Mayeux, and J. A. Luchsinger. 2006. Mediterranean diet, Alzheimer disease, and vascular mediation. *Arch Neurol* 63 (12): 1709–1717.

Schulz, R., and L. M. Martire. 2004. Family caregiving of persons with dementia: Prevalence, health effects, and support strategies. *AJGP* 12 (3): 240–249.

Seidler, A., T. Bernhardt, A. Nienhaus, and L. Frolich. 2003. Association between the psychosocial network and dementia—A case-control study. *J Psychiatr Res* 37 (2): 89–98.

Skoog, I. 2009. Antihypertensive treatment and dementia. *Pol Arch Med Wewn* 119 (9): 524–525.

Skoog, I., H. Lithell, L. Hansson, D. Elmfeldt, A. Hofman, B. Olofsson, P. Trenkwalder, and A. Zanchetti. 2005. Effect of baseline cognitive function and antihypertensive treatment on cognitive and cardiovascular outcomes: Study on Cognition and Prognosis in the Elderly (SCOPE). *Am J Hypertens* 18 (8): 1052–1059.

Snowdon, D. A., L. H. Greiner, J. A. Mortimer, K. P. Riley, P. A. Greiner, and W. R. Markesbery. 1997. Brain infarction and the clinical expression of Alzheimer disease. The Nun Study. *JAMA* 277 (10): 813–817.

Snowdon, D. A., S. K. Ostwald, and R. L. Kane. 1989. Education, survival, and independence in elderly Catholic sisters, 1936–1988. *Am J Epidemiol* 130 (5): 999–1012.

Sofi, F., F. Cesari, R. Abbate, G. F. Gensini, and A. Casini. 2008. Adherence to Mediterranean diet and health status: meta-analysis. *BMJ* 337:a1344.

Stern, Y. 2009. Cognitive reserve. *Neuropsychologia* 47 (10): 2015–2028.

Trompet, S., P. van Vliet, A. J. de Craen, J. Jolles, B. M. Buckley, M. B. Murphy, I. Ford, et al. 2009. Pravastatin and cognitive function in the elderly. Results of the PROSPER study. *J Neurol* 257 (1): 85–90.

Unverzagt, F. W., L. Kasten, K. E. Johnson, G. W. Rebok, M. Marsiske, K. M. Koepke, J. W. Elias, et al. 2007. Effect of memory impairment on training outcomes in ACTIVE. *J Int Neuropsychol Soc* 13 (6): 953–960.

van de Rest, O., J. M. Geleijnse, F. J. Kok, W. A. van Staveren, C. Dullemeijer, M. G. Olderikkert, A. T. Beekman, and C. P. de Groot. 2008. Effect of fish oil on cognitive performance in older subjects: A randomized, controlled trial. *Neurology* 71 (6): 430–438.

van den Berg, E., G. J. Biessels, A. J. de Craen, J. Gussekloo, and R. G. Westendorp. 2007. The metabolic syndrome is associated with decelerated cognitive decline in the oldest old. *Neurology* 69 (10): 979–985.

van Gelder, B. M., M. Tijhuis, S. Kalmijn, and D. Kromhout. 2007. Fish consumption, n-3 fatty acids, and subsequent 5-y cognitive decline in elderly men: The Zutphen Elderly Study. *Am J Clin Nutr* 85 (4): 1142–1147.

Vanhanen, M., K. Koivisto, L. Moilanen, E. L. Helkala, T. Hanninen, H. Soininen, K. Kervinen, Y. A. Kesaniemi, M. Laakso, and J. Kuusisto. 2006. Association of metabolic syndrome with Alzheimer disease: A population-based study. *Neurology* 67 (5): 843–847.

Warburton, D. E., C. W. Nicol, and S. S. Bredin. 2006. Health benefits of physical activity: The evidence. *CMAJ* 174 (6): 801–809.

Weuve, J. H., J. E. Manson, M. M. Breteler, J. H. Ware, and F. Grodstein. 2004. Physical activity, including walking, and cognitive function in older women. *JAMA* 292 (12): 1454–1461.

Whitmer, R. A. 2007. Type 2 diabetes and risk of cognitive impairment and dementia. *Curr Neurol Neurosci Rep* 7 (5): 373–380.

Whitmer, R. A., E. P. Gunderson, E. Barrett-Connor, C. P. Quesenberry Jr., and K. Yaffe. 2005. Obesity in middle age and future risk of dementia: A 27-year longitudinal population based study. *BMJ* 330 (7504): 1360.

Whitmer, R. A., A. J. Karter, K. Yaffe, C. P. Quesenberry Jr., and J. V. Selby. 2009. Hypoglycemic episodes and risk of dementia in older patients with type 2 diabetes mellitus. *JAMA* 301 (15): 1565–1572.

Williamson, J. D., M. E. Miller, R. N. Bryan, R. M. Lazar, L. H. Coker, J. Johnson, T. Cukierman, K. R. Horowitz, A. Murray, and L. J. Launer. 2007. The Action to Control Cardiovascular Risk in Diabetes Memory in Diabetes Study (ACCORD-MIND): Rationale, design, and methods. *Am J Cardiol* 99 (12A): 112i–122i.

Wilson, R. S., D. A. Bennett, J. L. Bienias, N. T. Aggarwal, C. F. Mendes De Leon, M. C. Morris, J. A. Schneider, and D. A. Evans. 2002. Cognitive activity and incident AD in a population-based sample of older persons. *Neurology* 59 (12): 1910–1914.

Wu, C., D. Zhou, C. Wen, L. Zhang, P. Como, and Y. Qiao. 2003. Relationship between blood pressure and Alzheimer's disease in Linxian County, China. *Life Sci* 72 (10): 1125–1133.

Yaffe, K. 2007. Metabolic syndrome and cognitive disorders: Is the sum greater than its parts? *Alzheimer Dis Assoc Disord* 21 (2): 167–171.

Yaffe, K., E. Barrett-Connor, F. Lin, and D. Grady. 2002. Serum lipoprotein levels, statin use, and cognitive function in older women. *Arch Neurol* 59 (3): 378–384.

Yaffe, K., T. Blackwell, A. M. Kanaya, N. Davidowitz, E. Barrett-Connor, and K. Krueger. 2004. Diabetes, impaired fasting glucose, and development of cognitive impairment in older women. *Neurology* 63 (4): 658–663.

Yaffe, K., T. E. Clemons, W. L. McBee, and A. S. Lindblad. 2004. Impact of anti-oxidants, zinc, and copper on cognition in the elderly: A randomized, con-trolled trial. *Neurology* 63 (9): 1705–1707.

Yaffe, K., M. Haan, T. Blackwell, E. Cherkasova, R. A. Whitmer, and N. West. 2007. Metabolic syndrome and cognitive decline in elderly Latinos: Findings from the Sacramento Area Latino Study of Aging study. *J Am Geriatr Soc* 55 (5): 758–762.

Chapter 5

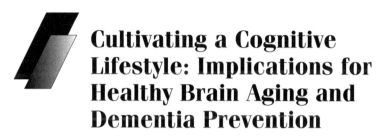

Cultivating a Cognitive Lifestyle: Implications for Healthy Brain Aging and Dementia Prevention

Michael J. Valenzuela

The concept of *brain reserve capacity* is most often invoked when explaining individual differences in clinical outcomes from brain injury or disease (Satz 1993). When used as a "black box" in this fashion it is intuitively appealing. Ever since formal investigation of head-injured patients began in times of war, clinicians and researchers have been amazed at the possible diversity of personal outcomes. Sometimes relatively small contusions can lead to devastating consequences; in others massive brain injury does not in the end produce a discernable difference in day-to-day function. Indeed, the volume of disrupted brain tissue is but a poor predictor of clinical symptoms (Grafman et al. 1986). Similar neuroclinical discordance occurs in stroke injury as well (Desmond et al. 2000).

So while most neuroscientists and clinicians would agree that the brain has some form of reserve capacity that differs significantly between individuals, the nature of this capacity has remained frustratingly difficult to define. A large part of this difficulty is because the notion of "reserve" can be analyzed at many levels. This is most apparent in the field of dementia, where arguably "reserve" has undergone the most research (Valenzuela 2008; Stern 2002).

In the following section, different interpretations of reserve in dementia-related research will be contrasted, with the caveat that a clinical effect should not be confused with the action of several potential mediating mechanisms. "Reserve" is a singular term, but it is highly unlikely that only a single mode of action underlies the brain's remarkable variability in clinical response to insult. Multiple, as yet undefined, interacting "reserve capacities" are therefore at play, and so the term risks losing explanatory power. Anchoring the phenomena at the behavioral level is suggested as perhaps the most tractable strategy. *Cognitive lifestyle* is introduced as one objective approach. This has already been shown to predict longitudinal changes in cognitive function and brain morphology.

Next a brief review of the possible neuronal mediators of cognitive lifestyle will follow and more specifically address how these could lead to the well-established finding that those with a more active cognitive lifestyle benefit from a significant reduction in dementia risk. The main theme here is that all the ingredients of a rich cognitive lifestyle stimulate *neuroplasticity* in the brain, ranging from activity-dependent gene expression to the adaptation of large-scale cortical networks. Given dementia is, in the end, a failure of neuroplasticity, this has significant consequences for potential preventative strategies. In the third and final section of this chapter, whether neuroplasticity can be co-opted for preventative purposes against dementia is critically assessed. Trials of structured complex mental activity training in the form of cognitive brain training are assessed in the areas of normal healthy aging and mild cognitive impairment (MCI), and shown to have great promise. These themes are brought together with clinical recommendations as well as views on how the field can continue to grow and shed light on this most interesting of brain-behavior interactions.

DEFINITION AND IMPLICATIONS OF COGNITIVE LIFESTYLE

Neurocentric Perspectives on Brain Reserve

Since the time of Tomlinson, Blessed, and Roth's (1970) pioneering dementia studies, there has existed a central paradox for the field: why do some individuals who died with significant levels of Alzheimer disease (AD) pathology have intact cognition immediately prior to death? While initially considered to be clinical rarities (Roth 1986), more recent population-based studies have shown that 33% of individuals with nontrivial AD at death were not demented in life (Neuropathology Group 2001). Obviously there is something unique about these individuals, but what could this be?

Katzman et al. (1988) were the first to propose a possible explanation for these cases. These individuals were observed to manifest three main differences compared to individuals who had clinically succumbed to their disease. First, they contained a greater number of large pyramidal neurons throughout the neocortex. Second, they had heavier brain weights, and third, they had performed at the highest levels on antemortem cognitive tests. Overall, these individuals "had incipient Alzheimer's disease but did not show it clinically because of this greater reserve" (144).

Given these observations and since neurons cannot be counted in life, early brain reserve research focused primarily on gross brain parameters. Intracranial volume (ICV), head circumference (Borenstein et al. 2001), and even head width (Jorm et al. 1997) have been used as basic proxies for maximal brain weight, which in turn was suggested to provide an estimate of neuronal numbers. This position has a number of problems. First, whether maximal brain volume or weight is highly correlated with neuronal number is debatable. Second, since a more sophisticated model has been missing for specifying *which* neurons and *where* in the brain numerical differences may be most important, aggregate numbers and therefore volume has been overemphasized. There is a long and ignoble history of attempts to link gross brain volume or weight to general cognitive features (Gould 1991). But most important, the key test for a putative neuronal corollary of reserve is that variations in this quantity can account for variance in a clinical outcome, in this case incident dementia. Studies have in general failed to show an inverse linear association between dementia incidence and the full range of ICV; an increased risk appears to be restricted to the low to very low ICV ranges (Schofield et al. 1997), or when in the presence of an additional risk factor such as APOE ε4 (Borenstein et al. 2001).

Another straightforward problem for a "hard" neurocentric interest in maximal brain volume is that it restricts the explanatory variable to a nonmodifiable property. Maximum ICV and head circumference are generally achieved by puberty (Mortimer 1997) and reflect genetic variance in neuronal quantum as well as developmental, nutritional and environmental factors in early life (Altman et al. 1968). More important, since these measures do not generally change after the onset of adulthood, does this mean that our underlying brain reserve is fixed? As will be reviewed in the next section, the weight of evidence from the epidemiological, clinical, and experimental literature suggests quite the opposite.

Cognitive Perspective

Katzman and colleagues had of course noted both *cognitive* and *neurological* differences in their sample. So another perspective of reserve has been to focus on "how well we use what has been left behind" rather than how much of it we had in the first place (Stern 2002; Mortimer 1988). Two distinctions are possible. If we substitute "neuronal numbers" with "neuropsychological competence" or "IQ," a threshold model can be applied whereby high *cognitive reserve* individuals simply perform better on cognitive tests to start with and therefore require a larger decrement before crossing a diagnostic threshold (Satz 1993). This model suggests no interaction with the underlying disease process and predicts no differential rates in cognitive decline. Only neuropsychological starting points differ. It has therefore been termed a *passive* version of reserve (Stern 2002), and identified as a potential source of systematic error in longitudinal studies (Tuokko et al. 2003). In the context of aging and dementia, any systematic definition of reserve must account for this passive effect, which in practical terms means demonstrating differential rates of neurological or cognitive change over time.

A more *active* form of cognitive reserve contends that individuals who have developed a range of deliberate cognitive strategies for solving complex problems are more likely to remain within normal functional limits for longer. This dynamic account predicts that two individuals may begin at the same cognitive starting point, suffer the same progressive burden of disease, but due to increased use of strategic coping mechanisms one may perform better at follow-up testing or experience less day-to-day functional limitations. While certainly an important clinical phenomena that captures part of the ecological nature of how individuals differ, this notion of reserve is surprisingly difficult to measure. Simply asking subjects about their use of deliberate strategies while performing cognitive tasks can produce more questions than answers (Naveh-Benjamin, Brav, and Levi 2007). This active and deliberative form of cognitive reserve therefore suffers from a lack of feasible operationalization.

Computational Perspective

More recent incarnations of *reserve capacity* have focused on computational processes such as network redundancy and flexibility (Valenzuela, Breakspear, and Sachdev 2007). In this case, individuals may not only vary on their range of deliberative strategies but also possess differences in the diversity of neural pathways available for execution of these cognitive processes. Having multiple neural pathways for instantiation of the same computational problem (redundancy), or an enhanced ability to reorganize pathways after "network attack" (in computational terms "degeneracy"; see Tononi, Sporns, and Edelman 1999), is theorized to facilitate maintenance of function after neurological insult. While this approach benefits from a unification of brain *and* cognitive reserve via an explicit mechanism, outside of computational simulations operationalization is again problematic (Rubinov et al. 2009).

A Behavioral Perspective: Defining Cognitive Lifestyle

The alternative pursued in our group has been to simply ask how mentally active and engaged has a person been over his or her lifespan in comparison to the average? Relevant information here includes level and duration of formal education from young adulthood to the present day, the nature and complexity of occupations throughout his or her working life, and the diversity, frequency and cognitive challenge of past and present leisure activities. This has been combined into a validated assessment tool, the Lifetime of Experience Questionnaire (LEQ) (Valenzuela and Sachdev 2007). Higher LEQ scores independently predict not only attenuated cognitive decline over time, but also a reduced rate of hippocampal atrophy (Valenzuela et al. 2008) (see Figure 5.1). This straightforward approach has the main advantage of providing a working operational definition that is clinically relevant.

The behavioral perspective inherent in the LEQ does not identify itself with a specific neurological quantity, computational property, or cognitive process. Participation in complex mental activities throughout the lifespan is assumed to lead to changes in a number of interacting mechanisms at different temporal and spatial scales (Valenzuela, Breakspear, and Sachdev 2007). Together these alter an individual's risk for dementia and cognitive dysfunction. Indeed, we have suggested elsewhere that perhaps there is no *one* brain or cognitive reserve, but a *number of reserves* (Valenzuela 2008). For too long researchers have seemed to confuse a single potential reserve *mechanism*, of which there are certainly a plurality, with the apparent unity of the reserve *effect* (i.e., clinical protection). The approach of using behavioral anchor points for the assessment of cognitive lifestyle is reliable and clinically predictive, and so it is hoped that more powerful and meaningful mechanistic studies will follow.

Cognitive Lifestyle and Dementia Risk

Cognitive lifestyle and dementia are linked. Highly consistent connections between complex mental activity and reduced dementia risk have been found across large-scale prospective studies of dementia incidence. Our meta-analysis of the area combined data from 22 international cohort studies and showed that overall individuals with more active cognitive

Figure 5.1

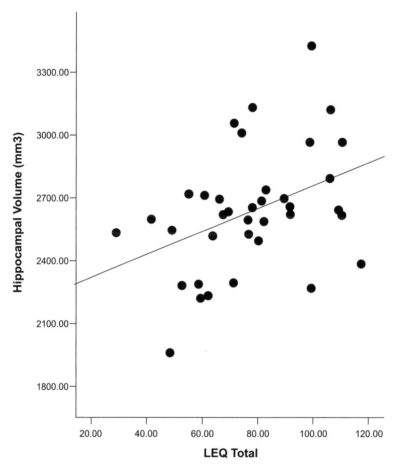

Scatterplot showing a positive relationship between the Lifetime of Experiences Questionnaire on the *x*-axis (a validated measure of cognitive lifestyle) and hippocampal volume on the *y*-axis. Insets show examples from individuals with high (left) and low (right) LEQ scores along with volumes of their hippocampus.

lifestyles were at 46% reduced risk for incident dementia (CI: 0.49–0.59) (Valenzuela and Sachdev 2006). In this systematic review, the effects of education (OR = 0.53), occupational complexity (OR = 0.56), and late-life leisure activities (OR = 0.50) were each individually highly consistent.

Similar protective effects of 40–50% risk reduction are also found when specifically isolated to cognitive lifestyle in late life (i.e., after 60 years of age), independent of earlier exposures to education or occupational complexity (Scarmeas et al. 2001). This has now been replicated internationally (Wang et al. 2002; Fratiglioni et al. 2000; Wilson et al. 2002). There is furthermore evidence for a dosage effect (Valenzuela et al. 2006). Verghese et al. (2003), for example, found a 50 percent risk reduction for incident dementia over five years in those with a moderate number of cognitive lifestyle activities compared to those with low numbers, while those with the highest degree of participation had a 67 percent reduction in incident dementia.

Protective effects in individuals with a more active cognitive lifestyle in later life even after controlling for earlier life experiences gives great hope that interventions implemented at this time can still be effective for helping prevent dementia. Yet despite such convergent epidemiological data, the *underlying reasons for the relationship* remain unclear. A brief review of possible mediating mechanisms is therefore presented next.

MECHANISMS UNDERLYING BENEFITS OF COGNITIVE LIFESTYLE

Both the structure and function of the brain can change in response to environmental complexity. Thirty years of research has now been amassed on the effects of environmental enrichment in rodents, a relatively simple intervention that involves moving animals from standard housing to a home environment with additional toys, mazes, wheels, and littermates (for a review see Nithianantharajah and Hannan 2006). Enrichment is therefore a multiplex intervention that increases animals' cognitive, physical, and social activity. This of course makes precise isolation of the mechanisms' underlying *solely* mental activity, in contradistinction to physical exercise or socialization, quite challenging. Yet rodent studies suggest more similarities than differences when comparing mechanisms involved in voluntary running (Cotman, Berchtold, and Christie 2007) to cognitive stimulation (Nithianantharajah and Hannan 2006). Similar principles may also apply in humans, but as yet we lack the tools to probe the brain *in vivo* at sufficient spatial and temporal resolution. Despite these limitations, neuroimaging studies are beginning to chart the nature of activity-dependent brain changes. Overall, human and animal research indicates that mental stimulation induces a complex web of biological mechanisms at different spatial and temporal scales. An active cognitive lifestyle therefore more than likely contributes to a stronger defense against dementia by a number of different means.

Molecular Mechanisms

Long-term potentiation (LTP) and depression (LTD) are important cellular and molecular processes implicated in memory (Malenka and Bear 2004). Both of these depend on activity-dependent changes to excitatory AMPA and NMDA receptors, which in effect change the probability that a postsynaptic neuron will fire in response to presynaptic stimulation. It is therefore significant that as little as five days of enrichment can upregulate AMPA receptors (Naka et al. 2005), and thereafter alter LTP and LTD (Artola et al. 2006).

Upstream to these effects in both space and time are molecular changes to gene expression. Remarkably, microarray analysis has shown dozens of gene expression changes, including those implicated in regulating synaptic plasticity, following as little as three hours of environmental stimulation (Rampon et al. 2000).

However, arguably the most important molecular changes occur in relation to brain derived neurotrophic factor (BDNF). BDNF is a "master molecule" of sorts, implicated in a wide range of neuroplastic processes including, neural stem cell survival, synaptogenesis, neurogenesis, dendritic arborisation, and synaptic plasticity (Fumagalli, Racagni, and Riva 2006). Enrichment causes profound increases in BDNF production throughout the brain, particularly in the hippocampus (Mohammed et al. 2002; Ickes et al. 2000). There is therefore increasing interest in BDNF as an "enviromimetic" (McOmish and Hannan 2007), although much further research is needed to understand the pathways involved in its regulation and differential effects.

Disease Modification

A number of studies of transgenic Alzheimer mice have now investigated the effects of environmental enrichment, with mixed findings. One study found a 50% reduction in amyloid burden subsequent to five months of enrichment, with a suggestion this was due to increased plaque breakdown (Lazarov et al. 2005). Another study found increased plaque load, but paradoxically, improved behavioral outcomes (Janowsky et al. 2005). A third group also noted cognitive improvements, along with evidence for both amyloid-dependent and -ndependent mechanisms (Arendash et al. 2004; Costa et al. 2006). Interestingly, for the optimal triple-pronged effect of decreased AD burden, increased synaptic density, and improved memory performance, all three aspects of enrichment were needed, that is, cognitive, social, and physical activity (Cracchiolo et al. 2007). Whether this disease modification is relevant to humans is of course difficult to determine given the wide gulf between transgenic models and humans. Clinical studies using amyloid imaging are therefore eagerly anticipated.

Cellular Mechanisms

Synaptogenesis is arguably the most robust neuroplastic change, with enrichment leading to increases in synaptic density in the order of 150–300% (Levi et al. 2003). Changes in synaptic density of this sort are highly correlated to memory function in the rat (Frick and Fernandez 2003). Moreover, this finding is relevant to human brain aging and dementia, since post mortem synaptophysin levels are strongly correlated to cognitive and clinical status before death: Two independent laboratories have found correlations between 0.7–0.8 (Terry et al. 1991; Scheff and Price 2003). One of the key mechanisms by which an active cognitive lifestyle leads to reduced dementia risk may be through upregulation of synaptogenesis in important memory-dependent areas of the brain.

Experience-dependent changes in neurogenesis (Kempermann 2006) and angiogenesis (Black et al. 1990) also occur, which in combination may explain why enrichment seems to lead to increased gross brain volume (Altman et al. 1968). However, the functional significance of neurogenesis remains highly controversial—correlations between neurogenesis and spatial memory performance in older animals have for example been contradictory (Kempermann 2006; Drapeau et al. 2003; Bizon and Gallagher 2005). Whether cognitive lifestyle modulates dementia risk through neurogenesis is not clear.

Cortical Network Mechanisms

Glucose-labeled PET studies can estimate the brain's overall rate of metabolic consumption as well as its regional variation. Using this approach, repeated cognitive exercise was found to lead to increased efficiency in the shape of a 25–30% reduction in global resting metabolism (Haier et al. 1988). On the other hand, cognitive exercise also results in selective and temporary increases in hemodynamic responsivity in those same brain areas engaged by the tasks (Olesen, Westerberg, and Klingberg 2004; Moore, Cohen, and Ranganath 2006).

Cortical compensatory processes are also important and refer to an enhanced ability to adapt against progressive disease in one part of the brain, through functional reorganization in another part of the brain. Studies have, for example, shown that elders with preserved memory ability—behaviorally equivalent to that of younger individuals—engage bilateral prefrontal brain areas in comparison to older memory-deficient peers, who continue to only activate a unilateral brain network like younger individuals (Cabeza 1997; Grady et al. 2003; Rosen et al. 2002; Scarmeas et al. 2003). Successful brain aging may therefore not only involve the continued deployment of the same neural processing pathways, but also the recruitment of new brain networks better suited to the aged brain.

More recent neuroimaging studies have focused on characterizing changes in direct response to mental and physical training. In general these have found evidence for expansion of cortical grey matter after several weeks of training (Draganski et al. 2004; Boyke et al. 2008; Colcombe et al. 2006), as well as improvements in cerebral blood flow (Mozolic, Hayaska, and Laurienti 2010; Colcombe et al. 2004). Training may therefore at least partially counteract age-related and disease-related atrophy in different brain regions; however, more research is required since these findings appear to be highly dependent on analytical approach (Thomas et al. 2009). Memory training can also lead to specific increments in phosphocreatine concentration in the hippocampus as revealed by magnetic resonance spectroscopy (Valenzuela et al. 2003), of interest since AD leads to phosphocreatine depletion (Valenzuela and Sachdev 2001) and dietary supplementation is neuroprotective in animal models (Brustovetsky, Brustovetsky, and Dubinsky 2001). While more research is required, initial neuroimaging reports suggest that mental and physical training can have positive effects on the brain.

How Does This Delay or Prevention Dementia?

Complex mental activity is evidently a strong stimulator of the brain's myriad neuroplastic mechanisms. By contrast, the degenerative conditions that underlie dementia—including age-related degeneration, AD, and cerebrovascular disease—all combine to severely reduce neuroplasticity (Mesulam 1999). In a simplistic sense, an active cognitive lifestyle may therefore help protect against dementia by counteracting negative disease-related effects on neuroplasticity. More precise models and detailed human data are required to better understand these important therapeutic and preventative mechanisms.

Theoretical considerations also reveal a more fundamental link between cognitive lifestyle and dementia. For several decades we have considered dementia to simply represent the endpoint of a gradual buildup of pathology and associated neuronal loss. This view assumes a unidirectional relationship, implies a high level of clinicopathologic determinism, and is the basis for the search for better disease "biomarkers" based on amyloid imaging, hippocampal structural modeling, and so forth.

However, as reviewed above, clinical symptoms do no arise in almost a third of cases with supra-threshold pathological AD at post mortem. These individuals have benefited in life from some as-yet-undefined countervailing factors and, for reasons outlined above, individual differences in neuroplasticity may be implicated. For example, the great variability witnessed in cortical compensation and reorganization suggests that dementia may be better conceptualized as a "compensatory failure" (Valenzuela, Breakspear, and Sachdev 2007). This view suggests that disease burden is not the only salient factor when attempting to make sensible predictions and judgments about dementia, but that an assessment of an individual's neuroplastic capacities is also needed (see Figure 5.2). Dementia onset therefore becomes a dynamic tension between a progressive disease and the brain's limited but ever-surprising ability to adapt, react, and regenerate.

An important consequence of this paradigm is that interventions and practice that can enrich our neuroplastic capacities also help to subvert the clinical effects of neurodegenerative disease. In the next section we will therefore move from theory to practice and review the evidence base for interventions designed to augment cognitive lifestyle.

CAN ENRICHMENT OF COGNITIVE LIFESTYLE HELP PREVENT DEMENTIA?

Despite the strong epidemiological links between cognitive lifestyle and reduced dementia risk, and a wealth of potential explanatory mechanisms, important questions remain over the *arrow of causality*: does preceding mental activity reduce or delay expression of future dementia, or is preclinical dementia causing a reduction in participation in activities prior to formal diagnosis? In order to disentangle this complex "chicken or egg" problem, data from clinical trials of *cognitive training* are most important.

When reviewing a potentially vast literature, a specific type of cognitive lifestyle activity has been chosen for pragmatic reasons: cognitive training. Given the sometimes unclear usage of the term and possible overlap with other cognitive interventions such as cognitive remediation, cognitive rehabilitation, and cognitive stimulation, we have striven to use an explicit definition. *Cognitive training* is any intervention aimed at improving, maintaining, or restoring mental function through the repeated and structured practice of tasks that pose an inherent problem or mental challenge and that target specific cognitive domains (Gates and Valenzuela 2010). This definition does not include training in strategies to compensate

Figure 5.2

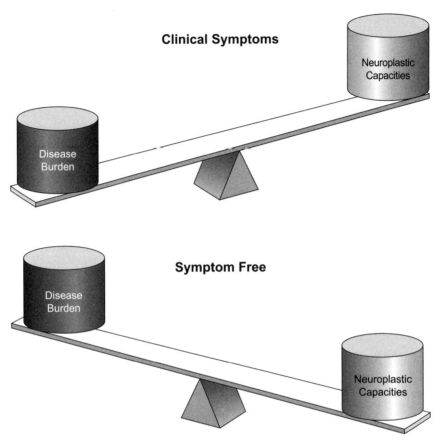

A framework for conceptualizing dementia as a dynamic balance between disease burden and neuroplastic capacities. Above, an individual with a given disease burden expresses cognitive symptoms in the context of relatively low neuroplastic capacities. Below, the same disease burden leads to no clinical symptoms due to greater neuroplastic capacities. The aim of interventions based on boosting cognitive lifestyle is to shift individuals at risk for dementia to the lower scenario.

for deficits, traditionally a rehabilitative or remedial approach (Sitzer, Twamley, and Jeste 2006).

Theoretical Issues

Repetitive cognitive training undoubtedly improves performance *on the trained task*— there is indeed more than 20 years of cognitive psychology research on this topic (Rebok, Carlson, and Langbaum 2007). To determine whether cognitive training could potentially help reduce or delay the incidence of dementia, two major issues need to be addressed.

Generalization or Transfer of Effect

Does the cognitive training intervention only lead to improvement in the trained task, or does it also transfer to nontrained tasks? We have proposed a hierarchy of generalization of increasing clinical relevance (Gates and Valenzuela 2010) (see Figure 5.3):

1. Transfer to nontrained tasks in same cognitive domain
2. Transfer to nontrained tasks in other cognitive domains
3. Transfer to global measures of general cognitive ability (e.g, Alzheimer's Disease Assessment Scale–Cognitive, tests for general intellectual ability, etc.)
4. Transfer to measures of general function (e.g., Instrumental Activities of Daily Living, Quality of Life, Mood, etc.)

Improvement on the same tasks as covered in training are therefore clinically trivial, while generalization of training to include better overall cognitive function, day-to-day abilities, and quality of life should be considered benchmark tests when evaluating clinical efficacy.

Persistence or Durability of Effect

Does the effect of cognitive training intervention last beyond the immediate posttraining period, or is continual cognitive training required? Longitudinal follow-up of cognitive training efficacy is required to answer this question. In the following brief review, a summary of randomized controlled trials (RCTs) in the healthy aging and MCI areas is provided.

RCTs in Healthy Aging

We have recently published a systematic review of RCTs of cognitive training in healthy older individuals in which longitudinal follow-up was a critical design feature (Valenzuela and Sachdev 2009). A total of seven trial outcomes suggested that a discrete program of cognitive training in the order of 2–3 months can have long-lasting and persistent protective effects on cognition. The overall weighted mean difference was strong in magnitude, estimated at 1.07 (CI: 0.32–1.83) and the nonweighted average relative effect size was Cohen's d = 0.5.

Figure 5.3

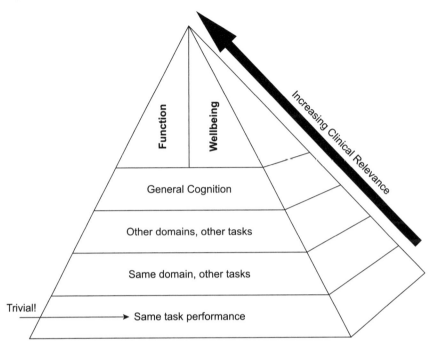

Hierarchy of generalization whereby change on the trained task is clinically
trivial, while improvements in day-to-day function and subjective measures of
well-being are the most clinically valuable.

   The ACTIVE study is the largest trial in the area (Ball et al. 2002) and
examined the effects of 10 sessions of cognitive training on 2832 healthy
older individuals. Participants completed three different intervention
groups: memory training, reasoning training, and processing speed training. Two years later, each intervention improved cognitive ability only
in the targeted area, an effect of limited clinical value. Follow up at five
years, however, found that reasoning training protected against functional
decline compared to any of the other interventions or the control wait-and-
see condition, albeit with very a modest effect size (Willis et al. 2006). This
is therefore the first large clinical trial to demonstrate potentially clinically
relevant transfer effects.
   There is also a high degree of community and commercial interest in
computer-based cognitive training. One group has conducted a RCT with
such a product (Mahncke et al. 2006). The attraction of computerized cognitive training is that training can be standardized and allows a gradient in task difficulty to be automatically incorporated as individuals' skill

levels progress. Neuropsychological tests immediately after the end of the training period found verbal memory performance improved by up to 25% of a standard deviation, and testing three months later showed that short term memory performance remained enhanced.

The combination of both cognitive and physical exercise is also of great interest. This has yet to be tested in a rigorous RCT. The Sim-A study investigated the effects of cognitive, physical, and combined training in healthy older individuals over a five-year period (Oswald et al. 2006). Thirty paper-and-pencil cognitive training sessions produced a significant effect over both the 12-month and five-year follow-up periods. Moreover, this effect seemed to transfer to a measure of general cognition. The group that did both cognitive and physical training experienced a larger effect size than the simple addition of those who completed just one type of training, suggestive of a potential synergistic action. Other smaller studies with samples of less than 100 individuals have found positive trends but have lacked power (Derwinger, Stigsdotter Neely, and Backman 2005; Scogin and Bienias 1988).

The overall effect size and consistency across longitudinal trials of cognitive training in the healthy elderly is therefore promising, yet many questions remain. There has been a wide variety of primary outcome measures across the trials, and details of the applied cognitive exercises also varied. Quality of trial design and reporting has in general been low. However, it is encouraging that those studies with longer-term follow-up showed no evidence of less potent effects. A durable long-term effect from cognitive training may therefore be realistic. Significantly, two of the more recent clinical studies have also shown that their training protocols generalize to domains beyond the narrow focus of the trained tasks (Willis et al. 2006; Oswald et al. 2006).

RCTs in Mild Cognitive Impairment

Mild cognitive impairment (MCI) may be an optimal stage at which to intervene for the purpose of prevention and delay of progression to bona fide dementia. A nonsystematic review of cognitive training in MCI has suggested potential efficacy for cognitive outcomes (Belleville 2008). At least three RCTs have been reported which adhere to our definition of cognitive training and are summarized below.

A small study (n=8) of community-based individuals with MCI tested a multifaceted memory enhancement training with a no-treatment control (Rapp, Brenes, and Marsh 2002). Training comprised of six two-hour meetings held weekly and also involved education, relaxation skills, and homework practice. Both cognitive training and rehabilitative strategies were therefore combined. Initially, there were no group differences; however, at the six month follow-up the treatment group had superior delayed list recall than the controls, suggestive of durable effects. No relative improvements in other cognitive domains or global cognitive function were evident.

Olazaran et al. (2004) studied a mixed sample of 12 individuals with MCI plus 72 people with AD, randomly assigned to a psychosocial control group or a cognitive motor intervention that included cognitive training. Results across diagnostic groups were combined, so it is impossible to isolate the effect size in the MCI group. Overall, Alzheimer's Disease Assessment Scale–Cognitive (ADAS-Cog) scores remained stable in the treatment group while it declined in controls. There was also a significantly positive effect of depression scores.

The most rigorous study to date has been by Rozzini et al. (2007) who conducted a RCT with individuals diagnosed solely with MCI (n=59). Participants were allocated into one of three groups: treatment with cholinesterase inhibitors (ChEI), ChEI plus cognitive training, or no treatment control. Cognitive training was based on a computerized software package and targeted multiple cognitive functions with increasing complexity. Participants completed 60 one-hour sessions of training over a period of nine months. Three months after the end of training, episodic memory and abstract reasoning were significantly increased in the combined ChEI+CT group, with a moderate relative effect size of 0.7 (in comparison to ChEI alone). This study therefore suggests an enduring effect of training in two areas of cognitive function above and beyond medical treatment. Transfer to general functioning was assessed with a mood scale and both treatment groups demonstrated reduced levels of depressive symptoms. The combined treatment group was also notable for a significant reduction in behavioral disturbance. This trial therefore provides clinically relevant evidence that cognitive training may be useful in MCI, an effect that is durable for at least three months and which seems to transfer to general daily function.

Research Challenges for the Field

The last 10 years has seen intense medical, community, and commercial interest in trying to harness the power of neuroplasticity for the prevention of age-related cognitive dysfunction. Perhaps the greatest influence has been a sociological trend away from pharmacological agents and toward behavioral and lifestyle modification and positivistic health attitudes. Yet this enthusiasm should not obscure our demand for rigorous scientific evidence when attempting to translate preclinical findings to individual and community interventions.

The greatest challenge for the field of cognitive training and dementia prevention is in the domain of clinical trials. No trial has, for example, definitively shown that cognitive training reduces the incidence of dementia, as opposed to the rate of cognitive decline. Higher-caliber RCTs are therefore required, with close attention to implementation of active control groups, longitudinal evaluation, choice of cognitive training protocol and outcome measures, and recruitment of relevant samples. While the optimal dose, nature, and frequency of cognitive training in MCI is unclear, a trend that does emerge is that training across multiple cognitive domains leads to better long-term cognitive outcomes (Gunther et al. 2003; Rozzini et al. 2007). A basic recommendation for maximum efficacy is therefore to trial cognitive training protocols that exercise a broad range of cognitive domains using the drill-and-practice approach.

This information will then need to inform wider community programs, and many more questions arise. For example, is starting a new cognitively demanding hobby as good as so many hours of computer-based cognitive training (Carlson et al. 2009)? If so, are all activities equally effective or only some? How often and what intensity of engagement is required? Is group participation better than individual practice at home? Generic issues of scalability, accessibility, economy and accountability will also need to be addressed.

Clinical Recommendations

In the meantime, the general public needs to be well informed about the links between cognitive lifestyle and reduced dementia risk. Given the negligible potential for harm, it is sensible to encourage all individuals to increase their levels of complex, enjoyable, and engaging cognitive activity for optimal brain health, particularly after retirement. Activities that combine cognitive, social, and physical exercise are likely to be the most powerful, and popular examples include learning to dance (Verghese et al. 2003), tai chi, learning a language and then traveling with it, among many others. Individuals should be encouraged to use their own preferences for participating in a new activity that combines these three key ingredients.

There is of course a clinical obligation to also realistically manage expectations, for no intervention can guarantee the absolute prevention of dementia. An active cognitive lifestyle may help prevent dementia and minimize risk, but as yet there is no strategy that can fully eliminate this risk. An active cognitive lifestyle should therefore be part of a holistic risk-reduction strategy that includes blood pressure control, minimization of other cardiac risk factors, and a healthy diet.

CONCLUSIONS

An active cognitive lifestyle involves a lifespan interest and engagement in cognitively complex pursuits, including formal and informal education, a preference for cognitively demanding work, and cognitively loaded leisure activities. There is now consistent epidemiological evidence showing that an active cognitive lifestyle is a protective factor against dementia. The neurobiological basis for this is complex and potentially involves stimulation of several interacting neuroplastic processes. Yet most important, these mechanisms can be exploited even well into later life, such that interventions like cognitive training that boost cognitive lifestyle, appear to slow the rate of cognitive decline. There are therefore good grounds to expect that interventions based around an enhanced cognitive lifestyle may contribute to the primary prevention of dementia, but much more research is required. In the meantime, we should encourage individuals to stay mentally active, particularly after retirement, for the promotion of brain health.

REFERENCES

Altman, J., R. Wallace, W. Anderson, and G. Das. 1968. Behaviourally induced changes in length of cerebrum in rat. *Developmental Psychobiology* 1: 112–117.

Arendash, G., et al. 2004. Environmental enrichment improves cognition in aged Alzheimer's transgenic mice despite stable β-amyloid deposition. *Neuroreport* 15: 1751–1754.

Artola, A., J. von Frijtag, P. Fermont, W. Gispen, L. Schrama, A. Kamal, et al. 2006. Long-lasting modulation of the induction of LTD and LTP in rat hippocampal CA1 by behavioural stress and environmental enrichment. *European Journal of Neuroscience* 23: 261–272.

Ball, K., D. Berch, K. Helmers, J. Jobe, M. Leveck, M. Marsiske, et al. 2002. Effect of cognitive training interventions with older adults—a randomised control trial. *JAMA* 288: 2271–2281.

Belleville, S. 2008. Cognitive training for persons with mild cognitive impairment 3. *International Psychogeriatrics* 20: 57–66.

Bizon, J., and M. Gallagher. 2005. More is less: Neurogenesis and age-related cognitive decline in Long-Evans rats. *Science, Aging, Knowledge and Environment* 2005 (7): re2.

Black, J., K. Isaacs, B. Anderson, A. Alcantara, and W. Greenough. 1990. Learning causes synaptogenesis, whereas motor activity causes angiogenesis, in cerebellar cortex of adult rats. *Proceedings of the National Academy of Sciences of the United States of America* 87: 5568–5572.

Borenstein, G. A., J. A. Mortimer, J. D. Bowen, W. C. McCormick, S. M. McCurry, G. D. Schellenberg, et al. 2001. Head circumference and incident Alzheimer's disease: Modification by apolipoprotein E. *Neurology* 57: 1453–1460.

Boyke, J., J. Driemeyer, C. Gaser, C. Buchel, and A. May. 2008. Training-induced brain structure changes in the elderly. *Journal of Neuroscience* 28: 7031–7035.

Brustovetsky, N., T. Brustovetsky, and J. Dubinsky. 2001. On the mechanisms of neuroprotection by creatine and phosphocreatine. *Journal of Neurochemistry* 76: 425–434.

Cabeza, R. 1997. Age-related differences in neural activity during memory encoding and retrieval: A positron emission tomography study. *Journal of Neuroscience* 17: 391–400.

Carlson, M., K. Erickson, A. Kramer, M. Voss, N. Bolea, M. Mielke, et al. 2009. Evidence for neurocognitive plasticity in at-risk older adults: The Experience Corps Program. *Journal of Gerontology A: Biological Science Medical Science* 64A: 1275–1282.

Colcombe, S., E. Eriksson, P. Scalf, J. Kim, R. Prakash, E. McAuley, et al. 2006. Aerobic exercise training increases brain volume in aging humans. *Journal of Gerontology: Medical Sciences* 61A: 1166–1170.

Colcombe, S., A. Kramer, K. Erickson, P. Scalf, E. McAuley, N. Cohen, et al. 2004. Cardiovascular fitness, cortical plasticity, and aging. *Proceedings of the National Academy of Sciences of the United States of America* 101: 3316–3321.

Costa, D., J. Cracchiolo, A. Bachstetter, T. Hughes, K. Bales, S. Paul, et al. 2006. Enrichment improves cognition in AD mice by amyloid-related and unrelated mechanisms. *Neurobiology of Aging* 28: 831–844.

Cotman, C. W., N. Berchtold, and L. Christie. 2007. Exercise builds brain health: Key roles of growth factor cascades and inflammation. *Trends in Neuroscience* 30: 465–472.

Cracchiolo, J., T. Mori, S. Nazian, J. Tan, H. Potter, and G. Arendash. 2007. Enhanced cognitive activity—over and above social or physical activity—is required to protect Alzheimer's mice against cognitive impairment, reduce Aβ deposition, and increase synaptic immunostaining. *Neurobiology of Learning and Memory* 88: 277–294.

Derwinger, A., A. Stigsdotter Neely, and L. Backman. 2005. Design your own memory strategies! Self-generated strategy training versus mnemonic training in old age: An 8-month follow-up. *Neuropsychological Rehabilitation* 15: 37–54.

Desmond, D. W., J. Moroney, M. Paik, M. Sano, E. Mohr, S. Aboumatar, et al. 2000. Frequency and clinical determinants of dementia after ischemic stroke. *Neurology* 54: 1124–1131.

Draganski, B., C. Gaser, V. Busch, G. Schuierer, U. Bogdahn, and A. May. 2004. Neuroplasticity: Changes in grey matter induced by training. *Nature* 427: 311–312.

Drapeau, E., W. Mayo, C. Aurousseau, M. Le Moal, P. Piazza, and D. Abrous. 2003. Spatial memory performances of aged rats in the water maze predict levels of hippocampal neurogenesis. *Proceedings of the National Academy of Sciences of the United States of America* 100: 14385–14390.

Fratiglioni, L., H. X. Wang, K. Ericsson, M. Maytan, and B. Winblad. 2000. Influence of social network on occurrence of dementia: A community-based longitudinal study. *Lancet* 355: 1315–1319.

Frick, K. and S. Fernandez. 2003. Enrichment enhances spatial memory and increases synaptophysin levels in aged female mice. *Neurobiology of Aging* 24: 615–626.

Fumagalli, F., G. Racagni, and M. Riva. 2006. The expanding role of BDNF: A therapeutic target for Alzheimer's disease. *Pharmacogenomics Journal* 6: 8–15.

Gates, N. and M. Valenzuela. 2010. Cognitive exercise and its role in cognitive function in the elderly. *Current Psychiatry Reports* 12: 20–27.

Gould, S. J. 1991. *The Mismeasure of Man.* New York: Norton.

Grady, C., A. McIntosh, S. Beig, M. Keightley, H. Burian, and S. Black. 2003. Evidence from functional neuroimaging of a compensatory prefrontal network in Alzheimer's disease. *Journal of Neuroscience* 23: 986–993.

Grafman, J., A. Salazar, H. Weingartner, S. Vance, and D. Amin. 1986. The relationship of brain-tissue loss volume and lesion location to cognitive deficit. *Journal of Neuroscience* 6: 301–307.

Gunther, V., P. Schafer, B. Holzner, and G. Kemmler. 2003. Long-term improvements in cognitive performance through computer-assisted cognitive training: A pilot study in a residential home for older people. *Aging and Mental Health* 7: 200–206.

Haier, R., B. Siegel, K. Nuechterlein, E. Hazlett, J. Wu, J. Paek, et al. 1988. Cortical glucose metabolic rate correlates of reasoning and attention studied with positron emission tomography. *Intelligence* 12: 199–217.

Ickes, B., T. Pham, L. Sanders, D. Albeck, A. Mohammed, and A. Granholm. 2000. Long-term environmental enrichment leads to regional increases in neurotrophin levels in rat brain. *Experimental Neurology* 164: 45–52.

Janowsky, J., et al. 2005. Environmental enrichment mitigates cognitive deficits in a mouse model of Alzheimer's disease. *Journal of Neuroscience* 25: 5217–5224.

Jorm, A. E., H. Creasey, A. Broe, M. Sulway, S. Kos, and O. Dent. 1997. The advantage of being broad-minded: brain diameter and neuropsychological test performance in elderly war veterans. *Personality and Individual Differences* 23: 371–377.

Katzman, R., R. Terry, R. DeTeresa, T. Brown, P. Davies, P. Fuld, et al. 1988. Clinical, pathological and neurochemical changes in dementia: A subgroup with preserved mental status and numerous neocortical plaques. *Annals of Neurology* 23: 138–144.

Kempermann, G. 2006. *Adult Neurogenesis.* New York: Oxford University Press.

Lazarov, O., J. Robinson, Y. Tang, I. Hairston, Z. Korade-Mirnics, V. Lee, et al. 2005. Environmental enrichment reduces Aß levels and amyloid deposition in transgenic mice. *Cell* 120: 701–713.

Levi, O., A. Jongen-Relo, J. Feldon, A. Roses, and D. Michaelson. 2003. ApoE4 impairs hippocampal plasticity isoform-specifically and blocks the environmental stimulation of synaptogensis and memory. *Neurobiology of Disease* 13: 273–282.

Mahncke, H., B. Connor, J. Appelman, O. Ahsanuddin, J. Hardy, R. Wood, et al. 2006. Memory enhancement in healthy older adults using a brain plasticity-based training program: A randomised, controlled study. *Proceedings of the National Academy of Sciences of the United States of America* 103: 12523–12528.

Malenka, R., and M. Bear. 2004. LTP and LTD: An embarrassment of riches. *Neuron* 44: 5–21.

McOmish, C., and A. Hannan. 2007. Enviromimetics: exploring gene environment interactions to identify therapeutic targets for brain disorders. *Expert Opinion on Therapeutic Targets* 11: 899–913.

Mesulam, M. 1999. Neuroplasticity failure in Alzheimer's disease: Bridging the gap between plaques and tangles. *Neuron* 24: 521–529.

Mohammed, A. H., S. Zhu, S. Darmopil, J. Hjerling-Leffler, P. Ernfors, B. Winblad, et al. 2002. Environmental enrichment and the brain. *Progress in Brain Research* 138: 109–133.

Moore, C., M. Cohen, and C. Ranganath. 2006. Neural mechanisms of expert skills in visual working memory. *Journal of Neuroscience* 26: 11187–11196.

Mortimer, J. 1988. Do psychosocial risk factors contribute to Alzheimer's disease? In *Etiology of dementia of Alzheimer's type*, ed. A. Henderson and J. Henderson, 39–52. Chichester: Wiley and Sons.

Mortimer, J. A. 1997. Brain reserve and the clinical expression of Alzheimer's disease. *Geriatrics* 52 (Suppl 2): S50–S53.

Mozolic, J., S. Hayaska, and P. Laurienti. 2010. A cognitive training intervention increases resting cerebral blood flow in healthy older adults. *Frontiers in Neuroscience Human Neuroscience* 4: 16.

Naka, F., N. Narita, N. Okado, and M. Narita. 2005. Modification of AMPA receptor properties following environmental enrichment. *Brain and Development* 27: 275–278.

Naveh-Benjamin, M., T. Brav, and O. Levi. 2007. The associative memory deficits of older adults: The role of strategy utilization. *Psychology and Aging* 22: 202–208.

Neuropathology Group. 2001. Pathological correlates of late-onset dementia in a multicentre, community-based population in England and Wales. Neuropathology Group of the Medical Research Council Cognitive Function and Ageing Study MRC CFAS. *Lancet* 375: 169–175.

Nithianantharajah, J., and A. Hannan. 2006. Enriched environments, experience-dependent plasticity and disorders of the nervous system. *Nature Reviews Neuroscience* 7: 697–709.

Olazaran, J., R. Muniz, B. Reisberg, J. Pena-Casanova, T. Del Ser, et al. 2004. Benefits of cognitive-motor intervention in MCI and mild to moderate Alzheimer disease. *Neurology* 63: 2348–2353.

Olesen, P., H. Westerberg, and T. Klingberg. 2004. Increased prefrontal and parietal activity after training of working memory. *Nature Neuroscience* 7: 75–79.

Oswald, W., T. Gunzelmann, R. Rupprecht, and B. Hagen. 2006. Differential effects of single versus combined cognitive and physical training with older adults: The SimA study in a 5-year perspective. *European Journal of Ageing* 3: 179–192.

Rampon, C., C. H. Jiang, H. Dong, Y. P. Tang, D. J. Lockhart, P. G. Schultz, et al. 2000. Effects of environmental enrichment on gene expression in the brain. *Proceedings of the National Academy of Sciences of the United States of America* 97: 12880–12884.

Rapp, S., G. Brenes, and A. Marsh. 2002. Memory enhancement training for older adults with mild cognitive impairment: A preliminary study. *Aging and Mental Health*, 5–11.

Rebok, G., M. Carlson, and J. Langbaum. 2007. Training and maintaining memory abilities in healthy older adults: traditional and novel approaches. *Journal of Gerontology Series B: Psychological Sciences and Social Sciences* 62B: 53–61.

Rosen, A., M. Prull, R. O'Hara, E. Race, J. Desmond, G. Glover, et al. 2002. Variable effects of aging on frontal lobe contributions to memory. *NeuroReport* 13: 2425–2428.

Roth, M. 1986. The association of clinical and neurological findings and its bearing on the classification and aetiology of Alzheimer's disease. *British Medical Bulletin* 42: 42–50.

Rozzini, L., D. Costardi, V. Chilovi, S. Franzoni, M. Trabucchi, and A. Padovani. 2007. Efficacy of cognitive rehabilitation in patients with mild cognitive impairment treated with cholinesterase inhibitors. *International Journal of Geriatric Psychiatry* 22 (4): 356–360.

Rubinov, M., A. McIntosh, M. Valenzuela, and M. Breakspear. 2009. Simulation of neuronal death and network recovery in a computational model of distributed cortical activity. *American Journal of Geriatric Psychiatry* 17: 210–217.

Satz, P. 1993. Brain reserve capacity on symptom onset after brain injury: A formulation and review of evidence for threshold theory. *Neuropsychology* 7: 273–295.

Scarmeas, N., G. Levy, M. Tang, J. Manly, and Y. Stern. 2001. Influence of leisure activity on the incidence of Alzheimer's disease. *Neurology* 57: 2236–2242.

Scarmeas, N., E. Zarahn, K. Anderson, C. Habeck, J. Hilton, J. Flynn, et al. 2003. Association of life activities with cerebral blood flow in Alzheimer disease. *Archives of Neurology* 60: 359–365.

Scheff, S. and D. A. Price. 2003. Synaptic pathology in Alzheimer's disease: A review of ultrastructural studies. *Neurobiology of Aging* 24: 1029–1046.

Schofield, P., G. Logroscino, H. Andrews, S. Albert, and Y. Stern. 1997. An association between head circumference and Alzheimer's disease in a population-based study of aging and dementia. *Neurology* 49: 30–37.

Scogin, F., and J. Bienias. 1988. A three-year follow-up of older adult participants in a memory-skills training program. *Psychology and Aging* 3: 334–337.

Sitzer, D., E. Twamley, and D. Jeste. 2006. Cognitive training in Alzheimer's disease: A meta-analysis of the literature. *Acta Psychiatrica Scandinavica* 114: 75–90.

Stern, Y. 2002. What is cognitive reserve? Theory and research application of the reserve concept. *Journal of the International Neuropsychological Society* 8: 448–460.

Terry, R. D., E. Masliah, D. P. Salmon, N. Butters, R. DeTeresa, R. Hill, et al. 1991. Physical basis of cognitive alterations in Alzheimer's disease: Synapse loss is the major correlate of cognitive impairment. *Annals of Neurology* 30: 572–580.

Thomas, A., S. Marrett, Z. Saad, D. Ruff, A. Martin, and P. Bandettini. 2009. Functional but not structural changes associated with learning: An exploration of longitudinal Voxel-based morphometry VBM. *NeuroImage* 48: 117–125.

Tomlinson, B., G. Blessed, and M. Roth. 1970. Observations on the brains of demented old people. *Journal of the Neurological Sciences* 11: 205–242.

Tononi, G., O. Sporns, and G. Edelman. 1999. Measures of degeneracy and redundancy in biological networks. *Proceedings of the National Academy of Sciences of the United States of America* 96: 3257–3262.

Tuokko, H., D. Garrett, I. McDowell, N. Silverberg, and B. Kristjansson. 2003. Cognitive decline in high-functioning older adults: reserve or ascertainment bias? *Aging and Mental Health* 7: 259–270.

Valenzuela, M., M. Breakspear, and P. Sachdev. 2007. Complex mental activity and the ageing brain: Molecular, cellular and cortical network mechanisms. *Brain Research Reviews* 56: 198–213.

Valenzuela, M., and P. Sachdev. 2001. Magnetic resonance spectroscopy in AD. *Neurology* 56: 592–598.

Valenzuela, M., and P. Sachdev. 2009. Can cognitive exercise prevent the onset of dementia? A systematic review of randomized clinical trials with longitudinal follow up. *American Journal of Geriatric Psychiatry* 17: 179–187.

Valenzuela, M., P. Sachdev, T. Rundeck, and D. Bennett. 2006. Cognitive leisure activities, but not watching TV, for future brain benefits. *Neurology* 67: 729.

Valenzuela, M., P. Sachdev, W. Wen, X. Chen, and H. Brodaty. 2008. Lifespan mental activity predicts diminished rate of hippocampal atrophy. *PLoS One* 3: e2598.

Valenzuela, M. J. 2008. Brain reserve and the prevention of dementia. *Current Opinion in Psychiatry* 21: 296–302.

Valenzuela, M. J., M. Jones, W. Wen, C. Rae, S. Graham, R. Shnier, et al. 2003. Memory training alters hippocampal neurochemistry in healthy elderly. *NeuroReport* 14: 1333–1337.

Valenzuela, M. J., and P. Sachdev. 2006. Brain reserve and dementia: A systematic review. *Psychological Medicine* 36: 441–454.

Valenzuela, M. J., and P. Sachdev. 2007. Assessment of complex mental activity across the lifespan: Development of the Lifetime of Experiences Questionnaire. *Psychological Medicine* 37: 1015–1025.

Verghese, J., R. Lipton, M. Katz, C. Hall, C. Derby, G. Kuslansky, et al. 2003. Leisure activities and the risk of dementia in the elderly. *New England Journal of Medicine* 348: 2508–2516.

Wang, H., A. Karp, B. Winblad, and L. Fratiglioni. 2002. Late-life engagement in social and leisure activities is associated with a decreased risk of dementia: A longitudinal study from the Kungsholmen Project. *American Journal of Epidemiology* 12: 1081–1087.

Willis, S., S. Tennstedt, M. Marsiske, K. Ball, J. Elias, et al. 2006. Long-term effects of cognitive training on everyday functional outcomes in older adults. *JAMA* 296: 2805–2814.

Wilson, R. S., C. F. Mendes De Leon, L. L. Barnes, J. A. Schneider, J. L. Bienias, D. A. Evans, et al. 2002. Participation in cognitively stimulating activities and risk of incident Alzheimer disease. *JAMA* 287: 742–748.

Chapter 6

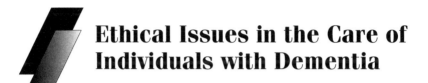

Ethical Issues in the Care of Individuals with Dementia

Art Walaszek

THE PRINCIPLES OF MEDICAL ETHICS

Three ethical principles are fundamental to medical care in general and the care of individuals with dementia in particular: autonomy, welfare, and social justice (ABIM Foundation 2002). The principle of autonomy dictates that individuals must be allowed to make decisions about their own medical care and about their overall welfare, and to act independently and without coercion; in turn, clinicians must respect these decisions and thereby support their patients' autonomy. Maintaining autonomy is a challenge for individuals with dementia: cognitive, emotional, behavioral, and functional impairments interfere with one's ability to comprehend, to reason, to recall, and to have a coherent sense of self. As will be discussed in detail below, clinicians are often called upon to assess the capacity of older adults to make medical decisions, to live independently, and to manage their affairs.

Clinicians are obligated to provide treatment that serves the best interests of their patients—thus the principle of patient welfare (or beneficence). In dementia care, a number of issues arise in this area: diagnosing dementia early and using biomarkers appropriately; ensuring that individuals who do not have the capacity to make decisions receive appropriate care; prescribing antipsychotic medications for behavioral and psychological symptoms of dementia; protecting vulnerable older adults from physical, emotional, and financial exploitation; and ensuring comfort at the end of life.

The principle of social justice calls for a fair distribution of healthcare resources and an elimination of discrimination in health care (ABIM Foundation 2002). The aging population and ever-escalating costs of health care will test this principle as society debates the equitable use of scarce resources. The debatable cost-effectiveness of cognitive enhancers and the appropriate role of palliative approaches in advanced dementia are also issues of social justice.

ETHICAL CHALLENGES IN THE DIAGNOSIS OF DEMENTIA

The diagnosis of dementia remains essentially a clinical one, using established criteria that are reasonably accurate when compared with the gold standard, pathological examination at autopsy. Early concerns about the utility of diagnosing an irreversible, terminal condition such as Alzheimer's disease (AD) have waned as effective treatments have emerged (Walaszek 2009). In fact, the ethical principle of truth-telling dictates that patients must be informed of their diagnosis. Early diagnosis allows an individual to prepare advance directives and designate a power of attorney, to consider participating in research, to participate in support groups, and to decide whether or not to take a cognitive enhancer (Post 2000). Great interest now exists in biological markers that would either result in more definitive diagnosis and appropriate treatment, or that could identify individuals at risk of dementia so that preventive measures can be developed.

Nevertheless, there has been understandable concern that testing for such markers in young, asymptomatic individuals, in the absence of effective preventive measures, may result in psychological distress, stigma, discrimination, and difficulty with employability. This is in particular true for genetic polymorphisms associated with AD: the ε4 allele of apolipoprotein E and mutations in the PS1, PS2, and APP genes. A 1997 position statement argued that apolipoprotein E testing should have a limited role in diagnosis and no place in screening asymptomatic individuals; PS1, PS2 and APP testing may be useful in evaluating individuals with early-onset dementia (Post et al. 1997).

Several recent studies have further refined this issue. The REVEAL (Risk Evaluation and Education for Alzheimer's Disease) study examined the effect of genetic disclosure on adult children of patients who had autopsy-confirmed AD. The subjects randomly assigned to learn their apolipoprotein E status, including those who carried the ε4 allele, did not become more depressed or anxious than those who did not learn their status; also, subjects who learned their status became more engaged in activities (such as physical exercise) that may lower the risk of developing AD (Roberts et al. 2005). All subjects had extensive genetic counseling, suggesting that genetic testing in asymptomatic relatives of patients who have AD may be ethical if proper supports are in place. Consistent with this finding, the Alzheimer's Association argues that genetic testing should only be done when coupled with comprehensive pre- and post-test genetic counseling (Alzheimer's Association 2008). Because genetic risk varies by ethnicity, genetic counseling must be tailored to each individual's ethnic background (Christensen et al. 2008).

An extension of the REVEAL study to subjects tested for the PS1 or PS2 mutation (which confers a vastly greater risk of developing AD than the ε4 allele) also found that subjects who learned their genetic status experienced no greater psychological distress than those who did not (Cassidy et al. 2008). Longitudinal follow-up of the REVEAL study (six weeks, six months and one year after disclosure or nondisclosure of genetic status) confirmed that disclosure did not result in excessive distress, though a baseline high level of emotional distress was predictive after greater distress after disclosure (Green et al. 2009).

Concern remains about disclosure of genetic test results. The Alzheimer's Association asserts that anonymous testing should be available, that is, the test result should not enter a patient's medical record (Alzheimer's Association 2008). In the United States, the Genetic Information Nondiscrimination Act (GINA) of 2008 prohibits discrimination in health coverage and employment based on genetic information, which may help allay some of these concerns (National Human Genome Research Institute 2008).

In summary, asymptomatic individuals receiving a positive result of genetic testing for AD may not be subject to as many psychological and other consequences as initially thought and may in fact alter their behavior in ways that could lower their risk of developing AD. Nevertheless, until effective preventive measures are developed, caution should be exercised when testing AD biomarkers in asymptomatic individuals, in particular as new biomarkers (e.g., functional neuroimaging with positron emission tomography) become available.

THE ASSESSMENT OF CAPACITY IN INDIVIDUALS WITH DEMENTIA

By definition, dementia results in a decline in cognition and functioning, which in turn diminishes one's capacity to make personal choices and to care for oneself. Clinicians are often called upon to assess the capacity of an individual with dementia to make medical decisions. Legal systems become involved to determine if an individual is incompetent, that is, unable to make decisions about one's welfare. Such situations involve balancing the ethical principles of autonomy and patient welfare.

An individual's ability to provide informed consent requires that information relevant to the decision is available, that the individual is free to make a choice without coercion or manipulation (voluntarism), and that the individual has the ability to make a decision (decisional capacity). Dementia can impair both voluntarism and decisional capacity. Voluntarism may be affected by illness-related considerations (e.g., executive dysfunction, apathy, inattention, memory loss, poor impulse control), psychological issues (e.g., depression, loneliness, impulsivity, anxiety, paranoia), cultural values (e.g., discomfort questioning authority), and external pressures (e.g., pressure from or coercion by caregivers) (Roberts 2002). An individual with apathy due to dementia may appear to consent to an intervention without actually having the capacity to do so (Grimes et al. 2000), thus it behooves a clinician to consider the possibility of incapacity not only when an individual refuses but also when one assents. Concerns about voluntarism are especially relevant when an individual with dementia must rely on a caregiver for assistance and when one is a resident of a long-term care facility.

Having decisional capacity requires an individual to be able to express a preference, understand relevant information about a situation and the choice to be made, manipulate the relevant information and thereby reason about the situation, and appreciate how the situation is personally relevant (Roberts and Dyer 2004, 54–56). A "sliding scale" approach is widely accepted; that is, the higher the risk of accepting or refusing an intervention, the higher the threshold required for consent or refusal (Drane 1984).

Although a diagnosis of dementia does not in and of itself mean that an individual has lost decisional capacity, dementia is a powerful contributor to incapacity. For example, a prospective study of subjects with mild AD found them to have, when compared to healthy older adults, impairments in the capacity domains of understanding, reasoning and appreciation that worsened over the course of two years. At baseline, 70% of AD subjects were deemed capable of reasoning, but at two-year follow-up, only 30% were; interestingly, no AD at baseline were thought to be fully capable of understanding, presumably due to deficits in short-term memory and executive function (Huthwaite et al. 2006). Another prospective study comparing 53 subjects with dementia to 53 older adult controls without dementia showed that 9.4% of subjects had incapacity at baseline, but only nine months later, 26.4% had incapacity, primarily due to declining ability to reason (Moye et al. 2006). Performance on neuropsychological testing has been shown to account for a significant amount of the variance in the decisional capacity among subjects with dementia, including 77.8% of the variance in understanding (Gurrera et al. 2006).

Though the specifics of assessing capacity and addressing incapacity vary among jurisdictions (and clinicians should be aware of local laws and regulations), a general framework has been proposed. A clinician asks an individual with dementia a series of questions to assess her or his understanding, appreciation, reasoning and ability to express a choice (Karlawish 2008):

1. After disclosing relevant information (e.g., the risks and benefits of a treatment), the clinician asks the individual to repeat the information in her or his own words.
2. The clinician asks about the individual's beliefs about the diagnosis of dementia (i.e, whether s/he believes s/he has dementia) and about possible benefits to her or him of treatment.
3. The clinician ascertains if the individual can compare options and can infer how a choice will affect her or him, testing for logic and consistency.
4. The individual must be able to communicate a consistent decision.

Multiple instruments are available to standardize and/or augment the assessment of decisional capacity. In a review of 15 capacity assessment instruments, Dunn et al. (2006) argued that the MacArthur Competence Assessment Tool for Treatment (MacCAT-T) is the best studied and has the broadest application to various clinical situations. The MacCAT-T is based on the gold standard MacArthur capacity model. Training is required to ensure inter-rater reliability. The assessment begins with a discussion of the clinical situation, including the diagnosis, the proposed treatment, and its risks, benefits and alternatives. The interviewer asks multiple questions to assess the components of decisional capacity: understanding, reasoning and appreciation. The patient makes a choice and explains her or his reasoning. Finally, the interviewer comes to a conclusion about whether or not the patient has capacity to make the decision (Grisso, Appelbaum, and Hill-Fotouhi 1997). It has been suggested that the MacCAT-T and similar competency assessment tools are best used as adjuncts to the clinical assessment described above.

Studies assessing the utility of bedside cognitive tests have yielded mixed results. Kim, Karlawish, and Caine (2002), in their review of this literature, argue that a Mini-Mental State Exam (MMSE) (Folstein et al. 1975) score of greater than 24 is predictive of capacity, less than 18 predictive of incapacity, with intermediate scores requiring further assessment to determine capacity. A subsequent study of 37 subjects with mild-to-moderate AD found the specificity for incapacity to be 92.9% for an MMSE cutoff of 19, and the sensitivity for incapacity to be 91.3% for a cutoff of 26 (Kim and Caine 2002). However, no bedside cognitive test alone can accurately predict capacity; rather, a clinician may incorporate such testing as part of a comprehensive capacity assessment.

Whereas the preceding discussion has focused on the assessment of capacity to make medical decisions, there are a number of other capacities that may be affected by dementia.

Everyday Decisionmaking and the Ability to Live Independently

At some point in the course of their illness, individuals with dementia will require assistance with their basic and instrumental activities of daily living, and they may eventually lose the ability to live independently. Individuals with AD perform poorly on standardized measures of everyday problem-solving (Willis et al. 1998). Executive dysfunction in particular has been associated with worsening functional status. Structured assessments of executive function such as the Executive Interview and of functional abilities such as the Kohlman Evaluation of Living Skills (KELS) may help identify individuals needing higher levels of care. The KELS may in particular be useful in suspected cases of self-neglect (Royall, Chiodo, and Polk 2005; Pickens et al. 2007).

Finances

Difficulty managing finances is an early disruption in AD in the instrumental activities of daily living. Patients with dementia and their caregivers frequently misestimate the patients' financial abilities, suggesting that an objective evaluation tool may be useful (Okonkwo et al. 2008). For example, the Financial Capacity Instrument has been used to determine that individuals with mild AD had high rates of impaired financial capacity (47–87%), and those with moderate AD were almost uniformly incapacitated (90–100%) (Marson et al. 2000). Concerns that arise in this setting include the risk of financial exploitation of the elder, and the need to identify a proxy to manage finances (either by invoking a durable power of attorney or by appointing a guardian).

Driving

Another early functional impairment in AD is the ability to drive, which raises the possibility of harm of self and others. The American Academy of Neurology recommends that individuals with mild cognitive impairment or mild AD should be monitored closely and should be considered for a formal evaluation of driving skills. Those with moderate or severe AD should not drive (Dubinsky, Stein, and Lyons 2000). Clinicians should familiarize themselves with local laws regarding their obligation to report potentially dangerous driving.

Sexual Relations

Many older adults with cognitive impairment remain sexually active. Of particular ethical interest are situations wherein one partner in a relationship has developed dementia and the other is cognitively intact. Unfortunately, the capacity of individuals with dementia to consent to sexual relations has been poorly studied. One model suggests that having any deficits in awareness of the relationship, in the capacity to avoid exploitation, or in the awareness of potential risks of sex indicates that the individual does not have the capacity to consent to a sexual relationship (Lichtenberg and Strzepek 1990).

Voting

A standard for assessing the capacity to vote has only recently been developed (Karlawish et al. 2004). Though most individuals with mild dementia retain the capacity to vote, those with severe dementia typically do not have that capacity (Appelbaum, Bonnie, and Karlawish 2005). In the United States, surrogate decision-makers are not allowed to cast votes for those who do not have capacity (Karlawish et al. 2004). On the other hand, individuals with capacity who reside in long-term care facilities may be at risk of being disenfranchised because of procedural problems (Karlawish, Bonnie, et al. 2008).

Testamentary Capacity

One of the rationales for early diagnosis in dementia is that the individual is more likely to have the capacity to make decisions about her or his future, including creating an advance directive, identifying powers of attorney, and executing a will. The International Psychogeriatric

Association has developed guidelines for the assessment of testamentary capacity (Shulman et al. 2009).

ADDRESSING INCAPACITY

A finding of incapacity should lead to (a) the identification and addressing of any reversible causes of incapacity; (b) attempts to improve capacity by means of cognitive and educational strategies; and/or (c) surrogate decision-making.

Although most causes of dementia are irreversible, there may be other contributions to incapacity, including depression, anxiety, delirium, and polypharmacy (Walaszek 2009). Given that cognitive enhancers may improve cognition and functioning in a subset of individuals with dementia, it is possible that treatment with a cognitive enhancer may improve capacity—although this hypothesis has yet to be tested, and it presupposes that an individual has capacity to consent to treatment with a cognitive enhancer in the first place.

A variety of strategies have been developed to improve capacity in older adults to make medical decisions, including simplifying information, providing it in the form of a story book or video, disclosing information in parts, using health educators, and quizzing subjects (Sugarman, McCrory, and Hubal 1998). As described below, an "enhanced written consent procedure" has been developed to improve the capacity of individuals with dementia to participate in research (Mittal et al. 2007). Roberts and Dyer (2004, 70) recommend a stepwise approach for consent in individuals with deficits in decisional capacity: seek consent to simply begin treatment; then, as the individual's symptoms (and presumably capacity) improve, discuss more substantive or challenging choices.

When capacity cannot be restored, a surrogate or proxy decisionmaker must step in. The identity of the decisionmaker depends on whether or not the incapacitated individual had previously designated a surrogate, namely, a power of attorney. Often individuals have not designated a power of attorney; in such cases, most jurisdictions have laws that describe the sequence of which family members (e.g., spouse, adult children, siblings, and so on) become surrogate decisionmakers.

The "best interest" and "substituted judgment" standards govern the behavior of surrogate decisionmakers. In the former, the surrogate makes a decision based on what the surrogate perceives is in the best interest of the individual with dementia. In the latter, the surrogate makes a decision based on the choice the individual would have made, if the individual had been able to do so; in some cases, the individual may have created an advance directive to express future preferences and thereby guide this decision-making. A combined approach has been recommended, wherein the substituted judgment standard is applied when it is clear what the individual would have decided; otherwise, the best interest standard is used (Gutheil and Appelbaum 2000, 232–233).

A capacity assessment yields a dichotomous outcome: an individual is deemed able or not able to make a medical decision. In reality, however, individuals with dementia often collaborate with family members and other caregivers in decisionmaking. This has been referred to as a "shared decisionmaking" model, wherein the individual can make a decision with assistance or the responsibility for decisionmaking is shared among the parties; unfortunately, legal procedures are generally not available to support this pragmatic approach (Kapp 2002).

When an individual has been found incapable of making everyday decisions, managing her or his affairs, and living independently, a court will declare her or him incompetent and appoint a guardian. Clinicians should be aware of local laws governing guardianship proceedings, especially because they may be called upon to testify regarding the individual's mental state and decisional capacity. Moye et al. (2007) have reviewed the process of evaluating an individual for guardianship.

ETHICAL CHALLENGES IN THE USE OF COGNITIVE ENHANCERS

Diagnosing dementia, especially early in the course of the illness, offers individuals the opportunity to decide on treatment with cognitive enhancers. Although currently available cognitive enhancers (donepezil, rivastigmine, galantamine, and memantine) do not reverse cognitive losses or modify the course of dementia, a subset of patients may benefit from a clinically significant delay in cognitive decline (Qaseem et al. 2008). However, a number of ethical concerns have been raised about the use of these agents.

First, an individual with dementia may have diminished capacity to consent to treatment with a cognitive enhancer. A study of 48 subjects with mild or moderate AD found that only 40% had the capacity to consent to cognitive enhancing treatment (Karlawish et al. 2005). Anosognosia, or lack of recognition that one has dementia, interferes with capacity as well. Even if an individual initially consents, it is possible that, due to cognitive decline, s/he will no longer be able to consent to continued treatment. Thus, clinicians may need to assess to capacity of an individual with dementia to provide informed consent, as described above.

Post et al. (2001), citing qualitative data from focus groups of patients, caregivers, and clinicians, raised the possibility of instilling false hope among patients and caregivers regarding the outcome of treatment with cognitive enhancers. However, a more recent study employing semi-structured interviews of 12 caregivers of patients who had used cognitive enhancers failed to replicate this finding. Interestingly, the authors noted that "some hope is necessary to continue to live through the situation" (Huizing et al. 2006).

If cognitive enhancers prolong morbidity or extend life, then treatment will increase suffering rather than decrease suffering (Post and White-house 1998). However, there is no evidence that the use of cholinesterase inhibitors alone or in combination with memantine is associated with a change in time to death. This study also replicated earlier findings that the use of cognitive enhancers is associated with delayed time to nursing home placement (Lopez et al. 2009).

The cost-effectiveness of cognitive enhancers is uncertain, raising concerns about social justice and the appropriate use of limited resources. The cost of donepezil may be over US$120,000 per quality-adjusted year of life, and the savings resulting from delayed institutionalization may not offset the cost of medication (Loveman et al. 2006). The National Institute for Health and Clinic Excellence (NICE) in the United Kingdom has responded to these concerns by limiting the use of cholinesterase inhibitors to patients with moderately severe AD (MMSE score between 10 and 20) and recommending against the use of memantine (NICE 2007). A review of the accessibility of cognitive enhancers in 23 of 26 European Union nations revealed widely varying criteria for use, with upper limits of MMSE ranging between 20 and 30 and lower limits of MMSE between 10 and 13 for cholinesterase inhibitors; for memantine, the respective ranges were 11–26 and 0–13. There were also marked differences in policies regarding who could prescribe cognitive enhancers (general practitioners versus specialists) and reimbursement for cognitive enhancers (Oude Voshaar, Burns, and Olde Rikkert 2006). It is unlikely that such variability is solely due to different interpretations of the research literature regarding cost-effectiveness; rather, local political and financial considerations probably contribute to the variability. The combined use of a cholinesterase inhibitor and memantine may further increase costs, though a clinical trial is currently underway to determine the cost-effectiveness of combination therapy (Jones et al. 2009).

Finally, it is not clear when to discontinue treatment with cognitive enhancers. In addition to evidence of modest benefit in severe dementia for cholinesterase inhibitors (Winblad et al. 2009) and memantine (Thomas and Grossberg 2009), there are reports of declines in cognition, functioning, or behavior with discontinuation of cognitive enhancers (e.g., Daiello et al. 2009). Blass et al. (2008) found that 30% of nursing home residents with advanced dementia were prescribed cognitive enhancers, though the prevalence decreased to 10% by the time of death. A consensus panel of geriatricians at the University of Chicago concluded that the use of cholinesterase inhibitors and memantine was "never appropriate" in the palliative care of advanced dementia (Holmes et al. 2008), yet a study of 10,065 individuals with advanced dementia admitted to U.S. hospices found that 21% were prescribed a cognitive enhancer (Weschules, Maxwell, and Shega 2008).

Clinicians, patients, and proxy decisionmakers should closely collaborate in the on-going monitoring of the risks and benefits of continued treatment with cognitive enhancers. Further research is required to determine at what point to discontinue treatment with cognitive enhancers.

ETHICAL CHALLENGES IN THE TREATMENT OF BEHAVIORAL AND PSYCHOLOGICAL SYMPTOMS OF DEMENTIA

Although dementia is defined in terms of cognitive impairment and functional decline, emotional and behavioral symptoms are also very common. In fact, at least 80% of individuals with dementia will experience behavioral and psychological symptoms of dementia (BPSD) such as depression, anxiety, psychosis, and agitation (Lyketsos et al. 2002). These symptoms may lead to poor patient quality of life, increased caregiver burden, concerns about patient safety, and higher risk of institutionalization. Atypical antipsychotics, the pharmacological agents most likely to be effective in addressing these symptoms, are associated with significant morbidity and mortality (Schneider, Dagerman, and Insel 2006). A meta-analysis of trials of atypical antipsychotics in dementia found a mortality rate of 3.5% versus 2.3% for placebo, with an odds ratio of 1.54 (95% confidence interval, 1.06–2.23) (Schneider, Dagerman, and Insel 2005). In April 2005 the U.S. FDA added a black-box warning advising against the use of antipsychotics in older adults with dementia. Clinical treatment guidelines (e.g., Lyketsos et al. 2006) recommend a sequential strategy to addressing BPSD that includes:

- first identifying and addressing possible medical causes (delirium, pain, dehydration, urinary tract infection, and so on);
- then using evidence-based nonpharmacologic interventions (behavioral management, cognitive stimulation, socialization);
- then considering pharmacological interventions if BPSD cause significant distress or are potentially dangerous.

Additional safeguards exist in nursing homes by means of U.S. federal regulations limiting the initiation of psychotropic medications to specific indications, requiring regular review of medications by pharmacists, and requiring trials of drug discontinuation (Kapp 2009, 478); see below for details.

Nevertheless, pending the development of more effective treatments, antipsychotic medications will likely remain the mainstay of managing severe BPSD. Clinicians thus face the ethical dilemma of recommending a treatment that may hasten death. A further complication is that the patients themselves rarely have the capacity to consent to treatment with antipsychotics, and so a surrogate decisionmaker must be involved. Thus, a clinician considering prescribing an antipsychotic medication for BPSD must very carefully review the risks, benefits, and alternatives of such treatment with patients and their surrogates, emphasizing that these medications are not appropriate long-term solutions (Lyketsos et al. 2006).

As a result of behavioral disturbances that are imminently dangerous to self or others, an individual with dementia may require a higher level of supervision and care, for example, a psychiatric hospitalization. Local regulations regarding involuntary psychiatric treatment vary tremendously, and the clinician must be familiar with the standards and laws in her or his own jurisdiction. In general, criteria for involuntary commitment include that the patient must, as a result of being mentally ill, pose an imminent danger to self, pose an imminent danger to others, or be unable to care for self; some jurisdictions allow for involuntary hospitalization if, in the absence of treatment, severe deterioration in the patient's condition is likely (Gutheil and Appelbaum 2000, 52–53). Voluntary psychiatric hospitalization is complicated by the high rates of incapacity to make medical decisions among individuals with dementia. For example, a study of 379 older adults admitted to general medical units and then assessed for capacity found that 59% lacked medical decisionmaking capacity, with dementia and delirium being major contributors to incapacity (Mujic et al. 2009). Maxmin et al. (2009) interviewed 99 older adult psychiatric inpatients, only 52.5% of whom had capacity for admission and 38.4% for treatment decisions; again, dementia was associated with incapacity. It has been suggested that a lower threshold for capacity for admission is acceptable as long as patients agree to "enter the hospital and some in-hospital review process [is] available to pass [judgment] on the appropriateness of their decision" (Gutheil and Appelbaum 2000, 48).

Because medical causes of BSPD, including delirium, are common, it is critical that a patient admitted to the hospital receive an appropriate medical evaluation, either by admission to a medical unit initially or by medical consultation on a psychiatric unit.

ELDER ABUSE AND SELF-NEGLECT

Individuals with dementia are vulnerable to victimization by others or, more commonly, to self-neglect. Types of elder abuse include physical abuse, emotional or psychological abuse, sexual abuse, material abuse (i.e., financial exploitation), neglect, abandonment, and self-neglect. Rates of elder abuse range from 4.5 to 14.6 per 1,000, with an estimated 1–2 million cases each year in the United States (Jogerst et al. 2003). A recent survey of American older adults indicated that 1 in 10 had experienced elder abuse in the last year (Acierno et al. 2010). Risk factors for elder abuse include a diagnosis of dementia, presence of BPSD, low social supports, need for help with activities of daily living, female gender, low socioeconomic status, African American ethnic background, declining physical function, caregiver burden and caregiver depression/anxiety (Cooper et al. 2010; Acierno et al. 2010). Family members are implicated in 90% of elder abuse cases. After self-neglect, financial exploitation is the most common type of elder abuse (see Tueth 2000 for a review of this topic).

All 50 states have laws to protect older adults from abuse and neglect, with four states (Colorado, New York, North Dakota, South Dakota) allowing for voluntary reporting and all other states requiring mandatory reporting when healthcare professionals suspect elder abuse (Walaszek 2009). Surveys of healthcare professionals indicate that 33.7–39.9% had detected elder abuse in the last year, but only half had reported suspected abuse (Cooper et al. 2009). Face-to-face training of health care professionals about the management of suspected abuse appears to increase knowledge and increase reporting rates (Cooper, Selwood, and Livingston 2009).

Clinicians should familiarize themselves with local laws regarding the reporting of elder abuse. Those working with patients with dementia should maintain a high index of suspicion of self-neglect. Self-neglect is the most common form of elder abuse and can be difficult to detect because individuals with dementia may not be able to provide accurate reports of their functioning; caregivers and family members are typically not available to report the self-neglect. Self-neglect has been associated with a marked increase in risk of mortality (Dong et al. 2009). Concern about self-neglect should lead to a clinician formally assessing the individual's capacity to live independently, as described above. Relevant local authorities tasked with addressing elder abuse may need to be contacted.

Clinicians face an ethical quandary when they suspect elder abuse, but the elder does not wish to have the abuse reported; this represents a tension between the ethical principles of beneficence and autonomy. In such situations, clinicians will need to carefully evaluate the reasons why the patient does not want abuse reported (e.g., fear of retaliation), determine if the patient believes s/he is abused, and assess the patient's capacity to refuse further intervention. Of course, if there is evidence that an individual is in immediate danger, local authorities must be contacted.

ETHICAL ISSUES RELEVANT TO LONG-TERM CARE FACILITIES

Among the most challenging transitions for an individual with dementia is the move from one's home into a long-term care facility. Ethically, institutionalization is a response to the changing balance between the principles of autonomy and beneficence. That is, as an individual with dementia becomes progressively less able to care for herself or himself, some autonomy may be lost in order to support her or his well-being. The individual with dementia may not have the capacity to make this decision or may actively refuse admission to a long-term care facility, thereby necessitating the involvement of surrogate decisionmakers or legal processes such as guardianship. The assessment of capacity to live independently is discussed above.

Clinicians and their patients appear to disagree frequently on the appropriateness of institutionalization (Bartels et al. 2003) and there are significant cross-cultural differences in attitudes toward long-term care (McCormick et al. 2002). Individuals in long-term care face substantial limitations on making personal choices, affecting their autonomy and voluntarism (Kapp 1998). Thus, when an individual with dementia is no longer able to live independently, careful consideration should be made of her or his beliefs and values when determining an appropriate next step. For example, alternatives to institutionalization may include increased services within one's home and increased support for family members serving as caregivers.

Though only 4% of individuals with dementia live in a long-term care facility at any one time (Matthews and Dening 2002), approximately 90% will eventually move to a long-term care facility, compared to 50% of nondemented older adults (Smith, Kokmen, and O'Brien 2000). The majority of nursing home residents (56% in one estimate) have dementia (Matthews and Dening 2002), and the rates of incapacity to make medical decisions are high (Moye and Marson 2007).

Extensive U.S. federal regulations (referred to collectively as OBRA 1987) govern the behavior of nursing homes (Kapp 2009, 466). Nursing homes must comply with Medicaid regulations (CMS, or Centers for Medicare and Medicaid Services), with the Americans with Disabilities Act and the Rehabilitation Act, with standards of accrediting bodies (e.g., the Joint Commission), and with state regulations. These measures are intended to insure the appropriate treatment of nursing home residents with neuropsychiatric issues, including dementia and BPSD. Screening must take place prior to admission to a nursing home to determine if a patient has mental-health needs and if that facility can offer appropriate services for those needs (Kapp 2009, 468, 469). Residential care and assisted living facilities have emerged as common alternatives to nursing homes; rates of dementia and BPSD are similar in these settings to nursing homes, but with less oversight and with regulation that varies from state to state (Gruber-Baldini et al. 2004).

The use of physical restraints has increasingly been recognized as often "unnecessary, improper, and even abusive." The CMS have encouraged the aggressive enforcement of federal regulations limiting the use of "any physical restraints imposed or psychoactive drug administered for purposes of discipline or convenience, and not required to treat the resident's medical symptoms" (Kapp 2009, 476, 477). In order to respect the autonomy and preserve the dignity of nursing home residents, facilities should address BPSD by employing nonpharmacologic interventions (as described above), improving the environment (e.g., more activities for residents to prevent boredom), and/or making administrative or staff changes. A randomized controlled trial in four Norwegian nursing homes of a two-day staff training followed by six monthly meetings was associated with decreased use of restraints at 6-month follow-up (though not at 12 months), and decreased BPSD among nursing home residents at both 6 months and 12 months (Testad et al. 2010). This suggests that training, regular monitoring and on-going guidance are necessary to promote and maintain changes in the use of restraints.

A goal of OBRA 1987 regulations has been to prevent the use of psychotropic medications as "chemical restraints" or for environmental control, though it is recognized that there are appropriate uses of psychotropic medications. OBRA 1987 has resulted in decreased use of antipsychotic medications and increased use of antidepressant medications, the former through strict guidelines about the use of antipsychotics and the latter through increased detection of depression (Lantz, Giambanco, and Buchalter 1996). As described above, antipsychotic medications may have a role in the treatment of severe BPSD, but this decision should be weighed carefully with proxy decisionmakers. OBRA 1987 requires that antipsychotic medications be given only if they are "necessary to treat a specific condition as diagnosed and documented in the clinical record." CMS considers a "dementing illness with associated behavioral symptoms" a valid indication for antipsychotic medications, but the symptoms must be dangerous to self or others or must result in severe distress or decline in functioning. The resident's record must include documentation of the decisionmaking process, including diagnostic evaluation of BPSD, alternative nonpharmacologic interventions, and risk-benefit analysis. Furthermore, efforts must be made to discontinue antipsychotic medications (unless clinically contraindicated) by means of gradual dose reductions and behavioral interventions (CMS 2009). Clinicians prescribing psychotropic medications in long-term care facilities should familiarize themselves with relevant regulations.

RESEARCH INVOLVING INDIVIDUALS WITH DEMENTIA

Clinical research is essential for developing effective preventive, diagnostic, and treatment strategies in dementia care. However, by virtue of their cognitive impairment, individuals with dementia may have diminished capacity to consent to participate in research. In this section, we discuss assessing the capacity of a potential research subject to provide informed consent, methods of increasing capacity to participate in research, the use of surrogate decisionmakers to provide informed consent, and advance directives for participation in research.

Dunn and Misra (2009) have reviewed the literature on ethical issues in research involving older adults with neuropsychiatric disorders, including dementia. They note that a research setting is inherently different from a clinical setting, as "participation is voluntary and the risk-to-benefit ratio is typically skewed toward more direct risk with less direct benefit." Individuals with AD have diminished capacity to consent to clinical research compared with older adults with schizophrenia or diabetes mellitus (Palmer et al. 2005). Capacity varies significantly among those with AD, though severity of cognitive impairment is a strong predictor of capacity and individuals with AD eventually lose capacity (Dunn and Misra 2009).

The MacArthur Competence Assessment Tool for Clinical Research (MacCAT-CR) (Appelbaum and Grisso 2001) is a widely accepted and well-validated instrument to measure capacity to participate in research (Grisso and Appelbaum 1995). This tool is analogous to the MacCAT-T described above. The MacCAT-CR is adapted for discussion of the specific research study; over the course of 15–20 minutes, information is gathered about the potential subject's understanding, appreciation, reasoning, and ability to express a choice. Though some element of subjectivity remains in the assessment of capacity using the MacCAT-CR, this systematic and structured approach may allow for specific impairments in decisional capacity to be identified and perhaps addressed (Dunn and Misra 2009).

Methods have been developed to enhance an individual's capacity to participate in research. Mittal and colleagues (2007) studied the effectiveness of a multimedia presentation describing a hypothetical clinical trial versus that of an "enhanced written consent procedure" in 35 subjects with AD or mild cognitive impairment. As assessed by the MacCAT-CR, subjects in both study groups demonstrated an improvement in their understanding of the trial. Further research is required in larger samples, in more diverse populations, and involving different types of hypothetical studies.

Surrogate decisionmakers may, under certain circumstances, provide consent for participation in research. According to an Alzheimer's Association position statement (1997), a proxy may provide consent in the following circumstances:

- if the research entails minimal risk to the individual with dementia;
- if the research entails greater than minimal risk, but there is also "a reasonable potential for benefit to the individual";
- if the research entails greater than minimal risk and there is no reasonable potential for benefit, but the individual had executed an advance directive for research (see below)—in which case, the role of the surrogate is to "monitor the individual's involvement in the research."

It should be noted, however, that standards vary significantly among organizations, regulatory bodies, and legal statutes, so individual institutional review boards have reached different conclusions regarding the appropriateness of surrogate consent.

Surveys of older Americans seem to indicate strong public support for surrogate consent for dementia research. Kim et al. (2009) surveyed a subset (N=1,515) of subjects from the Health and Retirement Study, a nationally representative study of persons 51 and older. Subjects were randomized to review one of four plausible AD research scenarios: a study involving lumbar puncture (LP), a randomized controlled trial (RCT) of a new drug, a vaccine study, or a gene transfer neurosurgical study. When subjects were asked to consider if they would allow a close family member to provide consent for them to participate in these hypothetical studies, 70.8% responded affirmatively to the LP study, 79.7% to the RCT, 57.4% to the vaccine study, and 68.7% to the gene transfer study. When subjects were asked if our society should allow families to consent for individuals who cannot consent themselves, the affirmative responses were, respectively, 72.0%, 82.5%, 70.5% and 67.5%. Predictors of assenting to proxy consent included a personal willingness to participate in research, female gender, being married (versus not married), and excellent self-related health; ethnic background was not a predictor, and support for proxy consent was strong among African Americans and Hispanics. Other studies (e.g., Karlawish et al. 2009) have similarly demonstrated strong public support for surrogate consent for dementia research.

The use of a surrogate begs the question of what method the surrogate should use when deciding whether or not to enroll an individual with dementia in a study. As noted above, there are two standards governing the behavior of surrogate decisionmakers: best interest and substituted judgment (Gutheil and Appelbaum 2000, 232). Studies investigating which standard surrogates follow in dementia research have generally yielded support for the best interest model. Karlawish, Kim, et al. (2008) surveyed the views of research subjects and their "study partners" enrolled in a randomized control trial of simvastatin for the treatment of AD; the results indicated that study partners (some of whom were also surrogate decisionmakers) followed the best-interest standard. Interestingly, study partners were highly involved in decisionmaking whether or not they were formally identified as surrogates, suggesting that a shared decision-making model, as described above, may apply in dementia research.

It is possible that an individual with intact decisionmaking capacity could execute an advance directive for participation in dementia research. However, a controlled trial of a research advanced directive in 149 subjects with dementia and their proxies did not demonstrate altered study enrollment rates, decision ease or proxy comfort and certainty compared to a control group (Stocking et al. 2007). Furthermore, concerns have been raised about the inability of a research advance directive to address the specific information required to consent to a particular study (Dunn and Misra 2009).

END-OF-LIFE CARE IN INDIVIDUALS WITH DEMENTIA

The terminal stage of dementia is marked by severe cognitive impairment and a high rate of morbidity and mortality. For example, a prospective

18-month study of nursing home residents with advanced dementia (mean MMSE score of 5) revealed a mortality rate of 54.8%; medical morbidities included poor eating in 85.5% of residents, a febrile episode in 52.6%, and pneumonia in 41.1%, each of which in turn increased the risk of death. Distressing symptoms were common: 46.0% of residents experienced dyspnea and 39.1% had pain. Advanced dementia has a life expectancy similar to metastatic breast cancer and stage IV congestive heart failure (Mitchell et al. 2009). It is therefore clinically and ethically appropriate to employ a palliative care approach for individuals who have severe dementia, including a focus on promoting patient comfort, avoiding hospitalization and surgery, respecting advance directives, and employing do-not-resuscitate orders (American Academy of Neurology Ethics and Humanities Subcommittee 1996). Post (2000) also presents this issue in terms of social justice: The cost to society of interventions to extend the life of patients who have advanced dementia may not be just or justifiable.

Whereas a terminally ill but cognitively intact individual may personally decide to receive care that is focused on comfort, a proxy decisionmaker must be involved in palliative-care decisions for individuals with dementia. Mitchell et al. (2009) found that only 18.0% of proxies had received prognostic information from a physician. Patients whose proxies believed that the patient had less than 6 months to live and understood the clinical complications of dementia were markedly less likely to undergo burdensome interventions (hospitalization, tube-feeding, parenteral therapy) (Mitchell at al. 2009). Thus, surrogate decisionmakers must receive adequate information and support in order to ensure that individuals with advanced dementia receive appropriate palliative care (Hertogh 2006). Interestingly, clinicians themselves may need further education in this regard: In a study of patients with advanced dementia admitted to nursing homes, only 1.1% were perceived to have a life expectancy of less than six months, whereas 71.0% died during that period (Mitchell, Kiely, and Hamel 2004).

Among the most challenging steps is the withholding of artificial hydration and nutrition. As noted above, stopping eating is often a precursor of death in individuals with dementia. Feeding tubes probably do not reduce a patient's suffering and may, in fact, cause suffering (Gillick 2000). An Alzheimer's Association position statement argues that it is ethically permissible to withhold nutrition and artificial hydration from individuals who refuse to eat or drink (Alzheimer's Association 1988).

Roberts and Dyer (2004, 186–191) provide a useful framework for ethical issues at the end of life, including addressing the patient's physical and psychological pain; ensuring that all decisions are consistent with the patient's values, preferences, and spiritual beliefs; addressing difficult issues with the patient and caregivers; and consulting all relevant parties, including family members, other healthcare providers, attorneys, and spiritual figures.

CONCLUSIONS

Many clinical decisions in the care of individuals with dementia are inherently ethical decisions. The very nature of dementia is to progressively rob an individual of her or his capacity to remember, to make personal decisions, and to care for oneself—thereby striking at the core of autonomy. Yet, each individual is unique in terms of her or his own beliefs, cultural background, personality, life experiences, relationships, and progression of illness. Thus, clinicians, patients, and their caregivers must work together to carefully review the risks and benefits of options related to the diagnosis and treatment of dementia, management of distressing symptoms, participation in research trials, institutionalization, and end-of-life issues. Because individuals with dementia are vulnerable to abuse and exploitation, clinicians must be especially vigilant for any evidence of elder abuse. Given aging world populations, discussions must take place at a societal level regarding the fair and just distribution of medical resources—while not forgetting that it is our moral obligation to address the suffering of individuals with dementia.

REFERENCES

ABIM Foundation. 2002. Medical professionalism in the new millennium: A physician charter. *Annals of Internal Medicine* 136: 243–246.

Acierno, R., M. A. Hernandez, A. B. Amstadter, H. S. Resnick, K. Steve, W. Muzzy, and D. G. Kilpatrick. 2010. Prevalence and correlates of emotional, physical, sexual, and financial abuse and potential neglect in the United States: The National Elder Mistreatment Study. *American Journal of Public Health* 100: 292–297.

Alzheimer's Association. 1988. Treatment of patients with advanced dementia. http://www.alz.org/national/documents/statements_advancedementia. pdf (accessed April 26, 2010).

Alzheimer's Association. 1997. Ethical issues in dementia research (with special emphasis on "informed consent"). http://www.alz.org/national/documents/ statements_ethicalissues.pdf (accessed April 24, 2010).

Alzheimer's Association. 2008. Genetic testing. http://www.alz.org/national/ documents/statements_genetictesting.pdf (accessed April 24, 2010).

American Academy of Neurology Ethics and Humanities Subcommittee. 1996. Ethical issues in the management of the demented patient. *Neurology* 46: 1180–1183.

Appelbaum, P. S., R. J. Bonnie, and J. H. Karlawish. 2005. The capacity to vote of persons with Alzheimer's disease. *American Journal of Psychiatry* 162: 2094–2100.

Appelbaum, P. S., and T. Grisso. 2001. *MacArthur Competence Assessment Tool for clinical research.* Sarasota, FL: Professional Resource Press.

Bartels, S. J., K. M. Miles, A. R. Dums, and K. J. Levine. 2003. Are nursing homes appropriate for older adults with severe mental illness? Conflicting consumer and clinician views and implications for the Olmstead decision. *Journal of the American Geriatrics Society* 51: 1571–1579.

Blass, D. M., B. S. Black, H. Phillips, T. Finucane, A. Baker, D. Loreck, and P. V. Rabins. 2008. Medication use in nursing home residents with advanced dementia. *International Journal of Geriatric Psychiatry* 23: 490–496.

Cassidy, M. R., J. S. Roberts, T. D. Bird, E. J. Steinbart, L. A. Cupples, C. A. Chen, E. Linnenbringer, and R. C. Green. 2008. Comparing test-specific distress of susceptibility versus deterministic genetic testing for Alzheimer's disease. *Alzheimer's and Dementia* 4: 406–413.

Centers for Medicare and Medicaid Services. 2009. State operation manual. Appendix PP: Guidance to surveys for long-term care facilities. http://www.cms.gov/manuals/Downloads/som107ap_pp_guidelines_ltcf.pdf (accessed April 27, 2010).

Christensen, K. D., J. S. Roberts, C. D. Royal, G. A. Fasaye, T. Obisesan, L. A. Cupples, P. J. Whitehouse, et al. 2008. Incorporating ethnicity into genetic risk assessment for Alzheimer disease: The REVEAL study experience. *Genetics in Medicine* 10: 207–214.

Cooper, C., A. Selwood, M. Blanchard, Z. Walker, R. Blizard, and G. Livingston. 2010. The determinants of family carers' abusive behaviour to people with dementia: Results of the CARD study. *Journal of Affective Disorders* 121: 136–142.

Cooper, C., A. Selwood, and G. Livingston. 2009. Knowledge, detection, and reporting of abuse by health and social care professionals: A systematic review. *American Journal of Geriatric Psychiatry* 17: 826–838

Daiello, L. A., B. R. Ott, K. L. Lapane, S. E. Reinert, J. T. Machan, and D. D. Dore. 2009. Effect of discontinuing cholinesterase inhibitor therapy on behavioral and mood symptoms in nursing home patients with dementia. *American Journal of Geriatric Pharmacotherapy* 7: 74–83.

Dong, X., M. Simon, C. Mendes de Leon, T. Fulmer, T. Beck, L. Hebert, C. Dyer, G. Paveza, and D. Evans. 2009. Elder self-neglect and abuse and mortality risk in a community-dwelling population. *JAMA* 302: 517–526.

Drane, J. F. 1984. Measuring decision-making capacity in cognitively impaired individuals. *JAMA* 252: 925–927.

Dubinsky, R. M., A. C. Stein, and K. Lyons. 2000. Practice parameter: risk of driving and Alzheimer's disease (an evidence-based review): Report of the quality standards subcommittee of the American Academy of Neurology. *Neurology* 54: 2205–2211.

Dunn, L. B., and S. Misra. 2009. Research ethics issues in geriatric psychiatry. *Psychiatric Clinics of North America* 32: 395–411.

Dunn, L. B., M. A. Nowrangi, B. W. Palmer, D. V. Jeste, and E. R. Saks. 2006. Assessing decisional capacity for clinical research or treatment: A review of instruments. *American Journal of Psychiatry* 163: 1323–1334.

Folstein, M. F., S. E. Folstein, and P. R. McHugh. 1975. "Mini-Mental State": A practical method for grading the cognitive state of patients for the clinician. *Journal of Psychiatric Research* 12: 189–198.

Gillick, M. R. 2000. Rethinking the role of tube feeding in patients with advanced dementia. *New England Journal of Medicine* 342: 206–210.

Green, R. C., J. S. Roberts, L. A. Cupples, N. R. Relkin, P. J. Whitehouse, T. Brown, S. L. Eckert, et al. 2009. Disclosure of APOE genotype for risk of Alzheimer's disease. *New England Journal of Medicine* 361: 245–254.

Grimes, A. L., L. B. McCullough, M. E. Kunik, V. Molinari, and R. H. Workman Jr. 2000. Informed consent and neuroanatomic correlates of intentionality and voluntariness among psychiatric patients. *Psychiatric Services* 51: 1561–1567.

Grisso, T, and P. S. Appelbaum. 1995. The MacArthur treatment competence study. III: Abilities of patients to consent to psychiatric and medical treatments. *Law and Human Behavior* 19: 149–174.

Grisso, T., P. S. Appelbaum, and C. Hill-Fotouhi. 1997. The MacCAT-T: A clinical tool to assess patients' capacities to make treatment decisions. *Psychiatric Services* 48: 1415–1419.

Gruber-Baldini, A. L., M. Boustani, P. D. Sloane, and S. Zimmerman. 2004. Behavioral symptoms in residential care/assisted living facilities: Prevalence, risk factors, and medication management. *Journal of the American Geriatrics Society* 52: 1610–1617.

Gurrera, R. J., J. Moye, M. J. Karel, A. R. Azar, and J. C. Armesto. 2006. Cognitive performance predicts treatment decisional abilities in mild to moderate dementia. *Neurology* 66: 1367–1372.

Gutheil, T. G., and P. S. Appelbaum. 2000. *Clinical Handbook of Psychiatry and the Law*, 3rd ed. Philadelphia: Lippincott Williams & Wilkins.

Hertogh, C. M. 2006. Advance care planning and the relevance of a palliative care approach in dementia. *Age and Ageing* 35: 553–555.

Holmes, H. M., G. A. Sachs, J. W. Shega, G. W. Hougham, H. D. Cox, and W. Dale. 2008. Integrating palliative medicine into the care of persons with advanced dementia: Identifying appropriate medication use. *Journal of the American Geriatrics Society* 56: 1306–1311.

Huizing, A. R., R. L. Berghmans, G. A. Widdershoven, and F. R. Verhey. 2006. Do caregivers' experiences correspond with the concerns raised in the literature? Ethical issues relating to anti-dementia drugs. *International Journal of Geriatric Psychiatry* 21: 869–875.

Huthwaite, J. S., R. C. Martin, H. R. Griffith, B. Anderson, L. E. Harrell, and D. C. Marson. 2006. Declining medical decision-making capacity in mild AD: A two-year longitudinal study. *Behavioral Sciences and the Law* 24: 453–463.

Jogerst, G. J., J. M. Daly, M. F. Brinig, J. D. Dawson, G. A. Schmuch, and J. G. Ingram. 2003. Domestic elder abuse and the law. *American Journal of Public Health* 12: 2131–2136.

Jones, R., B. Sheehan, P. Phillips, E. Juszczak, J. Adams, A. Baldwin, C. Ballard, et al. 2009. DOMINO-AD protocol: Donepezil and memantine in moderate to severe Alzheimer's disease—a multicentre RCT. *Trials* 10: 57.

Kapp, M. B. 1998. "A place like that": Advance directives and nursing home admissions. *Psychology, Public Policy and Law* 4: 805–828.

Kapp, M. B. 2002. Decisional capacity in theory and practice: legal process versus "bumbling through." *Aging and Mental Health* 6: 413–417.

Kapp, M. B. 2009. Ethical and medicolegal issues. In *Psychiatry in long-term care*, 2nd ed., ed. W. E. Reichman and P. R. Katz. Oxford: Oxford University Press.

Karlawish, J. 2008. Measuring decision-making capacity in cognitively impaired individuals. *Neurosignals* 16: 91–98.

Karlawish, J. H., R. J. Bonnie, P. S. Appelbaum, R. A. Kane, C. G. Lyketsos, P. S. Karlan, B. D. James, C. Sabatino, T. Lawrence, and D. Knopman. 2008. Identifying the barriers and challenges to voting by residents in nursing homes and assisted living settings. *Journal of Aging and Social Policy* 20: 65–79.

Karlawish, J. H., R. J. Bonnie, P. S. Appelbaum, C. Lyketsos, B. James, D. Knopman, C. Patusky, R. A. Kane, and P. S. Karlan. 2004. Addressing the ethical, legal, and social issues raised by voting by persons with dementia. *JAMA* 292: 1345–1350.

Karlawish, J. H., D. J. Casarett, B. D. James, S. X. Xie, and S. Y. Kim. 2005. The ability of persons with Alzheimer disease (AD) to make a decision about taking an AD treatment. *Neurology* 64: 1514–1519.

Karlawish, J., S. Y. Kim, D. Knopman, C. H. van Dyck, B. D. James, and D. Marson. 2008. The views of Alzheimer disease patients and their study partners on proxy consent for clinical trial enrollment. *American Journal of Geriatric Psychiatry* 16: 240–247.

Karlawish, J., J. Rubright, D. Casarett, M. Cary, T. Ten Have, and P. Sankar. 2009. Older adults' attitudes toward enrollment of non-competent subjects participating in Alzheimer's research. *American Journal of Psychiatry* 166: 131–134.

Kim, S. Y., and E. D. Caine. 2002. Utility and limits of the Mini Mental State Examination in evaluating consent capacity in Alzheimer's disease. *Psychiatric Services* 53: 1322–1324.

Kim, S. Y., J. H. Karlawish, and E. D. Caine. 2002. Current state of research on decision-making competence of cognitively impaired elderly persons. *American Journal of Geriatric Psychiatry* 10: 151–165.

Kim, S. Y., H. M. Kim, K. M. Langa, J. H. Karlawish, D. S. Knopman, and P. S. Appelbaum. 2009. Surrogate consent for dementia research: a national survey of older Americans. *Neurology* 72: 149–155.

Lantz, M. S., V. Giambanco, and E. N. Buchalter. 1996. A ten-year review of the effect of OBRA-87 on psychotropic prescribing practices in an academic nursing home. *Psychiatric Services* 47: 951–955.

Lichtenberg, P. A., and D. M. Strzepek. 1990. Assessments of institutionalized dementia patients' competencies to participate in intimate relationships. *Gerontologist* 30: 117–120.

Lopez, O. L., J. T. Becker, A. S. Wahed, J. Saxton, R. A. Sweet, D. A. Wolk, W. Klunk, and S. T. Dekosky. 2009. Long-term effects of the concomitant use of memantine with cholinesterase inhibition in Alzheimer disease. *Journal of Neurology, Neurosurgery and Psychiatry* 80: 600–607.

Loveman, E., C. Green, J. Kirby, A. Takeda, J. Picot, E. Payne, and A. Clegg. 2006. The clinical and cost-effectiveness of donepezil, rivastigmine, galantamine and memantine for Alzheimer's disease. *Health Technology Assessment* 10: 1–151.

Lyketsos, C. G., O. Lopez, B. Jones, A. L. Fitzpatrick, J. Breitner, and S. DeKosky. 2002. Prevalence of neuropsychiatric symptoms in dementia and mild cognitive impairment: results from the cardiovascular health study. *JAMA* 288: 1475–1483.

Lyketsos, C. G., C. C. Colenda, C. Beck, K. Blank, M. P. Doraiswamy, D. A. Kalunian, K. Yaffe, and Task Force of American Association for Geriatric Psychiatry. 2006. Position statement of the American Association for Geriatric Psychiatry regarding principles of care for patients with dementia resulting from Alzheimer disease. *American Journal of Geriatric Psychiatry* 14: 561–572.

Marson, D. C., S. M. Sawrie, S. Snyder, B. McInturff, T. Stalvey, A. Boothe, T. Aldridge, A. Chatterjee and L. E. Harrell. 2000. Assessing financial capacity in patients with Alzheimer disease: A conceptual model and prototype instrument. *Archives of Neurology* 57: 877–884.

Matthews, F. E., and T. Dening for the UK Medical Research Council Cognitive Function and Ageing Study. 2002. Prevalence of dementia in institutional care. *Lancet* 360: 225–226.

Maxmin, K., C. Cooper, L. Potter, and G. Livingston. 2009. Mental capacity to consent to treatment and admission decisions in older adult psychiatric inpatients. *International Journal of Geriatric Psychiatry* 24: 1367–1375.

McCormick, W. C., C. Y. Ohata, J. Uomoto, H. M. Young, A. B. Graves, W. Kukull, L. Teri, et al. 2002. Similarities and differences in attitudes toward long-term care between Japanese Americans and Caucasian Americans. *Journal of the American Geriatrics Society* 50: 1149–1155.

Mitchell, S. L, D. K. Kiely, and M. B. Hamel. 2004. Dying with advanced dementia in the nursing home. *Archives of Internal Medicine* 164: 321–326.

Mitchell, S. L., J. M. Teno, D. K. Kiely, M. L. Shaffer, R. N. Jones, H. G. Prigerson, L. Volicer, J. L. Givens, and M. B. Hamel. 2009. The clinical course of advanced dementia. *NEJM* 361: 1529–1538.

Mittal, D., B. W. Palmer, L. B. Dunn, R. Landes, C. Ghormley, C. Beck, S. Golshan, D. Blevins, and D. V. Jeste. 2007. Comparison of two enhanced consent procedures for patients with mild Alzheimer disease or mild cognitive impairment. *American Journal of Geriatric Psychiatry* 15: 163–167.

Moye, J., S. W. Butz, D. C. Marson, E. Wood, and ABA-APA. 2007. Capacity assessment of older adults working group: A conceptual model and assessment template for capacity evaluation in adult guardianship. *Gerontologist* 47: 591–603.

Moye, J., M. J. Karel, R. J. Gurrera, and A. R. Azar. 2006. Neuropsychological predictors of decision-making capacity over 9 months in mild-to-moderate dementia. *Journal of General Internal Medicine* 21: 78–83.

Moye, J., and D. C. Marson. 2007. Assessment of decision-making capacity in older adults: An emerging area of practice and research. *Journal of Gerontology Series B: Psychological Sciences and Social Sciences* 62: P3–P11.

Mujic, F., M. Von Heising, R. J. Stewart, and M. J. Prince. 2009. Mental capacity assessments among general hospital inpatients referred to a specialist liaison psychiatry service for older people. *International Psychogeriatrics* 21: 729–737.

National Human Genome Research Institute (NIH). 2008. Genetic Information Nondiscrimination Act (GINA) of 2008. http://www.genome.gov/24519851 (accessed April 25, 2010).

National Institute for Health and Clinical Excellence (NICE). 2007. Donepezil, galantamine, rivastigmine (review) and memantine for the treatment of Alzheimer's disease (amended). http://www.nice.org.uk/TA111 (accessed April 27, 2010).

Okonkwo, O. C., V. G. Wadley, H. R. Griffith, K. Belue, S. Lanza, E. Y. Zamrini, L. E. Harrell, et al. 2008. Awareness of deficits in financial abilities in patients with mild cognitive impairment: Going beyond self-informant discrepancy. *American Journal of Geriatric Psychiatry* 16: 650–659.

Oude Voshaar, R. C., A. Burns, and M. G. M. Olde Rikkert. 2006. Alarming arbitrariness in EU prescription and reimbursement criteria for anti-dementia drugs. *International Journal of Geriatric Psychiatry* 21: 29–31.

Palmer, B. W., L. B. Dunn, P. S. Appelbaum, S. Mudaliar, L. Thal, R. Henry, S. Golshan, and D. V. Jeste. 2005. Assessment of capacity to consent to research among older persons with schizophrenia, Alzheimer disease, or diabetes mellitus: Comparison of a 3-item questionnaire with a comprehensive standardized capacity instrument. *Archives of General Psychiatry* 62: 726–733.

Pickens, S., A. D. Naik, J. Burnett, P. A. Kelly, M. Gleason, and C. B. Dyer. 2007. The utility of the Kohlman Evaluation of Living Skills test is associated with substantiated cases of elder self-neglect. *Journal of the American Academy of Nurse Practitioners* 19: 137–142.

Post, S. G. 2000. Key issues in the ethics of dementia care. *Neurology Clinics* 18: 1011–1022.

Post, S. G., J. C. Stuckey, P. J. Whitehouse, S. Ollerton, C. Durkin, D. Robbins, and S. J. Fallcreek. 2001. A focus group on cognition-enhancing medications in Alzheimer disease: Disparities between professionals and consumers. *Alzheimer Disease and Associated Disorders* 15: 80–88.

Post, S. G., and P. J. Whitehouse. 1998. Emerging antidementia drugs: A preliminary ethical view. *Journal of the American Geriatrics Society* 46: 784–787.

Post, S. G., P. J. Whitehouse, R. H. Binstock, T. D. Bird, S. K. Eckert, L. A. Farrer, L. M. Fleck, et al. 1997. The clinical introduction of genetic testing for Alzheimer disease: an ethical perspective. *JAMA* 277 (1997): 832–836.

Qaseem, A., V. Snow, J. T. Cross Jr., M. A. Forciea, R. Hopkins Jr., P. Shekelle, A. Adelman, et al. 2008. Current pharmacologic treatment of dementia: A clinical practice guideline from the American College of Physicians and the American Academy of Family Physicians. *Annals of Internal Medicine* 148: 370–378.

Roberts, L. W. 2002. Informed consent and the capacity for voluntarism. *American Journal of Psychiatry* 159: 705–712.

Roberts, J. S., L. A. Cupples, N. R. Relkin, P. J. Whitehouse, R. C. Green, and REVEAL (Risk Evaluation and Education for Alzheimer's Disease) Study Group. 2005. Genetic risk assessment for adult children of people with Alzheimer's disease: The Risk Evaluation and Education for Alzheimer's Disease (REVEAL) study. *Journal of Geriatric Psychiatry and Neurology* 18: 250–255.

Roberts, L. W., and A. R. Dyer. 2004. *Concise Guide to Ethics in Mental Health Care.* Washington, DC: American Psychiatric Publishing.

Royall, D. R., L. K. Chiodo, and M. J. Polk. 2005. An empiric approach to level of care determinations: The importance of executive measures. *Journal of Gerontology Series A: Biological Sciences and Medical Sciences* 60: 1056–1064.

Schneider, L. S., K. Dagerman, and P. S. Insel. 2005. Risk of death with atypical antipsychotic drug treatment for dementia: Meta-analysis of randomized placebo-controlled trials. *JAMA* 294: 1934–1943.

Schneider, L. S., K. Dagerman, and P. S. Insel. 2006. Efficacy and adverse effects of atypical antipsychotics for dementia: Meta-analysis of randomized, placebo-controlled trials. *American Journal of Geriatric Psychiatry* 14: 191–210.

Shulman, K. I., C. Peisah, R. Jacoby, J. Heinik, and S. Finkel. 2009. Contemporaneous assessment of testamentary capacity. *International Psychogeriatrics* 21: 433–439.

Smith, G. E., E. Kokmen, and P. C. O'Brien. 2000. Risk factors for nursing home placement in a population-based dementia cohort. *Journal of the American Geriatrics Society* 48: 519–525.

Stocking, C. B., G. W. Hougham, D. D. Danner, M. B. Patterson, P. J. Whitehouse, and G. A. Sachs. 2007. Empirical assessment of a research advance directive for persons with dementia and their proxies. *Journal of the American Geriatrics Society* 55: 1609–1612.

Sugarman, J., D. C. McCrory, and R. C. Hubal. 1998. Getting meaningful informed consent from older adults: A structured literature review of empirical research. *Journal of the American Geriatrics Society* 46: 517–524.

Testad, I., C. Ballard, K. Brønnick, and D. Aarsland. 2010. The effect of staff training on agitation and use of restraint in nursing home residents with dementia: A single-blind, randomized controlled trial. *Journal of Clinical Psychiatry* 71: 80–86.

Thomas, S. J., and G. T. Grossberg. 2009. Memantine: A review of studies into its safety and efficacy in treating Alzheimer's disease and other dementias. *Clinical Interventions in Aging* 4: 367–377.

Tueth, M. J. 2000. Exposing financial exploitation of impaired elderly person. *American Journal of Geriatric Psychiatry* 8: 104–111.

Walaszek, A. 2009. Clinical ethics issues in geriatric psychiatry. *Psychiatric Clinics of North America* 32: 343–359.

Weschules, D. J., T. L. Maxwell, and J. W. Shega. 2008. Acetylcholinesterase inhibitor and N-methyl-D-aspartic acid receptor antagonist use among hospice enrollees with a primary diagnosis of dementia. *Journal of Palliative Medicine* 11: 738–745.

Willis, S. L., R. Allen-Burge, M. M. Dolan, R. M. Bertrand, J. Yesavage, and J. L. Taylor. 1998. Everyday problem solving among individuals with Alzheimer's disease. *Gerontologist* 38: 569–577.

Winblad, B., S. E. Black, A. Homma, E. M. Schwam, M. Moline, Y. Xu, C. A. Perdomo, J. Swartz, and K. Albert. 2009. Donepezil treatment in severe Alzheimer's disease: A pooled analysis of three clinical trials. *Current Medical Research and Opinion* 25: 2577–2587.

Chapter 7

Cognitive Screening and Neuropsychological and Functional Assessment: Contributions to Early Detection of Dementia

Mônica Sanches Yassuda, Mariana Kneese Flaks, and Fernanda Speggiorin Pereira

As the elderly population increases, dementia and depression have become the most prevalent neuropsychiatric disorders among aged individuals (Ferri et al. 2005). Considering the fact that dementia is a neurodegenerative disease with progressive neuronal loss, it becomes a medical and social problem in a large and growing scale. The final diagnosis of most dementia syndromes depends on neuropathologic examination. However, a thorough clinical examination including anamnesis, psychiatric evaluation, neuropsychological assessment, and physical and neurological examination, combined with biochemical tests and neuroimaging, could enhance the accuracy of early and differential diagnosis. Technological innovations that use structural and functional neuroimaging techniques as well as molecular biology and molecular genetics procedures have provided new tools that can facilitate the early diagnosis of dementias, especially of Alzheimer's disease (Ho et al. 2010; Hampel et al. 2008; Shaw et al. 2007).

The expected advances in pharmacological treatment, seeking to modify pathogenic processes, increase the need to identify the disease in its early stages, before dysfunctional and severe cognitive deficits are established

(Bischkopf, Busse, and Angermeyer 2002). As a result, differential diagnosis carries therapeutic and prognostic implications. Despite the important scientific progress related to imaging and biological markers, the diagnosis of dementia syndromes remains a clinical process, supplemented by relevant investigations such as cognitive testing (Portet et al. 2006).

Due to the difficulties in identifying the early signs of dementia only by means of clinical assessment and routine medical examination, cognitive assessment is a key tool that can improve diagnostic accuracy. In this context, cognitive screening tools, which are used at the beginning of the diagnostic process, and the neuropsychological instruments, which are used in more extensive investigations, are required.

Neuropsychological assessment can often point toward patterns of cognitive alteration that are typical of dementia. The tests are sensitive to brain dysfunction and identify damaged areas that are not yet evident in imaging and in an electroencephalogram. Neuropsychological testing may define the location and lateralization of brain dysfunction related to behavioral impairment by quantifying changes in sensory or motor functions and by examining more complex brain functions such as language, visual-spatial awareness, verbal and nonverbal memory (Lezak, Howieson, and Loring 2004).

Neuropsychological assessment is important when the clinical pattern is ambiguous or complex, making it possible to reliably identify different types of dementia early in the course of the disease, and to distinguish dementia from normal aging or from other illnesses. Additionally, it provides guidance to physicians and to family members with regards to deficit compensation strategies for a particular patient. It can also provide information concerning conduct and therapeutic options during the disease (Lezak, Howieson, and Loring 2004). Furthermore, consecutive cognitive testing presents objective data as to whether changes in the clinical profile are occurring as expected for a given diagnosis.

In what follows, we review a range of validated neuropsychological assessment tools that can facilitate accurate diagnosis of an early dementing process in aged individuals. We provide guidance on interpretive strengths and weakness of each of these tools. We emphasize our experience within the Brazilian context in order to provide a more global picture of the contributions of neuropsychological markers for the dementias, in addition to the standard North American account of this emerging area of study and practice.

According to criteria from the National Institute for Communicative Disorders and Stroke–Alzheimer's Disease and Related Disorders

Association (NINCDS-ADRDA Work Group—Dubois et al. 2007), before recommending extensive and often costly neuropsychological assessment, screening tools should be used to verify the need for this procedure in case of possible dementia. The purpose of the screening tool is different from that of the neuropsychological instrument. The screening process indicates the likelihood of dementia. If results from the screening are positive, the assessment may ratify or reject the diagnostic hypothesis.

COGNITIVE SCREENING TOOLS

Shulman and Feinstein (2003) state that the ideal screening test should be:

1. Brief
2. Well accepted by patients without giving rise to discomfort or defensive reactions
3. Easy to apply and to review
4. Relatively free of confounding elements such as schooling, culture and language
5. Have good psychometric properties such as reliability and validity regardless of the tester and in test-retest situations, sensitivity, specificity, and high positive and negative predictability
6. Cover a representative range of intellectual functions

On the other hand, screening tests should be used and interpreted with caution, considering that there is no flawless cognitive assessment tool. Special attention should be paid to the likelihood of a high percentage of false-negatives, when the screening is conducted in early stage dementia, or in individuals with high intellectual levels or with many years of schooling (Katzman 1993; Stern et al. 1994; Cummings et al. 1998). False-positive results may occur among healthy individuals with low schooling. Few years of schooling and illiteracy are associated with a greater prevalence of dementia (De Ronchi et al. 1998; Herrera et al. 2002; Bottino et al. 2008), yet many individuals who cannot read score within ranges typical of dementia even though their functions are completely preserved. This emphasizes the importance of tests that are less vulnerable to educational experience or for normative values corrected for education. Special attention should be paid to developing countries (Ferri et al. 2005; Yassuda et al. 2009), where underschooling is frequently observed among elders.

Some cognitive screening tools specifically designed for suspected dementia are described below. Diagnostic accuracy data is also reviewed.

Mini Mental State Examination

The Mini Mental State Examination (MMSE) (Folstein, Folstein, and McHugh 1975) is a widely used and studied screening tool to detect changes in cognition in geriatric patients in many countries. It is part of an array of neuropsychological batteries such as the CAMDEX-R (Cambridge Examination for Mental Disorders of the Elderly) (Roth et al. 1986) and the CERAD battery (The Consortium to Establish a Registry for Alzheimer's Disease) (Morris et al. 1989).

The MMSE provides objective assessment of cognition through questions clustered into seven categories:

1. Orientation to time
2. Orientation to place
3. Memorization of three words (immediate memory)
4. Attention and calculation (subtract the number 7 from 100 five consecutive times)
5. Recall of the previous three words (delayed memory)
6. Language (objects naming, repetition of a sentence, execute a verbal and a written command, write a sentence)
7. Visual construction (copy of a drawing)

The scores range from 0 to 30, and the overall score decreases as cognitive impairment increases. It takes little more than five minutes, a pencil, and a sheet of paper to administer.

In developing countries, where a wide range of educational profiles can be found, schooling must be taken into account before administering the test. In addition, when testing minorities in developed countries who may not have received more than a high school education, caution must be used when interpreting MMSE performance. Therefore, the cutoff scores for dementia syndromes may need to be adjusted according to the educational level.

Studies from different countries have been seeking to establish differential cutoff points for specific educational strata, for high and low educational levels, to improve accuracy in identifying possible cases of dementia (Ostrosky-Solis, Lopez-Arango, and Ardila 2000; Rosselli et al. 2000; Espino et al. 2001; de Silva and Gunatilake 2002; Brucki et al. 2003; Xu et al. 2003; Reyes-Beaman et al. 2004; Simpao et al. 2005; Crane et al. 2006; Laks et al. 2007; O'Bryant et al. 2008, Kohn et al. 2008). In addition, cross-cultural comparisons of the MMSE in different countries provide information regarding the cut-off scores in each population (Gibbons et al. 2002; Jones 2006; Dodge et al. 2009).

Clock Drawing Test

Spreen and Strauss (1998) wrote a thorough review on use of the Clock Drawing Test (CDT), indicating it has been widely used as part of short mental tests in neurological investigations. Moreover, its use is often recommended as a screening test in suspected dementia cases.

The first systematic use of the CDT was reported by Goodglass and Wingfield (1993), and the test was included as part of the Boston Aphasia Battery. Since then, different application and correction protocols for the CDT have been developed (Shulman 2000). Due to this fact, no specific CDT norms will be cited in this chapter.

Unlike most assessment tools for dementia, which emphasize memory and attention in verbal domains, the CDT is based on visuo-spatial skills, dependent upon motor execution skills (Sunderland et al. 1989). The test assesses, in addition to visuo-spatial functions, the executive ability needed to recreate the memory of a clock face from a verbal command and translate it into a graphic image (Spreen and Strauss 1998). This constructive *praxis* involves not only visuo-perceptual analysis but also motor execution, attention, language comprehension and understanding of numbers (Mendez, Ala, and Underwood 1992). The CDT can be carried out in a variety of ways regarding directions and scoring, based on the concepts devised by different authors. The needed tools to administer the CDT are just a sheet of paper and a pencil.

The CDT is considered a suitable tool to identify individuals with possible dementia, yet its accuracy may be reduced among individuals with limited education (Shulman 2000; Storey et al. 2002; Nishiwaki et al. 2004; Parker and Philp 2004; Fuzikawa et al. 2007; Atalaia-Silva and Lourenço 2008; Aprahamian et al. 2010).

Syndrom Kurztest—Short Cognitive Performance Test

The Syndrom Kurztest (SKT) (Erzigkeit 1992) is a screening tool to asses the magnitude of attentional deficits, taking into account information processing speed and memory deficits.

It comprises nine subtests; six are attention subtests and three are memory subtests. The attention tests measure simple attention, processing speed, concentration, inhibitory control, and working memory. Memory is assessed in its visual aspect involving immediate and delayed recall and recognition. The required time to administer this test is estimated at 10 minutes, and scoring at three minutes. SKT overall score ranges from 0 to 27 points, and the higher the score the more severe the cognitive deficit. The total score can be subdivided into attention and memory subscores, describing the contribution of each function to the final score. Special material is required, such as a board with numbers, a stimulus booklet, and a chronometer. The test presents five parallel versions that were developed to avoid learning effect in case of retesting. Its normative values take into consideration age and intelligence level (Erzigkeit 2001).

The SKT is most frequently used to detect mild cognitive impairment and mild to moderate stages of dementia (Erzigkeit 1992; Ihl et al. 1992; Overall and Schaltenbrand 1992; Kim, Nibbelink, and Overall 1993; Lehfeld and Erzigkeit 1997; Weyer et al. 1997; Flaks et al. 2006, 2009). The instrument loses its capacity for precise staging in cases of severe cognitive deficits when the understanding of instructions is markedly impaired (Erzigkeit 2001). Cross-cultural stability was found between several research centers (Lehfeld et al. 1997). However, the test is influenced by educational bias when applied in subjects with no or low educational level (Ostrosky-Solís et al. 1999; Flaks et al. 2009).

Frontal Assessment Battery

The Frontal Assessment Battery (FAB) (Dubois et al. 2000) is a more recent instrument designed to assess frontal lobe functions. It is a brief bedside cognitive and behavioral battery to screen for executive dysfunctions, more specifically, to assess functions related to the dorsolateral and medial frontal cortex (Guedj et al. 2008).

The FAB consists of six subtests that explore:

1. Conceptualization (abstraction taking into account similarities between two concepts)
2. Verbal fluency (mental flexibility)
3. Motor programming
4. Sensitivity to interference (tendency to distraction based on conflicting instructions)
5. Inhibitory control
6. Prehension behavior (environmental autonomy)

Scores range from 0 to 18, with higher scores indicating better test performance. It takes about 10 minutes to administer and only a chronometer is requested for test application.

Some research centers indicate that the FAB is a test capable of distinguishing frontotemporal dementia from Alzheimer's disease, as a measure of executive function (Slachevsky and Dubois 2004; Lipton et al. 2005; Castiglioni et al. 2006; Oguro et al. 2006; Kugo et al. 2007; Nakaaki et al.

2007). A recent research study regarding the performance of healthy aged individuals suggested the FAB may be influenced by schooling (Beato et al. 2007).

Verbal Fluency

The purpose of verbal fluency tests (VFT) is to assess the spontaneous production of words beginning with a given letter (phonemic association) or within one category (semantic association) for a limited 60-second time period.

These tests assess executive and language functions, and could also evaluate semantic memory (Spreen and Strauss 1998). A study conducted in healthy elderly indicated that a good performance in verbal fluency is related to the ability to quickly organize information and formulate effective recall strategies (Bolla et al. 2006). The needed tools to administer the verbal fluency tests are just a sheet of paper, a pencil, and a chronometer.

Lam et al. (2006), in a study of VFT, with semantic restriction, described the test as capable of discriminating different stages of cognitive impairment, and Libon et al. (2009) emphasized this characteristic in frontotemporal lobar degeneration patients.

Investigators found that special attention must be paid when the test is administered to subjects with low educational level, because results are clearly affected by schooling (Caramelli et al. 2007). Special attention should be given to the category used. Fruit category proved to be the best VFT as it may be less biased by education, being a more appropriate test across different educational groups (Rosselli et al. 2009).

Addenbrooke's Cognitive Examination—Revised

Addenbrooke's Cognitive Examination–Revised (ACE-R) (Mioshi et al. 2006) is a recent tool designed to detect early stage dementia, which may be especially useful to distinguish AD from frontotemporal dementia.

ACE-R assesses five cognitive domains, namely:

1. Orientation (time and space), attention, and concentration (subtract the number 7 from 100 five consecutive times and spell the word "world" backward)
2. Verbal memory (immediate and delayed recall of three words), episodic memory (remember a name and a address), and semantic memory (historical information)
3. Verbal fluency

4. Language (comprehension of an oral command, write a sentence, repeat words and phrase, name objects, and reading)
5. Visuo-spatial skills (copy drawings) and perceptual abilities

The total score ranges from 0 to 100, in that higher scores denote better performance. It takes approximately 10 to 15 minutes to administer. The needed tools to administer the ACE-R are just a sheet of paper, a pencil, and a chronometer.

Research studies suggest that the ACE-R is a valid dementia screening test that is sensitive to early cognitive dysfunction (Galton et al. 2005; Mioshi et al. 2006; Larner 2007). Different cut-off points are recommended for different educational levels (García-Caballero et al. 2006; Carvalho, Barbosa, and Caramelli 2010).

Other Brief Screening Tests

More recently two other screening tests have been proposed to detect early cognitive impairment. The Montreal Cognitive Assessment was designed to assist health professionals to detect mild cognitive impairment (Nasreddine et al. 2005), and several studies have suggested its validity to identify cognitive deficits associated with several neurologic conditions (for a full list of references about this instrument please refer to www.mocatest.org). The Test Your Memory (TYM) instrument has been designed as a cognitive screening test that can be self administered, in the waiting room, in about five minutes. Results have suggested it was accurate in detecting 93% of Alzheimer's disease patients compared to 52% when the MMSE was used. This screening test may also help to identify other types of dementia and mild cognitive impairment (Brown et al. 2009).

NEUROPSYCHOLOGICAL ASSESSMENT OF MAIN COGNITIVE FUNCTIONS IN THE DEMENTIAS

Memory and Learning Assessment

Memory comprises a multitude of subsystems and it is possible to observe an uneven age-related decline among them. Therefore, memory assessment requires the examination of different subsystems such as episodic memory, working memory, and prospective memory, among others. The assessment protocol should include tasks based on visual and auditory stimuli, which require immediate and delayed recall. The assessment of the learning curve in consecutive trials and the magnitude of information loss in delayed recalls are key aspects of the neuropsychological assessment of episodic memory when one is trying to differentiate age-related decline from early dementia.

Memory assessment involves the use of tools that require encoding new information, that is, the formation of new memory traces, with the primary aim of examining the integrity of the medial-temporal region, which includes the hippocampus and entorhinal cortex, directly involved in memory processes. Instruments that include multiple learning trials are of utmost importance, as they enable the assessment of the learning curve. Tests such as Word List from the Wechsler Memory Scale (WMS-III) (Wechsler, "Memory Scale" 1997) and Rey Auditory Verbal Learning Test (RAVLT) (Ivnik et al. 1990) provide five repetitions of the original word list. In the Selective Reminding Test (SRT) (Masur et al. 1990), which involves memorizing a list of 12 words, and in the Fuld Object-Memory Evaluation (FOME) (Fuld et al. 1990), which requires memorizing 10 objects placed in a bag, the examiner repeats only the nonrecalled items in each consecutive recall trial (for references and a detailed description of these instruments see Lezak, Howieson, and Loring 2004). Cognitively unimpaired older adults should improve performance in each trial, and in the delayed recall trial, after 30 minutes, they should remember most of the information recalled in the last trial (around 80%). Dementia patients, on the other hand, do not improve performance with re-exposure to the stimulus list and exhibit significant loss of information in delayed recall trials.

The Visual Reproduction and Logical Memory sub-tests, also from the WSM-III battery (Wechsler, "Memory Scale" 1997), are excellent options for assessing visual and auditory episodic memory respectively. In the former, the patient memorizes geometric figures, and in the latter he or she memorizes two stories. Both involve one immediate and one delayed recall, making it possible to examine short- and long-term memory.

The Rivermead Behavioral Memory Test (RBMT) (Wilson, Cockburn, and Baddeley 1985) is also a helpful tool in memory assessment, since it encompasses ecological tasks that are seldom explored in other batteries. It informs the examiner about possible difficulties subjects might encounter in their everyday lives, such as being oriented to time and place, recalling a name associated to a person's face, recalling a route the examiner walks in the room leaving an envelope at a certain spot, remembering to reclaim an object that was lent to someone, or asking a question at the sound of an alarm bell. In a recently published study, low performance in the RBMT screening score was found to be a significant predictor of conversion to Alzheimer's disease among normal controls and patients with amnestic mild cognitive impairment (Forlenza et al. 2010).

For working memory assessment, Digit Span Backward and the Letter-Number Sequencing from the Wechsler Adult Intelligence Scale (WAIS-III) battery (Wechsler, "Adult Intelligence" 1997) are useful in addition to a qualitative examination of the older individual's performance in the Arithmetic subtest from the same battery.

Results from memory tests are extremely important when exploring differential diagnosis in dementias. Alzheimer's disease is usually associated with a flat learning curve and significant loss in the delayed recall in episodic memory trials (Collie and Maruff 2000). Alzheimer's disease patients also frequently recall items that were not presented during learning trials. Dementias related to cerebrovascular diseases can often emerge with no mnestic dysfunction as executive dysfunction may be its most prominent marker (Gainotti et al. 2008). Memory preservation can also be observed in dementias in which the first affected areas are not the temporal-medial but the frontal areas, as can be observed in frontotemporal lobar degeneration associated with semantic dementia or in frontotemporal dementia (Rabinovici and Miller 2010).

Attention Assessment

Paying attention requires detecting changes in the outside world and simultaneously inhibiting interference from other competing stimuli (Posner and Raichle 1994). Attention is a multidimensional skill, and its components are intrinsically connected with other skills such as memory and executive functions; therefore, it is difficult to assess attention separately.

The following tests are simple to apply and can be used to assess different aspects of attention processes: Digit Span Forward and Digit Symbol from the WAIS-III battery (Wechsler, "Adult Intelligence" 1997); Trail A (Ashendorf et al. 2008); Stroop in its several formats; and letter, number, or symbol cancellation tests (Lezak, Howieson, and Loring 2004). The Mental Control subtest of the WMS-III battery can also be used (Wechsler, "Memory Scale" 1997).

Attentional deficits are common among aged patients with cerebrovascular diseases. Research studies suggest that a considerable number of subcortical white matter lesions are linked to poorer performance in visual and auditory attention tests and in executive function tests (Van Dijk et al. 2004), as well as to psychomotor slowing (Gainotti et al. 2008). Dementia with Lewy bodies, in turn, is characterized by significant cognitive fluctuation, especially in attention tests (Lezak, Howieson, and Loring 2004).

Attention tasks such as inhibitory and mental control (ability to focus) in the face of competing and concomitant stimuli, which are directly related to executive functions regarding storage and simultaneous processing of information, are described below.

Executive Function Assessment

The term *executive function* denominates a set of skills that are needed for complex behaviors. The executive system is a hypothetical cognitive principle involving planning tasks, organizational tasks, mental flexibility, abstract thinking, avoidance of inappropriate actions, and inhibition of irrelevant information processing. The executive system is also supposed to be in charge of adjusting one's behavior to solve day-to-day situations such as initiative, management of choices, consequence assessment, decisionmaking, action implementation and control, and course correction and adjustment when needed.

The examination of executive functions aims at assessing prefrontal cortex integrity. Several neuropsychological tests may be used to assess different aspects of cognition associated with executive functions. Some of the most frequently used are: (1) verbal fluency during a limited 60-second time frame, restricted semantically, for instance, by a category such as animal and fruit naming (Caramelli et al. 2007; Radanovic et al. 2009), or restricted phonemically, by using words starting with *F*, *A*, or *S* (Controlled Oral Word Association, COWA) (Lezak, Howieson, and Loring 2004) to assess information processing speed; (2) Clock Drawing Test, which assesses visuo-spatial functions as well as planning and self-regulation during execution, as previously described; (3) Trail B, as it demands coordination of two competing information systems (Ashendorf et al. 2008); and (4) Wisconsin Card Sorting Test (WCST) (Lezak, Howieson, and Loring 2004), possibly the most traditional executive function test, when the patient is required to combine 48 cards with one of four model cards that vary according to criteria such as color, shape and number of symbols to assess mental flexibility and abstraction capacity (Modified Card Sorting Test, MCST; Lezak, Howieson, and Loring 2004).

In order to assess complex decision making skills, the Iowa Gambling Task may be used as it has already been adjusted and validated for use with older populations (Bechara et al. 1994). The task entails choosing cards from four decks. As the individual verifies gains and losses associated with each card deck, she or he infers which decks are more advantageous and which are not. The subject's ability to evaluate choices to maximize gains, minimizing losses, is thus surveyed.

In recent years, an executive control assessment interview, EXIT-25 (Executive Interview, Royall, Mahurin, and Gray 1992) was developed, grouping traditional tests associated with frontal functions. The EXIT-25 is an important battery because performance in it is strongly correlated with activities of daily living (Royall et al. 2007; Pereira et al. 2008). In addition, decline in this scale significantly predicts dependence and need for care (Mann et al. 1992).

The Behavioral Assessment of the Dysexecutive Syndrome (BADS) (Lezak, Howieson, and Loring 2004) is also worth mentioning. It simulates daily challenges involving executive functions, such as removing a cork from inside a bottle using a few available tools, working out a route within a zoo, temporal judgment, and managing time for task completion. The advantage of this battery is its resemblance with challenges encountered in the subjects' everyday lives.

Language Assessment

Language functions tend to be preserved in healthy aged individuals. Vocabulary remains stable and can even expand with aging, slightly declining after the age of 70. Nevertheless, some language changes have been recorded in healthy elderly individuals. Difficulty in finding words or the "tip of the tongue" experience can be noted more often. From a qualitative standpoint, healthy older adults tend to: (1) use a greater number of words to describe something that could be expressed with only one; (2) describe the function of the object rather than name it; (3) less accurately identify objects due to sensory deficits; (4) make associative semantic errors, when something related to the object is mentioned instead of the object itself (Woodruff-Pak 1997). These changes could suggest difficulty or slowing in semantic access. Complex sentence comprehension and formulation, as well as speech organization and accuracy, could also moderately decline in healthy aged individuals.

The Vocabulary subtest from the WAIS-III battery (Wechsler, "Adult Intelligence" 1997) is among the tasks that are frequently used for language assessment among older adults, as it enables the examiner to verify whether the patients' word knowledge is compatible with his or her level of schooling. Qualitatively, the examiner may also notice if the definitions provided are accurate, and if access to these definitions is fast and easy. Another frequently used test is the Boston Naming Test (Steinberg et al. 2005), when the patient is asked to name 60 pictures, increasingly difficult, and the examiner may need to judge whether semantic and/or phonological clues are helpful. Vocabulary and naming trials are usually complemented by verbal fluency tasks, also used to measure executive function. An additional common practice is to ask the subject to complete and interpret proverbs. This task not only examines language comprehension but also assesses semantic memory and abstract thinking. In case of suspected aphasia, the Boston Diagnostic Aphasia Examination (BDAE) (Goodglass, Kaplan, and Barresi 2000) is commonly used. The traditional "cookie theft picture" of this battery can be used separately to examine the quality of oral and narrative speech.

Language assessment may be relevant in differential diagnosis of dementias. In the course of healthy aging, language abilities are expected to be preserved, with just mild changes typical of healthy aging (Woodruff-Pak 1997). Significant decline in this function may suggest that lesions in language-related regions (Broca's and Wernicke's areas) might be present, or that neurodegenerative disorders that manifest with losses in this function, such as semantic dementia or nonfluent progressive aphasia, might be present (Rabinovici and Miller 2010).

Visuo-Spatial Ability Assessment

Visuo-spatial abilities are needed to perform tasks such as copying figures, assembling objects, interpreting maps, dimensioning spatial relationships among objects. They also involve spatial orientation to perform complex actions, along with several other abilities (Woodruff-Pak 1997).

Among the most widely used trials to assess visuo-spatial ability in neuropsychological practice are the following: the above-mentioned Boston Naming Test, which in addition to naming capability also examines visual perception; the Hooper Visual Organization Test; the Rey-Osterrieth Complex Figure copying; the Necker Cube copying; and the Clock Drawing Test (for references and detailed description of these tools see Lezak, Howieson, and Loring 2004). The latter three instruments involve visuo-constructive abilities, as they require copying or drawing of complex figures. There are motor demands in addition to visual integration and organization. In addition, the Block Design subtest from the WAIS-III battery (Wechsler, "Adult Intelligence" 1997) is also regularly used to assess visual-perceptual and visuo-constructive abilities. In this subtest, the patient is asked to use blocks to form a three-dimensional representation of a bidimensional picture in a card.

Visuo-spatial ability loss can be observed in patients with dementias with different etiologies, usually in advanced stages. Patients with focal lesions in the parietal and occipital lobes tend to show significant impairment in visuo-spatial tasks. It must be pointed out that patients suffering from dementia with Lewy bodies display considerable visuo-spatial deficits even at early stages of the disease (Lezak, Howieson, and Loring

2004). Nevertheless, when assessing visuo-spatial abilities, the educational and occupational background of the older individual must be taken into account. In cases when the individual reports to have always performed poorly in visuo-constructive tasks, a below-average result should not be given much weight. On the other hand, for patients who used to sew, who used to develop carpentry projects, or with a history of complex crafts-manship, poor results in these tasks should be highlighted.

Neuropsychological tests are usually strongly influenced by educa-tional experience. Therefore, in developing countries, where older adults' education profile tends to be diverse, and when assessing minority seniors in developed nations, the assessment protocol should be planned care-fully. In a recent study (Yassuda et al. 2009) involving older adults with heterogeneous educational backgrounds, the RBMT, the FOME, and ver-bal fluency with animal category were not significantly influenced by edu-cation and therefore they should be used in such cases.

Functional Assessment in the Context of the Dementias

One vital aspect in the neuropsychological assessment of older indi-viduals concerns gathering proxy measures of performance in daily liv-ing tasks. In the context of aging, assessment of functionality is of utmost importance because it draws the line between normal and pathological cognitive aging.

The concept of functional status receives a variety of definitions and it is assessed in many different ways by health professionals. According to the World Health Organization (WHO), it is a key factor for the definition of physical and mental health. Due to the wide array of concepts and ter-minologies used, the WHO published in 2001 the International Classifica-tion of Functioning, Disability and Health, also known as ICF. According to this classification, functional status is considered a broad concept that encompasses a number of body functions and structures, as well as activ-ity and participation in a socio-environmental context (Buñuales, Diego, and Moreno 2002; WHO 2001).

Functional capacity concerns the ability to maintain the physical and mental skills needed for independent living, valuing autonomy and self-determination (Gordilho et al. 2000). Functional capacity is an index of how a given activity is carried out in everyday life, what people do in their environment, thus including involvement in real-life situations. It is a key aspect in the concept of independence, which implies the ability to function effectively without the help of others in activities of daily liv-ing. Functional disability can be denoted by the presence of difficulties in performing certain activities of daily living, or even by the complete inability to perform them unaided (Rosa et al. 2003).

Autonomy is related to the practice of self-governing and includes the following elements: individual freedom, privacy, free will, and harmony regarding one's own feelings and needs. The greater the independence, the greater the likelihood of having autonomy, though under partial dependency conditions the individual can keep his or her autonomy, depending on the social arrangements he or she manages to make.

Functional decline is the result of a complex interaction among several elements, and cognitive performance is one of the most important of them. The tools and batteries used to assess impairments in dementias focus primarily on cognitive performance. Usually there is less interest in apprehending how cognitive changes interfere with the person's functioning. However, functional assessment provides information about daily performance, which is vital for health professionals who constantly have to counsel family member regarding patients' ability to live independently. Functional assessment is also relevant as functional impairment distinguishes mild cognitive impairment (MCI) from dementia syndromes (Petersen et al. 2001).

Current studies have investigated whether MCI patients present functional deficits and which kind of functional loss is typical of older adults with MCI (Farias et al. 2006). Some researchers claim that a modest decline in functioning should be part of the set of criteria for MCI diagnosis (Perneczky et al. 2006). It is well established in the literature that functional decline in the dementias follows a gradient in which basic activities of daily living (BADL) are affected after more complex activities have already deteriorated. Among MCI patients, the focus of functional assessment is on complex instrumental activities of daily living (IADL). Following this line of research, international papers point out that decline in four IADLs as strong predictors of dementia: ability to use the telephone, use of means of transportation, management of one's own medications, and ability to handle finances (Barberger-Gateau et al. 1999), the latter usually being the first to be impaired (Griffith et al. 2007). In a Brazilian sample of older adults with heterogeneous cognitive profiles assessed with a direct measure of functional status (Direct Assessment of Functional Status, DAFS-BR), MCI patients had significantly lower scores in two domains, dealing with finances and shopping skills, compared to normal controls (Pereira et al. 2010).

Despite the clinical relevance of studying the relationship between cognitive and functional performance, few research studies have actually examined this relationship (Royall et al. 2007). It is not yet clear, for instance, to what extent functional performance fluctuation can be directly attributed to cognition, or whether both are dependent upon noncognitive variables, such as socioeconomic, cultural, or personal aspects (Mor et al. 1989). Rosa et al. (2003) found that the attributes that have the strongest association with functional decline in a sample of Brazilian older adults were illiteracy, retirement, being a pensioner, being a housewife, being over 65, having a multigenerational family structure, being hospitalized in the last six months, not having the habit of visiting friends or relatives, having visual disabilities and a history of stroke, and having a pessimistic view with regards to one's own health when compared to peers.

Executive functioning has been highlighted as the key factor regarding functional performance among older individuals with cognitive decline. It must be pointed out that the degree of the correlation between executive functions and functionality is greater than that observed between executive functions and memory. Executive dysfunction directly affects IADLs, whereas working memory may be preserved in early dementia, starting to be compromised only in more advanced stages (Royall et al. 2005; Pereira et al. 2008).

In the context of dementias, functional assessment may involve direct observation (performance trials) and the use of scales or questionnaires filled in by informants or the patient. Up to the present moment, no consensus has been reached regarding the best method to assess an older individual's functional performance (Royall et al. 2007). In clinical practice, functioning is assessed by reports of a family member or caregiver concerning the difficulties the patient has encountered in carrying out daily living activities. Even though this approach is often adopted, abundant empirical evidence suggests that information provided by third parties is possibly biased, for example, by mood, caregiver personality and burden, resulting in over- or underestimation of functional deficits (Onor et al. 2006; Tierney et al. 1996; Glass 1998; Loewenstein et al. 2001). Research suggests that objective functional assessments (based on observed performance) are more accurate in identifying functional limitations, in addition to making it possible to devise compensatory strategies (Mangone et al. 1993; Farias et al. 2006; Onor et al. 2006; Pereira et al. 2010).

The most frequently used tools to assess functional status are the Barthel Index (Mahoney and Barthel 1965), Activities of Daily Living Scale outlined by Katz et al. (1963), IADL Scales by Lawton and Brody (1969) and by Pfeffer et al. (1982), Brazilian OARS Multidimensional Functional Assessment Questionnaire (BOMFAQ) (Blay, Ramos, and Mary 1988), and Functional Independency Measurement (MIF) (Riberto et al. 2001).

Among other scales, objective functional assessment of aged individuals can be carried out with the use of the Direct Assessment of Functional Status–Revised (DAFS-R) (Loewenstein and Bates 2006). This assessment relies on direct observation of the individual while he or she undertakes activities that replicate IADLs—for instance, orientation to time, communication, ability to handle finances, aptitude to take care of shopping needs, and BADLs, for instance, dressing ability, personal hygiene, and nutrition. The DAFS-R is used in seven countries around the world (Loewenstein, Amigo, and Duara 1989). A recent paper (Pereira et al. 2008) found a strong correlation between executive control (EXIT-25, Royall et al. 1992) and performance in the DAFS-BR (the Brazilian version of DAFS-R). And as stated earlier, this instrument may help identify MCI cases (Pereira et al. 2010).

In conclusion, brief cognitive screening, neuropsychological assessment, and assessment of functional status may significantly contribute to the early diagnosis of cognitive impairment. Early diagnosis may facilitate the implementation of pharmacological and psychosocial interventions that might contribute to the stabilization of cognitive losses. Cognitive testing may also assist in evaluating the effectiveness of treatment protocols.

REFERENCES

Aprahamian, I., J. E. Martinelli, A. L. Neri, and M. S. Yassuda. 2010. The accuracy of the Clock Drawing Test compared to that of standard screening tests for Alzheimer's disease: Results from a study of Brazilian elderly with heterogeneous educational backgrounds *International Psychogeriatrics* 22 (1): 64–71.

Ashendorf, L., A. L. Jefferson, M. K. O'Connor, C. Chaisson, R. Green, and R. Stern. 2008. Trail Making Test errors in normal aging, mild cognitive impairment, and dementia. *Archives of Clinical Neuropsychology.* 23 (2): 129–137.

Atalaia-Silva, K. C., and R. A. Lourenço. 2008. Tradução, adaptação e validação de construto do Teste do Relógio aplicado entre idosos no Brasil [Adaptation and validation of the Clock Drawing Test among Brazilian elderly]. *Revista Saúde Pública* 42 (5): 930–937.

Barberger-Gateau, P., C. Fabrigoule, I. Rouch, et al. 1999. Neuropsychological correlates of self-reported performance in instrumental activities of daily living and prediction of dementia. *Journal of Gerontology Series B: Psychological Sciences and Social Sciences* 54: 293–303.

Beato, R. G., R. Nitrini, A. P. Formigoni, and P. Caramelli. 2007. Brazilian version of the frontal assessment battery (FAB): Preliminary data on administration to healthy elderly. *Dementia and Neuropsychologia* 1: 59–65.

Bechara, A., A. R. Damasio, H. Damasio, and S. W. Anderson. 1994. Insensitivity to future consequences following damage to human prefrontal cortex. *Cognition* 50 (1–3): 7–15.

Bischkopf, J., A. Busse, and M. C. Angermeyer. 2002. Mild Cognitive Impairment—A review of prevalence, incidence and outcome according to current approaches. *Acta Psychiatrica Scandinavica* 106: 403–414.

Blay, S. L., L. R. Ramos, and J. J. Mary. 1988. Validity of a Brazilian version of the Older Americans Resources and Services (OARS) mental-health screening questionnaire. *Journal of the American Geriatrics Society* 36: 687–692.

Bolla, K. I., K. N. Lindgren, C. Bonaccorsy, and M. L. Bleecker. 2006. Predictors of verbal fluency (FAS) in the healthy elderly. *Journal of Clinical Psychology* 46 (5): 623–628.

Bottino, C. M. C., D. Azevedo Jr., M. F. Tatsch, S. R. Hototian, M. A. Moscoso, J. C. Folquitto, A. Z. Scalco, M. C. Bazzarella, M. A. Lopes, and J. Litvoc. 2008. Estimate of dementia prevalence in a community sample from São Paulo, Brazil. *Dementia and Geriatric Cognitive Disorders* 26: 291–299.

Brown, J., K. Dawson, L. A. Brown, and P. Clatworthy. 2009. Self-administered cognitive screening test (TYM) for detection of Alzheimer's disease: Cross sectional study. *British Medical Journal* 338: b2030.

Brucki, S. M. D., R. Nitrini, P. Caramelli, P. H. F. Bertolucci, and I. H. Okamoto. 2003. Sugestões para o uso do Mini-Exame do Estado Mental no Brasil [Suggestions for the Mini-Mental State Examination in Brazil]. *Arquivos de Neuropsiquiatria* 61: 777–781.

Buñuales, M. T. J., P. G. Diego, and J. M. M. Moreno. 2002. La Classificación Internacional del Funcionamento de la Discapacidad y de la Salud (CIF). *Revista Española de Salud Pública* 6: 271–279.

Caramelli, P., M. T. Carthery-Goulart, C. S. Porto, H. Charchat-Fichman, and R. Nitrini. 2007. Category fluency as a screening test for Alzheimer's disease in illiterate and literate patients. *Alzheimer Disease and Associated Disorders* 21 (1): 65–67.

Carvalho, V. A., M. T. Barbosa, and P. Caramelli. 2010. Brazilian version of the Addenbrooke Cognitive Examination-revised in the diagnosis of mild Alzheimer disease. *Cognitive and Behavioral Neurology* 23: 8–13.

Castiglioni, S., O. Pelati, M. Zuffi, F. Somalvico, L. Marino, T. Tentorio, and M. Franceschi. 2006. The frontal assessment battery does not differentiate frontotemporal dementia from Alzheimer's disease. *Dementia and Geriatric Cognitive Disorders* 22 (2): 125–131.

Collie, A., and P. Maruff. 2000. The neuropsychology of preclinical Alzheimer's disease and mild cognitive impairment. *Neuroscience and Biobehavioral Reviews* 24: 365–374.

Crane, P. K., L. E. Gibbons, L. Jolley, G. van Belle, R. Selleri, E. Dalmonte, and D. De Ronchi. 2006. Differential item functioning related to education and age in the Italian version of the Mini-Mental State Examination. *International Psychogeriatrics* 18: 505–515.

Cummings, J. L., H. V. Vinters, G. M. Cole, and Z. S. Khachaturian. 1998. Alzheimer's disease: Etiologies, pathophysiology, cognitive reserve and treatment opportunities. *Neurology* 51 (Suppl 1): 2–7.

De Ronchi, D., L. Fratiglioni, P. Rucci, A. Paternicò, S. Graziani, and E. Dalmonte. 1998. The effect of education on dementia occurrence in an Italian population with mild to high socioeconomic status. *Neurology* 50: 1231–1238.

de Silva, H. A., and S. B. Gunatilake. 2002. Mini-Mental State Examination in Sinhalese: A sensitive test to screen for dementia in Sri Lanka. *International Journal of Geriatric Psychiatry* 17: 134–139.

Dodge, H., K. Meguro, H. Ishii, S. Yamaguchi, J. Saxton, and M. Ganguli. 2009. Cross-cultural comparisons of the Mini-Mental State Examination between Japanese and U.S. cohorts. *InternationalPsychogeriatrics* 21 (1): 113–122.

Dubois, B., H. Feldman, C. Jacova, S. DeKosky, P. Barberger-Gateau, J. Cummings, A. Delacourte, D. Galasko, S. Gauthier, and G. Jicha. 2007. Research criteria for the diagnosis of Alzheimer's disease: Revising the NINCDS–ADRDA criteria. *The Lancet Neurology* 6 (8): 734–746.

Dubois, B., A. Slachevsky, I. Litvan, and B. Pillon. 2000. The FAB: A Frontal Assessment Battery at bedside. *Neurology* 55: 1621–1626.

Erzigkeit, H. 1992. SKT: A short cognitive performance test for assessing memory and attention. *SKT Manual*. Erlangen, Germany: Beltz Test.

Erzigkeit, H. 2001. SKT: A short cognitive performance test for assessing deficits of memory and attention. *User's manual*. 23rd ed. Erlangen, Germany: Geromed GmbH.

Espino, D. V., M. J. Lichtenstein, R. F. Palmer, and H. P. Hazuda. 2001. Ethnic differences in Mini-Mental State Examination (MMSE) scores: Where you live makes a difference. *Journal of the American Geriatrics Society* 49 (5): 538–548.

Farias, S. T., D. Mungas, B. R. Reed, D. Harvey, D. Cahn-Weiner, and C. Decarli. 2006. MCI is associated with deficits in everyday functioning. *Alzheimer Disease and Associated Disorders* 20 (4): 217–223.

Ferri, C., M. Prince, C. Brayne, H. Brodaty, L. Fratiglioni, M. Ganguli, K. Hall, K. Hasegawa, H. Hendrie, and Y. Huang. 2005. Global prevalence of dementia: A Delphi consensus study. *The Lancet* 366 (9503): 2112–2117.

Flaks, M. K., M. S. Yassuda, A. C. B. Regina, C. G. Cid, C. H. P. Camargo, W. F. Gattaz, and O. V. Forlenza. 2006. The Short Cognitive Performance Test (SKT): A preliminary study of its psychometric properties in Brazil. *International Psychogeriatrics* 18 (1): 121–133.

Flaks, M. K., O. V. Forlenza, F. S. Pereira, L. F. Viola, and M. S. Yassuda. 2009. Short cognitive performance test: Diagnostic accuracy and education bias in older Brazilian adults. *Archives of Clinical Neuropsychology* 24 (3): 301–306.

Folstein, M. F., S. E. Folstein, and P. R. McHugh. 1975. Mini-Mental State: A practical method for grading the cognitive state of patients of the clinician. *Journal of Psychiatric Research* 12: 189–198.

Forlenza, O. V., B. S. Diniz, L. L. Talib, M. Radanovic, M. S. Yassuda, E. B. Ojopi, and W. F. Gattaz. 2010. Clinical and biological predictors of Alzheimer's disease in patients with amnestic mild cognitive impairment. *Revista Brasileira de Psiquiatria*, April 16 (Epub ahead of print).

Fuld, P., D. M. Masur, A. Blau, C. Howard, and M. Aronson. 1990. Object memory evaluation for prospective detection of dementia in normal functioning elderly: Predictive and normative data. *Journal of Clinical and Experimental Neuropsychology* 12 (4): 520–528.

Fuzikawa, C., M. F. Lima-Costa, E. Uchôa, and K. Shulman. 2007. Correlation and agreement between the Mini-Mental State Examination and the Clock Drawing Test in older adults with low levels of schooling: The Bambuí Health Aging Study (BHAS). *International Psychogeriatrics* 19 (4): 657–667.

Gainotti, G., M. Ferraciolli, M. G. Vita, and C. Marra. 2008. Patterns of neuropsychological impairment in MCI patients with small subcortical infarcts or hippocampal atrophy. *Journal of the International Neuropsychological Society* 14 (4): 611–619.

Galton, C. J., S. Erzinçlioglu, B. J. Sahakian, N. Antoun, and J. R. Hodges. 2005. A comparison of the Addenbrooke's Cognitive Examination (ACE), conventional neuropsychological assessment, and simple MRI-based medial temporal lobe evaluation in the early diagnosis of Alzheimer's disease. *Cognitive Behavioral Neurology* 18 (3): 144–150.

Garcia-Caballero, A., I. Garcia-Lado, J. Gonzalez-Hermida, et al. 2006. Validation of the Spanish version of the Addenbrooke's Cognitive Examination in a rural community in Spain. *International Journal of Geriatric Psychiatry* 21 (3): 239–245.

Gibbons, L. E., G. van Belle, M. Yang, C. Gill, C. Brayne, F. A. Huppert, E. Paykel, and E. Larson. 2002. Cross-cultural comparison of the Mini-Mental State Examination in United Kingdom and United States participants with Alzheimer's disease. *International Journal of Geriatric Psychiatry* 17: 723–728.

Glass, T. A. 1998. Conjugating the tenses of function: Discordance among hypothetical, experimental, and enacted function in older adults. *Gerontologist* 38: 101–112.

Goodglass, H., E. Kaplan, and B. Barresi. 2000. *The Boston Diagnostic Aphasia Examination* (BDAE-3). 3rd ed. Philadelphia: Lippincott.

Goodglass, H., and A. Wingfield. 1993. Selective preservation of a lexical category in aphasia: Dissociations in comprehension of body parts and geographical place names following focal brain lesion. *Memory* 1 (4): 313–328.

Gordilho, A., A. Sergio, J. Silvestre, L. R. Ramos, M. P. A. Freire, N. Espindola, et al. 2000. *Desafios a serem enfrentados no terceiro milênio pelo setor saúde na atenção integral ao idoso*. Rio de Janeiro: UnATI/UERI.

Griffith, H. R., K. Belue, A. Sicola, S. Krzywanski, et al. 2007. Impaired financial abilities in mild cognitive impairment: A direct assessment approach. *American Journal of Alzheimer's Disease and Other Dementias* 22 (3): 21–217.

Guedj, E., G. Allali, C. Goetz, I. Le Ber, M. Volteau, L. Lacomblez, P. Vera, et al. 2008. Frontal Assessment Battery is a marker of dorsolateral and medial frontal functions: A SPECT study in frontotemporal dementia. *Journal of the Neurological Sciences* 273 (1–2): 84–87.

Hampel, H., K. Bürger, S. Teipel, A. Bokde, H. Zetterberg, and K. Blennow. 2008. Core candidate neurochemical and imaging biomarkers of Alzheimer's disease. *Alzheimer and Dementia* 4 (1): 38–48.

Herrera, E., P. Caramelli, A. S. Silveira, and R. Nitrini. 2002. Epidemiologic survey of dementia in a community-dwelling Brazilian population. *Alzheimer Disease and Associated Disorders* 16: 103–108.

Ho, L., H. Fiveacoat, J. Wang, and G. M. Pasinetti. 2010. Alzheimer's disease biomarker discovery in symptomatic and asymptomatic patients: Experimental approaches and future clinical applications. *Experimental Gerontology* 45 (1): 15–22.

Ihl, R., L. Frölich, T. Dierks, E. M. Martin, and K. Maurer. 1992. Differential validity of psychometric tests in dementia of Alzheimer type. *Psychiatric Research* 44: 93–106.

Ivnik, R. J., J. F. Malec, E. G. Tangalos, R. C. Petersen, E. Kokmen, and L. T. Kurland. 1990. The auditory-verbal learning test (RAVLT): Norms for ages 55 years and older. *Psychological Assessment* 2: 304–312.

Jones, R. N. 2006. Identification of measurement differences between English and Spanish language versions of the Mini-Mental State Examination: detecting differential item functioning using MIMIC modeling. *Medical Care* 44: S124–133.

Katz, S., A. B. Ford, R. W. Moskowitz, N. B. A. Jackson, and M. W. Jaffe. 1963. Studies of illness in the aged. *Journal of the American Medical Society* 185 (12): 914–921.

Katzman, R. 1993. Education and prevalence of dementia and Alzheimer's disease. *Neurology* 43: 13–20.

Kim, Y. G., D. W. Nibbelink, and J. E. Overall. 1993. Factor structure and scoring of the SKT Test Battery. *Journal of Clinical Psychology* 49 (1): 61–71.

Kohn, R., B. Vicente, P. Rioseco, S. Saldivia, and S. Torres. 2008. The Mini-Mental State Examination: Age and education distribution for a Latin American population. *Aging and Mental Health* 12: 66–71.

Kugo, A., S. Terada, T. Ata, Y. Ido, Y. Kado, T. Ishihara, M. Hikiji, Y. Fujisawa, K. Sasaki, and S. Kuroda. 2007. Japanese version of the Frontal Assessment Battery for dementia. *Psychiatry Research* 153 (1): 69–75.

Laks, J., E. M. R. Batista, A. L. B. Contino, and E. Engelhardt. 2007. Mini-Mental State Examination norms in a community-dwelling sample of elderly with low schooling in Brazil. *Cadernos de Saúde Pública* (FIOCRUZ) 23: 315–319.

Lam, L. C., P. Ho, V. W. Lui, and C. W. Tam. 2006. Reduced semantic fluency as an additional screening tool for subjects with questionable dementia. *Dementia and Geriatric Cognitive Disorders* 22 (2): 159–164.

Larner, A. J. 2007. Addenbrooke's Cognitive Examination-Revised (ACE-R) in day-to-day clinical practice. *Age and Ageing* 36 (6): 685–686.

Lawton, M. P., and E. M. Brody. 1969. Assessment of older people: Self maintaining and instrumental activities of daily living. *Gerontologist* 9 (3): 179–186.

Lehfeld, H., and H. Erzigkeit. 1997. The SKT: A short cognitive performance test for assessing deficits of memory and attention. *International Psychogeriatrics* 9 (Suppl 1): 115–121.

Lehfeld, H., G. Rudinger, C. Rietz, C. Heinrich, V. Wied, L. Fornazzari, J. Pittas, I. Hindmarch, and H. Erzigkeit. 1997. Evidence of the cross-cultural stability of the factor structure of the SKT Short Test for assessing deficits of memory and attention. *International Psychogeriatrics* 9 (2): 139–153.

Lezak, M. D., D. B. Howieson, and D. W. Loring. 2004. *Neuropsychological Assessment*. New York: Oxford University Press.

Libon, D. J., C. McMillan, D. Gunawardena,, C. Powers, L. Massimo, A. Khan, B. Morgan, et al. 2009. Neurocognitive contributions to verbal fluency deficits in frontotemporal lobar degeneration. *Neurology* 73 (7): 535–542.

Lipton, A. M., K. A. Ohman, K. B. Womack, L. S. Hynan, E. T. Ninman, and L. H. Lacritz. 2005. Subscores of the FAB differentiate frontotemporal lobar degeneration from AD. *Neurology* 65: 726–731.

Loewenstein, D. A., E. Amigo, and R. Duara. 1989. A new scale for the assessment of functional status in Alzheimer's disease and related disorders. *Journal of Gerontology* 4: 114–121.

Loewenstein, D. A., S. Argüelles, M. Bravo, R. Q. Freeman, T. Argüelles, A. Acevedo, and C. Eisdorfer. 2001. Caregivers' judgments of the functional abilities of the Alzheimer's disease patient: A comparison of proxy reports and objective measures. *Journal of Gerontology Series B: Psychological Sciences and Social Sciences* 56: 78–84.

Loewenstein, D. A., and C. B. Bates. 2006. The Direct Assessment of Functional Status Revised (DAFS-R). *Manual for Administration and Scoring*. Miami: Neuropsychological Laboratories and the Wien Center for Alzheimer's Disease and Memory Disorders, Mount Sinai Medical Center.

Mahoney, F. I., and D. W. Barthel. 1965. Functional evaluation: The Barthel Index. *Maryland State Medical Journal* 14: 61–65.

Mangone, C. A., R. M. Sanguinetti, P. D. Baumann, R. C. Gonzalez, S. Pereyra, F. G. Bozzola, P. B. Gorelick, and R. E. Sica. 1993. Influence of feelings of burden on the caregiver's perception of the patient's functional status. *Dementia* 4 (5): 287–293.

Mann, U. M., E. Mohr, M. Gearing, and T. N. Chase. 1992. Heterogeneity in Alzheimer's disease: Progression rate segregated by distinct neuropsychological and cerebral metabolic profiles. *Journal of Neurology, Neurosurgery, and Psychiatry* 55: 956–959.

Masur, D. M., P. A. Fuld, A. D. Blau, H. Crystal, and M. K. Aronson. 1990. Predicting development of dementia in the elderly with the Selective Reminding Test. *Journal of Clinical and Experimental Neuropsychology* 12 (4): 529–538.

Mendez, M. F., T. Ala, and K. L. Underwood. 1992. Development of scoring criteria for the Clock Drawing Task in Alzheimer's disease. *Journal of the American Geriatrics Society* 40: 1095–1099.

Mioshi, E., K. Dawson, J. Mitchell, R. Arnold, and J. R. Hodges. 2006. The Adden-brooke's Cognitive Examination Revised (ACE-R): A brief cognitive test battery for dementia screening. *International Journal of Geriatric Psychiatry* 21 (11): 1078–1085.

Mor, V., J. Murphy, S. Masterson-Allen, C. Willey, A. Razmpour, M. E. Jacksin, et al. 1989. Risk of functional decline among well elders. *Journal of Clinical Epidemiology* 42: 895–904.

Morris, J. C., A. Heyman, R. C. Mohs, et al. 1989. The Consortium to Establish a Registry for Alzheimer's Disease (CERAD). Part I: Clinical and neuropsychological assessment of Alzheimer's disease. *Neurology* 39: 1159–1165.

Nakaaki, S., Y. Murata, J. Sato, Y. Shinagawa, T. Matsui, H. Tatsumi, and T. A. Furukawa. 2007. Reliability and validity of the Japanese version of the Frontal Assessment Battery in patients with the frontal variant of frontotemporal dementia. *Psychiatry and Clinical Neuroscience* 61 (1): 78–83.

Nasreddine, Z. S., N. A. Phillips, V. Bédirian, S. Charbonneau, V. Whitehead, I. Collin, J. L. Cummings, and H. Chertkow. 2005. The Montreal Cognitive Assessment (MoCA): A brief screening tool for mild cognitive impairment. *Journal of the American Geriatrics Society* 53: 695–699.

Nishiwaki, Y., E. Breeze, L. Smeeth, C. J. Bulpitt, R. Peters, and A. E. Fletcher. 2004. Validity of the Clock-Drawing Test as a screening tool for cognitive impairment in the elderly. *American Journal of Epidemiology* 160 (8): 797–807.

O'Bryant, S. E., J. D. Humphreys, G. E. Smith, R. J. Ivnik, N. R. Graff-Radford, R. C. Petersen, and J. A. Lucas. 2008. Detecting dementia with the Mini-Mental State Examination (MMSE) in highly educated individuals. *Archives of Neurology* 65 (7): 963–967.

Oguro, H., S. Yamaguchi, S. Abe, Y. Ishida, H. Bokura, and S. Kobayashi. 2006. Differentiating Alzheimer's disease from subcortical vascular dementia with the FAB test. *Journal of Neurology* 253 (11): 1490–1494.

Onor, M. L., M. Trevisiol, C. Negro, and E. Aguglia. 2006. Different perception of cognitive impairment, behavioral disturbances, and functional disabilities between persons with mild cognitive impairment and mild Alzheimer's disease and their caregivers. *American Journal of Alzheimer's Disease and Other Dementias* 21 (5): 333–338.

Ostrosky-Solís, F., G. Dávila, X. Ortiz, et al. 1999. Determination of normative criteria and validation of the SKT for use in a Spanish-speaking populations. *International Psychogeriatrics* 11: 171–180.

Ostrosky-Solis, F., G. Lopez-Arango, and A. Ardila. 2000. Sensitivity and specificity of the Mini-mental State Examination in a Spanish-speaking population. *Applied Neuropsychology* 7: 25–31.

Overall, J. E., and R. Schaltenbrand. 1992. The SKT neuropsychological test battery. *Journal of Geriatric Psychiatry and Neurology* 5: 220–227.

Parker, C., and I. Philp. 2004. Screening for cognitive impairment among older people in black and minority ethnic groups. *Age and Ageing* 33 (5): 447–452.

Pereira, F. S., M. S. Yassuda, A. M. Oliveira, and O. V. Forlenza. 2008. Executive dysfunction correlates with impaired functional status in older adults with varying degrees of cognitive impairment. *International Psychogeriatrics* 20 (6): 1104–1115.

Pereira, F. S., M. S. Yassuda, A. M. Oliveira, B. S. Diniz, M. Radanovic, L. L. Talib, W. F. Gattaz, and O. V. Forlenza. 2010. Profiles of functional deficits in mild cognitive impairment and dementia: benefits from objective measurement. *Journal of the International Neuropsychological Society* 16 (2): 297–305.

Perneczky, R., C. Pohl, C. Sorg, et al. 2006. Impairment of activities of daily living requiring memory or complex reasoning as part of de MCI syndrome. *International Journal of Geriatric Psychiatry* 35: 240–245.

Petersen, R. C., R. Doody, A. Kurz, R. C. Mohs, J. C. Morris, and P. V. Rabins. 2001. Current concepts in mild cognitive impairment. *Archives of Neurology* 58 (12): 1985–1992.

Pfeffer, R. I., T. T. Kurosaki, C. H. Harrah, J. M. Chance, and S. Filos. 1982. Measurement of functional activities in older adults in the community. *Journal of Gerontology* 37 (3): 323–329.

Portet, F., P. J. Ousset, P. J. Visser, G. B. Frisoni, F. Nobili, Ph. Scheltens, B. Vellas, and J. Touchon. 2006. Mild cognitive impairment (MCI) in medical practice: A critical review of the concept and new diagnostic procedure. Report of the MCI Working Group of the European Consortium on Alzheimer's Disease. *Journal of Neurology, Neurosurgery, and Psychiatry* 77: 714–718.

Posner, M. I., and M. Raichle. 2004. *Images of Mind.* New York: Scientific American Library.

Rabinovici, G. D., and B. L. Miller. 2010. Frontotemporal lobar degeneration: Epidemiology, pathophysiology, diagnosis and management. *CNS Drugs* 24 (5): 375–398.

Radanovic, M., B. S. Diniz, R. M. Mirandez, T. M. Novaretti, M. K. Flaks, M. S. Yassuda, and O. V. Forlenza. 2009. Verbal fluency in the detection of mild cognitive impairment and Alzheimer's disease among Brazilian Portuguese speakers: The influence of education. *International Psychogeriatrics* 21 (6): 1081–1087.

Reyes-Beaman, S., et al. 2004. Validation of a modified version of the Mini-Mental State Examination (MMSE) in Spanish. *Aging, Neuropsychology, and Cognition* 11: 1–11.

Riberto, M., M. H. Myazaki, D. J. Filho, H. Sakamoto, and L. R. Battistella. 2001. Reprotutibilidade da versão brasileira da Medida de Independência Funcional [Reproductibility of the Brazilian version of the Functional Independence Measure FIM]. *Acta Fisiatrica* 8: 41–52.

Rosa, T. E. C., M. H. Benício, M. O. Latorreb, and L. R. Ramos. 2003. Fatores determinantes da capacidade funcional entre idosos [Determinant factors of functional capacity among the elderly]. *Revista de Saúde Pública* 37 (1): 40–48.

Rosselli, D., A. Ardila, G. Pradilla, L. Morillo, L. Bautista, O. Rey, and M. Camacho. 2000. The Mini-Mental State Examination as a selected diagnostic test for dementia: A Colombian population study. *Revista Neurologia* 30 (5): 428–432.

Rosselli, M., R. Tappen, C. Williams, J. Salvatierra, and Y. Zoller. 2009. Level of education and category fluency task among Spanish speaking elders: Number of words, clustering, and switching strategies. *Neuropsychology Development and Cognition Section B: Aging Neuropsychology and Cognition* 16 (6): 721–744.

Roth, M., E. Tym, C. Q. Mountjoy, F. A. Huppert, H. Hendrie, S. Verma, and R. Goddard. 1986. CAMDEX: A standard instrument for the diagnosis of mental disorder in the elderly with special reference to the early detection of dementia. *British Journal of Psychiatry* 149: 698–709.

Royall, D. R., E. C. Lauterbach, D. Kaufer, P. Malloy, K. L. Coburn, and K. J. Black. 2007. The cognitive correlates of functional status: A review from the Committee on Research of the American Neuropsychiatric Association. *Journal of Neuropsychiatry and Clinical Neuroscience* 19 (3): 249–265.

Royall, D. R., R. K. Mahurin, and K. F. Gray. 1992. Beside assessment of executive impairment: The Executive Interview (EXIT). *Journal of the American Geriatrics Society* 40: 1221–1226.

Royall, D. R., R. Palmer, L. K. Chiodo, and M. J. Polk. 2005. Executive control mediates memory's association with change in instrumental activities of daily living: The Freedom House Study. *Journal of the American Geriatrics Society* 53: 1–11.

Shaw, L. M., M. Korecka, C. M. Clark, V. M. Y. Lee, and J. Q. Trojanowski. 2007. Biomarkers of neurodegeneration for diagnosis and monitoring therapeutics. *Nature Reviews Drug Discovery* 6: 295–303.

Simpao, M. P., D. V. Espino, R. F. Palmer, M. J. Lichtenstein, and H. P. Hazuda. 2005. Association between acculturation and structural assimilation and Mini-Mental State Examination–Assessed cognitive impairment in older Mexican Americans: Findings from the San Antonio Longitudinal Study of Aging. *Journal of the American Geriatrics Society* 53: 1234–1239.

Shulman K. 2000. I. Clock-drawing: Is it the ideal cognitive screening test? *International Journal of Geriatric Psychiatry* 15: 548–561.

Shulman, K., and A. Feinstein. 2003. *Quick Cognitive Screening for Clinicians*. London: Martin Dunitz.

Slachevsky, A., and B. Dubois. 2004. Frontal Assessment Battery and differential diagnosis of frontotemporal dementia and Alzheimer disease. *Archives of Neurology* 61 (7): 1104–1107.

Spreen, O., and E. Strauss. 1998. *A Compendium of Neuropsychological Tests: Administration, Norms, and Commentary*. 2nd ed. New York: Oxford University Press.

Steinberg, B. A., L. A. Bieliauskas, G. E. Smith, C. Langellotti, and R. J. Ivnik. 2005. Mayo's Older Americans Normative Studies: Age- and IQ-adjusted norms for the Boston Naming Test, the MAE Token Test, and the Judgment of Line Orientation Test. *Clinical Neuropsychology* 19 (3–4): 280–328.

Stern, Y., B. Gurland, T. K. Tatemichi, M. X. Tang, D. Wilder, and R. Mayeux. 1994. Influence of education and occupation on the incidence of Alzheimer's disease. *JAMA* 271: 1004–1010.

Storey, J. E., J. T. J. Rowland, D. Basic, and D. A. Conforti. 2002. Accuracy of the Clock Drawing Test for detecting dementia in a multicultural sample of elderly Australian patients. *International Psychogeriatrics* 14 (3): 259–271.

Sunderland, T., J. L. Hill, A. M. Mellow, et al. 1989. Clock drawing in Alzheimer's disease: A novel measure of dementia severity. *Journal of the American Geriatrics Society* 37: 725–729.

Tierney, M. C., J. P. Szalai, W. G. Snow, and R. H. Fisher. 1996. The prediction of Alzheimer disease: The role of patient and informant perceptions of cognitive deficits. *Archives of Neurology* 53 (5): 423–427.

Van Dijk, E. J., M. M. B. Breteler, R. Schmidt, K. Berger, L. G. Nilsson, M. Oudkerk, et al. 2004. The association between blood pressure, hypertension, and cerebral white matter lesions: Cardiovascular determinants of dementia study. *Hypertension* 44: 625–630.

Xu, G., J. S. Meyer, Y. Huang, F. Du, M. Chowdhury, and M. Quach. 2003. Adapting Mini-Mental State Examination for dementia screening among illiterate or minimally educated elderly Chinese. *International Journal of Geriatric Psychiatry* 18 (7): 609–616.

Wechsler, D. 1997. Wechsler Adult Intelligence Scale (WAIS-III). 3rd ed. San Antonio, TX: The Psychological Corporation.

Wechsler, D. 1997. Wechsler Memory Scale (WMS-III). 3rd ed. San Antonio, TX: The Psychological Corporation.

Weyer, G., H. Erzigkeit, S. Kanowski, R. Ihl, and D. Hadler. 1997. Alzheimer's Disease Assessment Scale: Reliability and validity in a multicenter clinical trial. *International Psychogeriatrics* 9: 123–138.

Wilson, B. A., J. Cockburn, and A. Baddeley. 1985. *The Rivermead Behavioural Memory Test*. Gaylord, MI: National Rehabilitation Services.

Woodruff-Pak, D. S. 1997. *The Neuropsychology of Aging*. Malden, MA: Blackwell.

World Health Organization. 2001. *International Classification of Functioning, Disability, and Health (ICF)*. Geneva: World Health Organization.

Yassuda, M. S., B. S. Diniz, L. F. Viola, F. S. Pereira, P. V. Nunes, and O. V. Forlenza. 2009. Neuropsychological profile of Brazilian older adults with heterogeneous educational backgrounds. *Archives of Clinical Neuropsychology* 24: 71–79.

Chapter 8

Does Poor Sleep Quality in Late Life Compromise Cognition and Accelerate Progression of the Degenerative Dementias?

Peter Engel

Cycles of sleep and wakefulness begin in utero and persist throughout life. As such, sleep is both a personally familiar experience and a biologically essential activity. At the same time, the fundamental links between sleep, health, and disease remain elusive. Several decades of sleep research now link rapid eye movement (REM) and non–rapid eye movement (nREM) sleep with new learning and consolidation of both motor and episodic memory. While other functions of sleep escape full understanding, sleep appears to be essential for survival through regulation of growth, development, maintenance, and repair of the brain as well as the entire organism (Diekelmann and Born 2010; Garcia-Rill et al. 2008; Vassalli and Dijk 2009). Hence, the connections between sleep, learning, and memory may have implications for brain development and maintenance during early and mid-life, and cognitive decline associated with aging and degenerative brain disease in late life. These potential late life relationships will be the principal focus of this chapter.

Over the lifespan crisp transitions between wakefulness and sleep and their tight circadian regulation diminish in intensity and precision. Sleep-stage transitions become more fragmented, sleep efficiency diminishes, and slow-wave sleep declines with age (Redline et al. 2004; Ohayon et al. 2004; Bloom et al. 2009; Dijk et al. 2010) (see Figure 8.1). These changes are enhanced in dementing disorders that are characterized by profound impairments of learning and memory. In some cases of dementia in which sleep disturbances are profound, components of wakefulness may infiltrate sleep (Cajochen et al. 2006; Espiritu 2008; Gagnon et al. 2008).

In Alzheimer's disease (AD), the dementia in which sleep and circadian disturbances are best studied, the major components of REM and nREM sleep appear to be relatively preserved despite progressive fragmentation of sleep architecture and varying degrees of cell loss in sleep-regulating regions of the brainstem, basal forebrain and hypothalamus. In Lewy body dementia (LBD), sleep and arousal mechanisms may be profoundly disturbed and REM sleep may be disrupted by intrusion of components of the waking state. In REM sleep behavior disorder (RBD), the profound hypotonia of REM sleep fails to occur and patients appear to act out their dreams, often with violent gestures and vocalizations. In LBD and Parkinson's disease, a related synucleopathy, RBD may precede the dementing illness by 10 years or more (Mahowald, Schenck, and Bornemann 2007; McKeith et al. 2005; Boeve et al. 2007; Iranzo, Santamaria, and Tolosa 2009; Postuma et al. 2009).

In this chapter we will consider two possible associations between decrements in sleep quality, age-related memory decline, and dementia: first, that age and dementia-related loss of sleep integrity directly contribute to cognitive impairment, and second, that age and disease-associated circadian and sleep disturbances enhance brain injury and accelerate disease progression. To address these questions the discussion will concentrate on AD, the most thoroughly studied dementia for which animal models are available, and LBD, given ample data on RBD and cognitive deficits associated with this disorder.

To investigate this broad area, identify gaps, and suggest future directions we will begin by examining sleep architecture in relation to aging, AD, and LBD and relate these to neuroanatomical correlates of sleep mechanisms to the extent that they are understood. An exploration of human and animal research that links sleep to learning and memory consolidation will follow. This background will form the basis for an investigation of the hypotheses proposed above.

Three points deserve mention early in this discussion. First, this chapter represents an attempt to identify connections between several broad and disparate areas of research in sleep, learning, and dementia. Second, treatment of sleep disorders in dementia both pharmacological and otherwise are well considered elsewhere and will not be addressed here (Espiritu

Figure 8.1

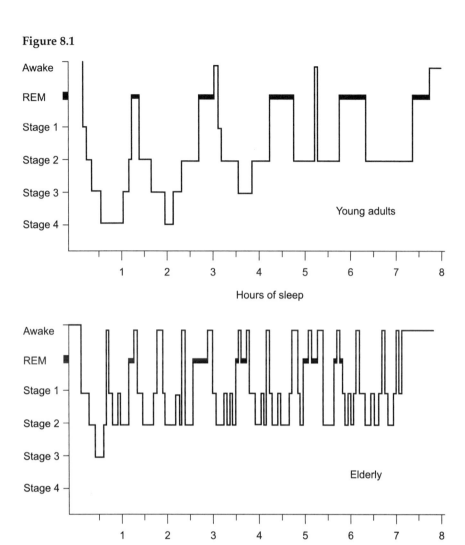

Hypnograms characteristic of young adults and elderly individuals. Decrements in sleep architecture in the elderly are characterized by delayed sleep onset, sleep fragmentation, early morning awakening, and decreased slow wave sleep (stages 3 and 4). (Reprinted with permission from "Sleep Problems in the Elderly," May 1, 1999, *American Family Physician.* Copyright ©1999 American Academy of Family Physicians. All rights reserved.)

2008; Boeve, "Update" 2008; Dauvillers 2007; Deschenes and McCurry 2009). Third, uncertainties related to the neuropathological and clinical features of AD and LBD point to the difficulties in the study of aging and dementia. The neuropathological differences between age-related change, Alzheimer's disease and Lewy body dementia are hardly distinct, and clinical variability in disease expression from one individual to another can be substantial. Alzheimer and Lewy body pathology commonly co-occur with the predominant features determining a specific diagnosis (Jellinger 2008; Kazee and Han 1995). These realities begin to frame the inherent limitations associated with any attempt to understand the relationships between sleep, aging, and the degenerative dementias. But such a caveat need not dissuade this exploration.

Since the earliest neuropathological change in AD begins in the allocortex and cortex with variable involvement of sleep and arousal systems in brainstem and midbrain, sleep disturbances in AD might be considered an exaggerated form of normal aging. These medial temporal lobe and cortical changes likely account for impairments of learning, memory, and abstract reasoning, and reduced fluency that characterize early stages of this disorder (Dubois et al. 2007; McKhann et al. 1984; American Psychiatric Association 2000; Braak and Braak 1991; Thal et al. 2002; Schneider et al. 2009).

LBD, in contrast, may be a "bottom up" dementia in which the earliest pathological changes occur in the brainstem, or systemically in the gut and spread rostrally with early involvement of sleep-regulating nuclei. This sequence may explain the presence of RBD as a common precursor of LBD with later evidence of deficits of attention, executive function, and visuospatial ability often with fluctuating cognition, visual hallucinations, and features of Parkinsonism (McKeith et al. 2005; Phillips et al. 2008; Braak et al. 2003). Memory may be spared early on in LBD, distinguishing this condition from AD. In relation to the two hypotheses under consideration, only the first, a possible relationship between sleep disturbances and cognitive impairment of LBD, will gain scrutiny here. Exploration of the second is precluded by an insufficient understanding of the factors that modulate the pathological processes associated with this disease.

SLEEP AND AROUSAL: NEUROBIOLOGY AND NEUROANATOMY

Arousal is mediated by the reticular activating system situated in the upper brainstem near the pons-midbrain junction where cholinergic and monaminergic cell groups constitute the central components. The cholinergic pedunculopointine (PPT) and laterodorsal (LDT) tegmental nuclei in the mesopontine tegmentum project to thalmocortical nuclei and the reticular nucleus to facilitate thalmocortical sensory transmission. Cholinergic basal forebrain projections to the cortex are implicated in waking and electroencephalographic (EEG) desynchronization. Lesions of the basal forebrain produce coma, underscoring the critical importance of this area in arousal.

The monoaminergic arousal system comprised of the noradrenergic locus coeruleus, dopaminergic ventral preaqueductal gray, serotoninergic raphe nuclei, and histaminergic tuberomammillary neurons project to the thalamus, lateral hypothalamus (LH), basal forebrain, and cortex. Orexin-secreting neurons in the LH project reciprocally to the brainstem monaminergic systems. Orexin, a peptide that promotes arousal and appetite increases firing rates in the monoaminergic arousal system while melanin-concentrating hormone neurons from LH inhibit the arousal system and mediate REM sleep homeostasis (Fuller, Gooley, and Saper 2006; Saper, Scammell, and Lu 2005; Schwartz and Roth 2008) (see Figure 8.2).

During sleep, the hypothalamic ventrolateral preoptic nucleus (VLPO) inhibits arousal circuits, an effect mediated by gamma amino buteric acid (GABA) and galanin. VLPO lesions produce profound insomnia in animals. Loss of VLPO neurons as occurs in aging and AD may contribute to insomnia and sleep fragmentation that can occur in these conditions. VLPO and arousal systems are mutually inhibitory with functions comparable to an electronic "flip-flop" switch imparting a degree of stability to either the waking or sleeping state (Saper and Scammell 2005). Cell loss also occurs in other sleep-modulating hypothalamic and brainstem nuclei in a variety of neurodegenerative diseases but shows no clear relationship with the associated sleep disturbances (Boeve et al. 2007; Benarroch et al. 2009; Jellinger 1988; Mufson, Mash, and Hersh 1988; Ransmayr, Faucheux, and Nowakowski 2000; Saper and German 1987; Schmeichel et al. 2008; Szymusiak, Gvilia, and McGinty 2007; Zhang et al. 2005; Zweig et al. 1989).

Transition from nREM to REM sleep is also mediated by a proposed "flip-flop" switch control of which appears to be progressively compromised by aging and degenerative neurological diseases. Mutually inhibitory cholinergic "REM-on" PPT neurons complement serotonergic dorsal raphe and noradrenergic locus coeruleus "REM-off" cells (Hobson 2009; Monti and Monti 2007). Dopaminergic and cholinergic nuclei are active during REM. In the rat REM-on activity in the subcoeruleus region is associated with electromyographic atonia and appears to effect this state through hyperpolarization of spinal cord anterior horn motor neurons during REM sleep. Loss of atonia as occurs in RBD suggests focal brainstem injury to these anterior horn cell inhibitory circuits (Boeve, "Update" 2008).

Figure 8.2

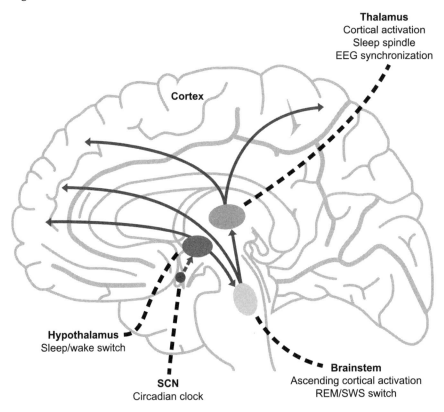

Simplified schematic of major sleep-regulating regions. Brainstem
nuclei for arousal and REM/slow-wave sleep regulation; locus coeruleus
(norepinephrine), raphe (serotonin), tuberomammilliary nucleus (histamine),
ventral periaqueductal grey (dopamine), pedunculopontine and laterodorsal
tegmental nuclei (acetylcholine). Hypothalamus; ventrolateral preoptic
nucleus promotes sleep (GABA, galanin, inhibitory transmitters). Orexin from
lateral hypothalamus promotes wakefulness. SCN, suprachiasmatic nucleus.
(Modified with permission from Macmillan Publishers, Ltd.: Emmanuel
Mignot, Shahrad Taheri, and Seiji Nishino, "Sleeping with the hypothalamus:
Emerging therapeutic targets for sleep disorders," *Nature Neuroscience* 5:
1071–1075. Copyright © 2002.)

In general, all cell groups fire more during wakefulness than nREM
sleep whereas REM sleep is a cholinergically hypermodulated and
aminergically demodulated state. Hence the cholinergic deficiency associated with both AD and LBD may contribute to the fragmentation of REM
sleep periods (Hobson 2009).

The suprachaismic nucleus of the hypothalamus exerts overall circadian control of sleep and wakefulness. In aging as well as AD and other degenerative dementias substantial cell loss occurs in the suprachaismic nucleus that is associated with reduction in the amplitude of various circadian rhythms and a phase advance, particularly for sleep. Reduction in sleep quality and increased sleep fragmentation are likely related to these changes (Braak and Braak 1992; Goudsmit et al. 1990; Mirmiran et al. 1992).

SLEEP ARCHITECTURE, AGING, AND ALZHEIMER'S DISEASE

Polysomnographic studies indicate that sleep efficiency and depth diminish with age, sleep becomes fragmented, and nocturnal arousals occur more frequently. These changes are more prominent in AD as are circadian disturbances in sleep-wake activity (Vassalli and Dijk 2009; Redline et al. 2004; Ohayon et al. 2004; Bloom et al. 2009; Dijk et al. 2010; Cajochen et al. 2006; Espiritu 2008; Gagnon et al. 2008; Bliwise 2004). Normal aging and AD are associated with diminished slow-wave sleep (SWS) and a reduced number of sleep spindles during stage 2 sleep (see Figure 8.1 above). Sleep spindles have been implicated in hippocampal-related learning. In addition, both human and animal studies indicate that sleep deprivation, sleep fragmentation, and reduction in REM or nREM sleep can impair motor and episodic learning (Chee and Chuah 2008; Walker 2008; Banks and Dinges 2007; Schabus et al. 2007; Sterpenich et al. 2007). None of these investigations included aged subjects.

Do Age-Related Changes in Sleep Produce Memory Impairment?

Age and AD-related changes in sleep are not readily comparable to sleep disturbances produced in experimental paradigms but several parallels may be of interest.

An extensive literature has defined the learning impairments associated with sleep deprivation and the need for sleep following learning for consolidation and enhancement of procedural and declarative memory. Both REM and nREM sleep enhance the consolidation of motor and episodic memory as well as other forms of learning. Current sleep research suggests that SWS supports system consolidation while REM sleep mediates synaptic consolidation. SWS slow oscillations, sleep spindles, and high-frequency hippocampal ripple oscillations are purported to coordinate reactivation and redistribution of hippocampal dependent memories to the neocortex, a phenomenon that occurs during low cholinergic states.

During REM, high cholinergic activity may promote synaptic consolidation. Optimum benefits of sleep for memory consolidation appear to occur when SWS is followed by REM sleep, the usual sequence in young humans and animals. Moreover, cholinergic activation strengthens long-term potentiation (LTP) in the hippocampal-medial prefrontal cortex pathway. These observations introduce the possibility that the cholinergic deficiency of AD and LBD combined with disruption of sleep architecture and loss of SWS compromise this dynamic of sleep-induced memory consolidation (Diekelmann and Born 2010; Walker 2009; Stickgold and Walker 2007).

Electrophysiological studies suggest that sleep spindles characteristic of stage 2 nREM sleep provide trains of depolarizations to cortex and hippocampus that are comparable to spike trains of in-vitro LTP, a synaptic mechanism implicated in learning (Steriade 1999). Such observations may be linked to impaired learning associated with the reduced number of sleep spindles both in aging and Alzheimer's disease, the smaller number of fast spindles in AD patients, and a positive correlation between the intensity of fast spindles and post-sleep immediate recall (Rauchs et al. 2008).

Two preliminary investigations suggest a relationship between sleep, learning, and aging. In the first, compared to their younger counterparts, middle-aged subjects demonstrated a decrement in declarative memory that correlated with reduced SWS time (Backhaus et al. 2007). The second showed that improved episodic memory tracked with total sleep time but not specific sleep stage in both young and old subjects (Aly and Moscovitch 2010).

Hence age-associated loss of sleep integrity that is exaggerated in Alzheimer's disease may be a direct contributor to clinically evident cognitive impairments through decrements in sleep-related memory consolidation and learning processes. Concurrently, age-related reduction in sleep quality combined with age-associated disease may accelerate the pathogenic processes of Alzheimer's disease. We will specifically explore this possibility by examining potential relationships between aging, age-related disorders, and the production of amyloid beta (A-beta).

Does the Loss of Sleep Integrity Accelerate Alzheimer's Disease Pathogenic Processes?

A predominant hypothesis of AD pathogenesis posits the toxicity of A-beta a 40-42 amino acid peptide produced by neurons as a fundamental pathogenic process. Substantial experimental evidence shows that A-beta 42 is neurotoxic, particularly in its soluble, oligameric forms and that A-beta is either produced in excess or inefficiently catabolized such that the peptide concentrations reach toxic levels. The neurotoxic effects of A-beta oligomers include depression of LTP, enhancement of long-term depression (LTD), inhibition of synaptogenesis, neuronal cell death and apoptosis (Yang, Hsu, and Kuo 2009). The relationship between A-beta and phosphorylated tau paired helical filaments that accumulate in dying Alzheimer disease neurons is less clear (Querfurth and LaFerla 2010).

A-beta is released into the synaptic space during depolarization, raising the possibility that it functions as a neuromodulator of LTP and synaptogenesis (Wasling et al. 2009). The assumption of a physiological function for A-beta is suggested by recent reports of enhanced memory retention and acetylcholine production in hippocampus in response to low doses of A-beta, impaired learning in normal mice following inhibition of A-beta expression, and in-vitro inhibition of hippocampal and dentate gyrus LTP in the presence of A-beta antibodies (Morley et al. 2010). In complementary studies, A-beta 42 in picomolar concentrations facilitated hippocampal LTP whereas nanomolar quantities had the opposite effect. Concurrently picomolar levels of A-beta improved reference and fear memory (Puzzo et al. 2008).

Other products of amyloid precursor protein have potential physiological functions. Knockout mice, deficient in neprilysin an amyloid degrading endopeptidase, showed increased A-beta concentrations in the brain. Aged NEP knockout animals demonstrated significantly improved learning and memory and improved LTP in hippocampus and amygdala. This improvement may reflect increased levels of A-beta or other neuropeptides usually metabolized by NEP (Walther et al. 2009). Secreted amyloid precursor protein alpha (sAPP), a product of alpha secretase that incorporates a portion of the A-beta peptide facilitates LTP in rat dentate gyrus in vitro. Preferred production of A-beta at the expense of sAPP alpha may be another potential contributor of the memory deficits of AD (Kim and Tsai 2009; Lauren et al. 2009; Taylor et al. 2008; Bissette 2009). A key point is that dysregulation of A-beta production may be the principal mediator of both immediate adverse effects on cognition through impairment of LTP and longer-term injury-inducing effects in brain areas with the greatest synaptic plasticity.

In AD the earliest pathological changes occur in the hippocampus and parahippocampal gyrus, regions that are critical for learning and memory and like the cortical association areas demonstrate considerable synaptic plasticity (Braak and Braak 1991). Disruption of the tightly regulated function of A-beta as a modulator of synaptic plasticity could result in toxic concentrations of this peptide through a variety of mechanisms, some of which may be related to disturbances of sleep integrity, others to age-associated diseases, brain injury by various mechanisms, and the aging process itself. The fact that Alzheimer neuropathology first evolves in brain areas of high synaptic plasticity representing components of the memory retrieval network (posterior cortical regions, including posterior cingulate, retrosplenial, and lateral parietal cortex) where atrophy is prominent in AD implicates the relative vulnerability of the most dynamic parts of the brain to AD-related injury (Buckner et al. 2005, 2009).

These observations lead to a second question: might age and dementia-related decrements in sleep integrity disrupt tightly regulated A-beta mechanisms, facilitate A-beta production, increase neurotoxicity, and promote disease progression? Preliminary information provides initial support for this idea. First, both wild type and Amyloid precursor protein Tg2576 transgenic mice demonstrate diurnal variation in A-beta levels as shown by brain in-vivo microdialysis. Comparable changes have been observed in the spinal fluid of human volunteers. Higher levels of A-beta occur during periods of wakefulness, an effect that is likely mediated by orexin. In transgenic mice sleep deprivation, a form of physiologic stress, results in increased A-beta levels and enhanced amyloid plaque deposition. Notably restraint stress acutely increases A-beta concentrations, an effect mediated by corticotrophin releasing factor (Kang et al. 2009).

Second, studies of sleep and circadian abnormalities in Tg2576 Alzheimer model mice show changes that mimic those in aged humans and patients with AD (Zhang et al. 2005; Bliwise 2004). These animals demonstrated a blunted increase in electroencephalographic delta power (i.e., a loss of slow-wave sleep EEG frequencies) following sleep deprivation, longer periods of wheel running activity during dark (wake) periods, and a shift in EEG power to higher frequencies during nREM sleep as compared to normal controls (Wisor et al. 2005; Volicer et al. 2001). Whether dysregulation of A-beta production in these animals accounts for these sleep changes or the other way around remains to be seen.

If we accept the possibility that excess A-beta is a significant participant in the pathogenesis of AD, that sleep disruption increases A-beta production, and that sleep becomes lighter and more fragmented with age then it may be of value to explore potential relationships between aging, sleep, cognitive decline and dementia. As previously discussed, both learning and memory consolidation occur during REM and SWS (Diekelmann and Born 2010; Walker 2009; Stickgold and Walker 2007). Disruption of normal sleep patterns compromises these functions. Sleep deprivation impairs hippocampal LTP and synaptic plasticity while enhancing LTD (Tadavarty, Kaan, and Sastry 2009; Kopp et al. 2006; Guzman-Marin et al.

2006; McDermott et al. 2006). Similar disturbances occur following REM sleep deprivation and sleep fragmentation (Ravassard et al. 2009; Ishikawa et al. 2006; Tartar et al. 2006).

These neurobiological effects are largely reiterated in studies of the effects of A-beta peptide on hippocampal function. Soluble oligomers of A-beta peptide inhibit LTP and enhance LTD in the CA1 region of rat hippocampus, an effect mediated in part by inhibition of glutamate reuptake, and by disruption of LTP through inhibition of the N-methyl-D-apartate receptor-dependent LTP induction (Li et al. 2009; Yamin 2009). A-beta induces dendritic spine loss, while A-beta protein fragments 25-35 and 31-35 potentiate hippocampal CA1 LTD in vivo (Hsieh et al. 2006; Cheng et al. 2009).

To date there is no direct evidence that decrements in sleep quality associated with aging and dementia directly contribute to deficits in learning and memory, depression of LTP, and acceleration of neurodegenerative processes that occur in sleep-deprived animals. Nonetheless, a potential connection may be more likely in late life if age-related change and age-associated disease enhance brain vulnerability. Of particular interest are age-related changes in the adrenal-hippocampal, pituitary axis, the proinflammatory state of late life, impaired cerebrovascular autoregulation, and age-related disorders such as sleep apnea, periodic leg movements during sleep, and restless leg syndrome.

COMPONENTS OF AGING AND AGE-RELATED DISEASE PROCESSES THAT MAY ENHANCE THE PRODUCTION OF A-BETA

Glucocorticoids

Basal cortisol levels increase with age, an effect that is enhanced in AD with the diurnal peak in serum cortisol occurring early in the morning. Hippocampal glucocorticoid receptors mediate the effects of cortisol on the hippocampus that include inhibition of LTP in response to acute elevations and atrophy following chronic elevations. The electrochemical response to glucocorticoids may be directly mediated by elevated A-beta levels, resulting from increased production and blunted metabolism of the peptide. Moreover, stress levels of glucocorticoids increase A-beta and tau pathology in a mouse model of Alzheimer's disease (Catania et al. 2009; Green et al. 2006; Kulstad et al. 2005; Magri et al. 2006; McAuley et al. 2009; Sotiropoulos et al. 2008; Yao et al. 2007). Notably, the elevations of cortisol, catecholamines, and inflammatory markers characteristic of aging are induced in younger individuals by sleep deprivation (Galvao Mde et al. 2009; Leproult and Van Cauter 2010; Mullington et al. 2009; Stamatakis and Punjabi 2010). These, in turn may be associated with increased A-beta production (Kang et al. 2009).

Immune Function, Sleep and A-beta Production

Intrinsic immunity becomes increasingly pro-inflammatory with age, as reflected by a shift in the mix of circulating cytokines from an anti-inflammatory Th-1 to a Th-2 pro-inflammatory pattern. A similar pro-inflammatory cytokine shift occurs in the aging brain where neuro-inflammation is marked by increased numbers of activated and primed microglia that are hyperresponsive to systemic inflammatory signals or a stressor (Goshen and Yirmiya 2009; Dilger and Johnson 2008; Godbout and Johnson 2009; Sparkman and Johnson 2008). Peripheral inflammatory activity may be enhanced by sleep deprivation although the effect of sleep deprivation or fragmentation on the CNS inflammatory response has not been clearly defined (Irwin et al. 2008; Yehuda et al. 2009).

Proinflammatory mediators increase brain A-beta production. Such is the case for systemic administration of lipopolysaccharide to APPswe transgenic mice in which A-beta production is increased threefold. Prostaglandin E2 stimulates A-beta production in vitro and possibly in vivo. In-vitro, glial interferon gamma and tumor necrosis factor enhance A-beta production, directly stimulate the beta-site APP cleaving enzyme (BACE 1), and suppress A-beta degradation (Sheng et al. 2003; Hoshino et al. 2009; Yamamoto et al. 2007; Hoshino et al. 2007).

While there are many gaps in the data, one might consider the possibility that inefficient, fragmented, slow-wave-deficient sleep of old age contributes to a chronic stress response that results in increased A-beta production, an effect that is exaggerated within systemic and central nervous system environments of inflammatory hyperresponsiveness.

Any type of brain injury enhances production of A-beta, raising the possibility that this or other APP-derived peptides have another physiologic function in the acute response to injury. The injury response includes activation of inflammatory mediators. Traumatic brain injury is a well-established risk factor for AD such that dysregulation of the injury response may facilitate later development of a neurodegenerative disease. The relationships between the neurophysiologic and neurotoxic effects of A-beta and dysregulation of A-beta function through age associated changes in sleep, stress and inflammatory responses suggest a link between these variables that deserves further investigation (Mattson et al. 1997; Truettner, Suzuki, and Dietrich 2005; Van Den Heuvel, Thornton, and Vink 2007; Uryu et al. 2007).

Do Age-Related Conditions Enhance Brain Vulnerability to Degenerative Changes?

Sleep apnea, restless leg syndrome (RLS), and periodic leg movements during sleep (PLMS) are common in late life (Tarasiuk et al. 2008; Al Lawati, Patel, and Ayas 2009; Karatas 2007). Episodic hypoventilation during sleep apnea may be associated with oxygen desaturation. RLS and PLMS delay sleep onset or disrupt sleep continuity. The recurrent hypoxia associated with sleep apnea may be related to animal studies of cerebral hypoperfusion and ischemia, both of which have been associated with depression of LTP as well as increased A-beta production (Zhang et al. 2007; Li et al. 2010; Gasparova, Jariabka, and Stolc 2008; Guglielmotto et al. 2009).

Cerebrovascular dysfunction that occurs in AD has been related to deposition of A-beta in blood vessels in cerebral amyloid angiopathy (CAA). CAA occurs to varying degrees in nearly all patients with Alzheimer's disease and in 60–75% of normal octogenarians. CAA results in impaired vasodilator as well as vasoconstrictor responses, capillary occlusions, and microbleeds, all of which could potentially accelerate A-beta production in vulnerable areas of the brain (Shin et al. 2007; Thal et al. 2008).

Virtually no convincing evidence links age-related elevations in glucocorticoids to accelerated brain aging, the proinflammatory state of aging to neurodegeneration, or age-related reductions in sleep efficiency to decrements in learning and memory. These intriguing possibilities deserve further experimental exploration.

REM SLEEP BEHAVIOR DISORDER AND LEWY BODY DEMENTIA

In contrast to AD, the neuropathological processes of LBD and the other synucleopathies are first evident in the brainstem and disseminate rostrally, although recent reports cite a considerable number of exceptions to this pattern (Jellinger 2008; Jost 2010; Braak et al. 2004). To date no pathologically confirmed case of AD has been associated with REM sleep behavior disorder (RBD). This is a remarkable contrast to LBD, Parkinson's disease, and other synnucleopathies in which RBD prevalence may reach 40%. Sleep architecture is little studied in LBD although preliminary information suggests sleep fragmentation and loss of sleep efficiency

(McKeith et al. 2005; Jellinger 2008; Boeve, "Polysomnographic evidence" 2008).

Many components of sleep-regulatory mechanisms are mediated by the brainstem, basal forebrain, and hypothalamus, but the degeneration of specific cholinergic neurons in the PPT and laterodorsal tegmental nuclei as well as dopamine cell loss in the periaqueductal gray in LBD and multiple system atrophy are not clearly associated with RBD (Benarroch et al. 2009; Schmeichel et al. 2008). Excess loss of dopamine cells may be related to daytime sleepiness observed in LBD.

Cognitive deficits are identified in RBD, including poorer working memory, attention, visual and verbal memory, and executive function. Semantic memory, language, and visual perception are preserved. These deficits are mild but significant and are probably unrelated to specific RBD episodes because these typically occur infrequently, once or several times a month (Gagnon et al. 2009; Postuma, Gagnon, and Montplaisir 2008; Terzaghi et al. 2008; Massicotte-Marquez et al. 2008; Plazzi et al. 2005). Limited published data suggests that sleep architecture and sleep efficiency are not significantly altered in RBD, although a single study demonstrated EEG slowing in RBD patients comparable to that occurring in Alzheimer's disease both in the waking and sleeping states (Wetter et al. 2001; Fantini et al. 2003). Thus relative sleep deprivation does not appear to be a reasonable explanation for RBD cognitive deficits. Alternatively these findings may reflect the early phase of a more generalized degenerative process.

The pattern of cognitive deficits in LBD patients that is distinguished by impairments in attention, executive tasks, and particularly in visuospatial and constructional abilities is more severe and somewhat different than that of RBD. Such differences are useful in distinguishing LBD from AD in which deficits of memory and language are prominent, but provide no obvious connection with the mild deficits of RBD (Tiraboschi et al. 2006).

The presumed integrity of sleep architecture in RBD suggests that other manifestations of LBD, particularly visual hallucinations and illusions, are not mediated by the intrusion of sleep states, particularly REM dream material into wakefulness. These distortions of visual perception more likely reflect reduction of cholinergic input and hypometabolism of visual association areas related to cholinergic deafferentation from the basal forebrain (Klein et al. 2010).

Similarly, links between the sleep disturbances of LDB and its pathological mechanisms remain unidentified. Alpha synuclein is a nuclear and presynaptic protein that in LBD, Parkinson's disease, and other synucleopathies aggregates in intracellular inclusions known as Lewy bodies. The means by which aggregated alpha synuclein contributes to neuronal injury and death is less well defined as compared to the neurotoxicity of A-beta in AD. It does appear that in common with aggregated A-beta, aggregated alpha synuclein triggers microglial activation, neuroinflammation, and neuronal loss. The common co-occurrence of LBD and AD pathology suggests that progression of both diseases may be mediated by similar inflammatory mediators. Virtually no information relates sleep disturbances, physiological stress, glucocorticoids, or other age-related conditions to cognitive decline and disease progression in LBD (Roodveldt, Christodoulou, and Dobson 2008; Mrak and Griffin 2007; Sawada, Imamura, and Nagatsu 2006; Mackenzie 2000).

SUMMARY AND CONCLUSIONS

The chapter addresses two hypotheses: first, age-related disruption of sleep architecture, depth and efficiency directly contributes to cognitive changes associated with aging and dementia, particularly memory loss; second these sleep disturbances, combined with aging effects and age-associated diseases, accelerate neuropathological processes of the degenerative dementias. Sleep contributes to learning and memory consolidation. Sleep disruption has the opposite effects and neurophysiologic studies suggest mechanisms such as inhibition of LTP. Parallel investigations of A-beta, a probable mediator of AD, indicate that many A-beta toxic effects are comparable to those associated with sleep disruption, sleep deprivation, in turn, increases A-beta production. The toxicity of A-beta may be enhanced by age-related diseases and the pro-inflammatory environment of an aged brain. A-beta likely has physiologic functions such as modulation of synaptogenesis. Dysregulation of such functions with excess A-beta production results in neurotoxicity. The relatively limited data supporting these ideas may be worthy of further experimental investigations.

These speculations are not readily extrapolated to LBD but its frequent association with RBD as the earliest symptom indicates initial involvement of brainstem and midbrain sleep and arousal systems. Such involvement may be reflected by fluctuating cognition and variable levels of arousal and awareness associated with this illness. Such a connection has yet to be verified. Lack of evidence linking visual hallucinations of LBD or fluctuations in cognition and arousal to disturbance in sleep-regulating mechanisms is somewhat surprising. These phenomena are frequently observed in other disorders of sleep regulation such as narcolepsy and in normal individuals with sleep paralysis and hypnagogic hallucinations (Wurtman 2006; Cheyne 2005). Further studies of

RBD and LBD are likely to clarify relationships between the instability and dysregulation of sleep states, arousal mechanisms, cognition, and other manifestations of LBD that are likely to be more varied and complex than currently appreciated (Mahowald and Schenck 1991; Vetrugno et al. 2009).

Even when considered in isolation, mechanisms of aging, functions of sleep, and the fundamental causes of the degenerative dementias escape full understanding. In life the three are related and interactive at various levels of biological organization. Considering them together may provoke new questions and testable hypotheses.

ACKNOWLEDGMENT: This chapter is supported in part by the GRECC, VA Boston Healthcare System, Geriatric Research, Educational and Clinical Center, 150 South Huntington Avenue, Boston, MA, 02130.

REFERENCES

Al Lawati, N. M., S. R. Patel, and N. T. Ayas. 2009. Epidemiology, risk factors, and consequences of obstructive sleep apnea and short sleep duration. *Prog Cardiovasc Dis* 51: 285–293.

Aly, M., and M. Moscovitch. 2010. The effects of sleep on episodic memory in older and younger adults. *Memory* 18: 327–334.

American Psychiatric Association, ed. 2000. *Diagnostic and Statistical Manual of Mental Disorders (IV-TR)*. 4th ed. rev. Washington, DC.

Backhaus, J., J. Born, R. Hoeckesfeld, S. Fokuhl, F. Hohagen, and K. Junghanns. 2007. Midlife decline in declarative memory consolidation is correlated with a decline in slow wave sleep. *Learn Mem* 14: 336–341.

Banks, S., and D. F. Dinges. 2007. Behavioral and physiological consequences of sleep restriction. *J Clin Sleep Med* 3: 519–528.

Benarroch, E. E., A. M. Schmeichel, B. N. Dugger, P. Sandroni, J. E. Parisi, and P. A. Low. 2009. Dopamine cell loss in the periaqueductal gray in multiple system atrophy and Lewy body dementia. *Neurology* 73: 106–112.

Bissette, G. 2009. Does Alzheimer's disease result from attempts at repair or protection after transient stress? *J Alzheimers Dis* 18: 371–380.

Bliwise, D. L. 2004. Sleep disorders in Alzheimer's disease and other dementias. *Clin Cornerstone* 6 (Suppl 1A): S16–28.

Bloom, H. G., I. Ahmed, C. A. Alessi, et al. 2009. Evidence-based recommendations for the assessment and management of sleep disorders in older persons. *J Am Geriatr Soc* 57: 761–789.

Boeve, B. F. 2008. Polysomnographic evidence of sleep fragmentation and poor sleep efficiency in dementia with Lewy bodies. *Alzheimer's and Dementia* 4: T435.

Boeve, B. F. 2008. Update on the diagnosis and management of sleep disturbances in dementia. *Sleep Med Clin* 3: 347–360.

Boeve, B. F., M. H. Silber, C. B. Saper, et al. 2007. Pathophysiology of REM sleep behaviour disorder and relevance to neurodegenerative disease. *Brain* 130: 2770–2788.

Braak, H., and E. Braak. 1991. Neuropathological stageing of Alzheimer-related changes. *Acta Neuropathol* 82: 239–259.

Braak, H., and E. Braak. 1992. Anatomy of the human hypothalamus (chiasmatic and tuberal region). *Prog Brain Res* 93: 3–14.

Braak, H., K. Del Tredici, U. Rub, R. A. de Vos, E. N. Jansen Steur, and E. Braak. 2003. Staging of brain pathology related to sporadic Parkinson's disease. *Neurobiol Aging* 24: 197–211.

Braak, H., E. Ghebremedhin, U. Rub, H. Bratzke, and K. Del Tredici. 2004. Stages in the development of Parkinson's disease-related pathology. *Cell Tissue Res* 318: 121–134.

Buckner, R. L., J. Sepulcre, T. Talukdar, et al. 2009. Cortical hubs revealed by intrinsic functional connectivity: Mapping, assessment of stability, and relation to Alzheimer's disease. *J Neurosci* 29: 1860–1873.

Buckner, R. L., A. Z. Snyder, B. J. Shannon, et al. 2005. Molecular, structural, and functional characterization of Alzheimer's disease: Evidence for a relationship between default activity, amyloid, and memory. *J Neurosci* 25: 7709–7717.

Cajochen, C., M. Munch, V. Knoblauch, K. Blatter, and A. Wirz-Justice. 2006. Age-related changes in the circadian and homeostatic regulation of human sleep. *Chronobiol Int* 23: 461–474.

Catania, C., I. Sotiropoulos, R. Silva, et al. 2009. The amyloidogenic potential and behavioral correlates of stress. *Mol Psychiatry* 14: 95–105.

Chee, M. W., and L. Y. Chuah. 2008. Functional neuroimaging insights into how sleep and sleep deprivation affect memory and cognition. *Curr Opin Neurol* 21: 417–423.

Cheng, L., W. J. Yin, J. F. Zhang, and J. S. Qi. 2009. Amyloid beta-protein fragments 25-35 and 31-35 potentiate long-term depression in hippocampal CA1 region of rats in vivo. *Synapse* 63: 206–214.

Cheyne, J. A. 2005. Sleep paralysis episode frequency and number, types, and structure of associated hallucinations. *J Sleep Res* 14: 319–324.

Dauvilliers, Y. 2007. Insomnia in patients with neurodegenerative conditions. *Sleep Med* 8 (Suppl 4): S27–34.

Deschenes, C. L., and S. M. McCurry. 2009. Current treatments for sleep disturbances in individuals with dementia. *Curr Psychiatry Rep* 11: 20–26.

Diekelmann, S., and J. Born. 2010. The memory function of sleep. *Nat Rev Neurosci* 11: 114–126.

Dijk, D. J., J. A. Groeger, N. Stanley, and S. Deacon. 2010. Age-related reduction in daytime sleep propensity and nocturnal slow wave sleep. *Sleep* 33: 211–223.

Dilger, R. N., and R. W. Johnson. 2008. Aging, microglial cell priming, and the discordant central inflammatory response to signals from the peripheral immune system. *J Leukoc Biol* 84: 932–939.

Dubois, B., H. H. Feldman, C. Jacova, et al. 2007. Research criteria for the diagnosis of Alzheimer's disease: Revising the NINCDS-ADRDA criteria. *Lancet Neurol* 6: 734–746.

Espiritu, J. R. 2008. Aging-related sleep changes. *Clin Geriatr Med* 24: 1–14, v.

Fantini, M. L., J. F. Gagnon, D. Petit, et al. 2003. Slowing of electroencephalogram in rapid eye movement sleep behavior disorder. *Ann Neurol* 53: 774–780.

Fuller, P. M., J. J. Gooley, and C. B. Saper. 2006. Neurobiology of the sleep-wake cycle: Sleep architecture, circadian regulation, and regulatory feedback. *J Biol Rhythms* 21: 482–493.

Gagnon, J. F., D. Petit, V. Latreille, and J. Montplaisir. 2008. Neurobiology of sleep disturbances in neurodegenerative disorders. *Curr Pharm Des* 14: 3430–3445.

Gagnon, J. F., M. Vendette, R. B. Postuma, et al. 2009. Mild cognitive impairment in rapid eye movement sleep behavior disorder and Parkinson's disease. *Ann Neurol* 66: 39–47.

Galvao Mde, O., R. Sinigaglia-Coimbra, S. E. Kawakami, S. Tufik, and D. Suchecki. 2009. Paradoxical sleep deprivation activates hypothalamic nuclei that regulate food intake and stress response. *Psychoneuroendocrinology* 34: 1176–1183.

Garcia-Rill, E., A. Charlesworth, D. Heister, M. Ye, and A. Hayar. 2008. The developmental decrease in REM sleep: The role of transmitters and electrical coupling. *Sleep* 31: 673–690.

Gasparova, Z., P. Jariabka, and S. Stolc. 2008. Effect of transient ischemia on long-term potentiation of synaptic transmission in rat hippocampal slices. *Neuro Endocrinol Lett* 29: 702–705.

Godbout, J. P., and R. W. Johnson. 2009. Age and neuroinflammation: A lifetime of psychoneuroimmune consequences. *Immunol Allergy Clin North Am* 29: 321–337.

Goshen, I., and R. Yirmiya. 2009. Interleukin-1 (IL-1): A central regulator of stress responses. *Front Neuroendocrinol* 30: 30–45.

Goudsmit, E., M. A. Hofman, E. Fliers, and D. F. Swaab. 1990. The supraoptic and paraventricular nuclei of the human hypothalamus in relation to sex, age and Alzheimer's disease. *Neurobiol Aging* 11: 529–536.

Green, K. N., L. M. Billings, B. Roozendaal, J. L. McGaugh, and F. M. LaFerla. 2006. Glucocorticoids increase amyloid-beta and tau pathology in a mouse model of Alzheimer's disease. *J Neurosci* 26: 9047–9056.

Guglielmotto, M., M. Aragno, R. Autelli, et al. 2009. The up-regulation of BACE1 mediated by hypoxia and ischemic injury: Role of oxidative stress and HIF1alpha. *J Neurochem* 108: 1045–1056.

Guzman-Marin, R., Z. Ying, N. Suntsova, et al. 2006. Suppression of hippocampal plasticity-related gene expression by sleep deprivation in rats. *J Physiol* 575: 807–819.

Hobson, J. A. 2009. REM sleep and dreaming: Towards a theory of protoconsciousness. *Nat Rev Neurosci* 10: 803–813.

Hoshino, T., T. Nakaya, T. Homan, et al. 2007. Involvement of prostaglandin E2 in production of amyloid-beta peptides both in vitro and in vivo. *J Biol Chem* 282: 32676–32688.

Hoshino, T., T. Namba, M. Takehara, et al. 2009. Prostaglandin E2 stimulates the production of amyloid-beta peptides through internalization of the EP4 receptor. *J Biol Chem* 284: 18493–18502.

Hsieh, H., J. Boehm, C. Sato, et al. 2006. AMPAR removal underlies A-beta-induced synaptic depression and dendritic spine loss. *Neuron* 52: 831–843.

Iranzo, A., J. Santamaria, and E. Tolosa. 2009. The clinical and pathophysiological relevance of REM sleep behavior disorder in neurodegenerative diseases. *Sleep Med Rev* 13: 385–401.

Irwin, M. R., M. Wang, D. Ribeiro, et al. 2008. Sleep loss activates cellular inflammatory signaling. *Biol Psychiatry* 64: 538–540.

Ishikawa, A., Y. Kanayama, H. Matsumura, H. Tsuchimochi, Y. Ishida, and S. Nakamura. 2006. Selective rapid eye movement sleep deprivation impairs the maintenance of long-term potentiation in the rat hippocampus. *Eur J Neurosci* 24: 243–248.

Jellinger, K. 1988. The pedunculopontine nucleus in Parkinson's disease, progressive supranuclear palsy and Alzheimer's disease. *J Neurol Neurosurg Psychiatry* 51: 540–543.

Jellinger, K. A. 2008. A critical reappraisal of current staging of Lewy-related pathology in human brain. *Acta Neuropathol* 116: 1–16.

Jost, W. H. 2010. Gastrointestinal dysfunction in Parkinson's Disease. *J Neurol Sci* 289: 69–73.

Kang, J. E., M. M. Lim, R. J. Bateman, et al. 2009. Amyloid-beta dynamics are regulated by orexin and the sleep-wake cycle. *Science* 326: 1005–1007.

Karatas, M. 2007. Restless legs syndrome and periodic limb movements during sleep: Diagnosis and treatment. *Neurologist* 13: 294–301.

Kazee, A. M., and L. Y. Han. 1995. Cortical Lewy bodies in Alzheimer's disease. *Arch Pathol Lab Med* 119: 448–453.

Kim, D., and L. H. Tsai. 2009. Bridging physiology and pathology in AD. *Cell* 137: 997–1000.

Klein, J. C., C. Eggers, E. Kalbe, et al. 2010. Neurotransmitter changes in dementia with Lewy bodies and Parkinson disease dementia in vivo. *Neurology* 74: 885–892.

Kopp, C., F. Longordo, J. R. Nicholson, and A. Luthi. 2006. Insufficient sleep reversibly alters bidirectional synaptic plasticity and NMDA receptor function. *J Neurosci* 26: 12456–12465.

Kulstad, J. J., P. J. McMillan, J. B. Leverenz, et al. 2005. Effects of chronic glucocorticoid administration on insulin-degrading enzyme and amyloid-beta peptide in the aged macaque. *J Neuropathol Exp Neurol* 64: 139–146.

Lauren, J., D. A. Gimbel, H. B. Nygaard, J. W. Gilbert, and S. M. Strittmatter. 2009. Cellular prion protein mediates impairment of synaptic plasticity by amyloid-beta oligomers. *Nature* 457: 1128–1132.

Leproult, R., and E. Van Cauter. 2010. Role of sleep and sleep loss in hormonal release and metabolism. *Endocr Dev* 17: 11–21.

Li, S., S. Hong, N. E. Shepardson, D. M. Walsh, G. M. Shankar, and D. Selkoe. 2009. Soluble oligomers of amyloid beta protein facilitate hippocampal long-term depression by disrupting neuronal glutamate uptake. *Neuron* 62: 788–801.

Li, S., W. Wang, C. Wang, and Y. Y. Tang. 2010. Possible involvement of NO/NOS signaling in hippocampal amyloid-beta production induced by transient focal cerebral ischemia in aged rats. *Neurosci Lett* 470: 106–110.

Mackenzie, I. R. 2000. Activated microglia in dementia with Lewy bodies. *Neurology* 55: 132–34.

Magri, F., L. Cravello, L. Barili, et al. 2006. Stress and dementia: The role of the hypothalamicpituitary-adrenal axis. *Aging Clin Exp Res* 18: 167–170.

Mahowald, M. W., and C. H. Schenck. 1991. Status dissociates—A perspective on states of being. *Sleep* 14: 69–79.

Mahowald, M. W., C. H. Schenck, and M. A. Bornemann. 2007. Pathophysiologic mechanisms in REM sleep behavior disorder. *Curr Neurol Neurosci Rep* 7: 167–172.

Massicotte-Marquez, J., A. Decary, J. F. Gagnon, et al. 2008. Executive dysfunction and memory impairment in idiopathic REM sleep behavior disorder. *Neurology* 70: 1250–1257.

Mattson, M. P., S. W. Barger, K. Furukawa, et al. 1997. Cellular signaling roles of TGF beta, TNF alpha and beta APP in brain injury responses and Alzheimer's disease. *Brain Res Brain Res Rev* 23: 47–61.

McAuley, M. T., R. A. Kenny, T. B. Kirkwood, D. J. Wilkinson, J. J. Jones, and V. M. Miller. 2009. A mathematical model of aging-related and cortisol induced hippocampal dysfunction. *BMC Neurosci* 10: 26.

McDermott, C. M., M. N. Hardy, N. G. Bazan, and J. C. Magee. 2006. Sleep deprivation-induced alterations in excitatory synaptic transmission in the CA1 region of the rat hippocampus. *J Physiol* 570: 553–565.

McKeith, I. G., D. W. Dickson, J. Lowe, et al. 2005. Diagnosis and management of dementia with Lewy bodies: Third report of the DLB Consortium. *Neurology* 65: 1863–1872.

McKhann, G., D. Drachman, M. Folstein, R. Katzman, D. Price, and E. M. Stadlan. 1984. Clinical diagnosis of Alzheimer's disease: Report of the NINCDS-ADRDA Work Group under the auspices of Department of Health and Human Services Task Force on Alzheimer's Disease. *Neurology* 34: 939–944.

Mirmiran, M., D. F. Swaab, J. H. Kok, M. A. Hofman, W. Witting, and W. A. Van Gool. 1992. Circadian rhythms and the suprachiasmatic nucleus in perinatal development, aging and Alzheimer's disease. *Prog Brain Res* 93: 151–162; discussion 162–153.

Monti, J. M., and D. Monti. 2007. The involvement of dopamine in the modulation of sleep and waking. *Sleep Med Rev* 11: 113–133.

Morley, J. E., S. A. Farr, W. A. Banks, S. N. Johnson, K. A. Yamada, and L. Xu. 2010. A physiological role for amyloid-beta protein: Enhancement of learning and memory. *J Alzheimers Dis* 19: 441–449.

Mrak, R. E., and W. S. Griffin. 2007. Common inflammatory mechanisms in Lewy body disease and Alzheimer disease. *J Neuropathol Exp Neurol* 66: 683–686.

Mufson, E. J., D. C. Mash, and L. B. Hersh. 1988. Neurofibrillary tangles in cholinergic pedunculopontine neurons in Alzheimer's disease. *Ann Neurol* 24: 623–629.

Mullington, J. M., M. Haack, M. Toth, J. M. Serrador, and H. K. Meier-Ewert. 2009. Cardiovascular, inflammatory, and metabolic consequences of sleep deprivation. *Prog Cardiovasc Dis* 51: 294–302.

Ohayon, M. M., M. A. Carskadon, C. Guilleminault, and M. V. Vitiello. 2004. Meta-analysis of quantitative sleep parameters from childhood to old age in healthy individuals: Developing normative sleep values across the human lifespan. *Sleep* 27: 1255–1273.

Phillips, R. J., G. C. Walter, S. L. Wilder, E. A. Baronowsky, and T. L. Powley. 2008. Alpha-synuclein-immunopositive myenteric neurons and vagal preganglionic terminals: Autonomic pathway implicated in Parkinson's disease? *Neuroscience* 153: 733–750.

Plazzi, G., R. Vetrugno, F. Provini, and P. Montagna. 2005. Sleepwalking and other ambulatory behaviours during sleep. *Neurol Sci* 26 (Suppl 3): s193–198.

Postuma, R. B., J. F. Gagnon, and J. Montplaisir. 2008. Cognition in REM sleep behavior disorder—A window into preclinical dementia? *Sleep Med* 9: 341–342.

Postuma, R. B., J. F. Gagnon, M. Vendette, and J. Y. Montplaisir. 2009. Idiopathic REM sleep behavior disorder in the transition to degenerative disease. *Mov Disord* 24: 2225–2232.

Puzzo, D., L. Privitera, E. Leznik, et al. 2008. Picomolar amyloid-beta positively modulates synaptic plasticity and memory in hippocampus. *J Neurosci* 28: 14537–14545.

Querfurth, H. W., and F. M. LaFerla. 2010. Alzheimer's disease. *N Engl J Med* 362: 329–344.

Ransmayr, G., B. Faucheux, C. Nowakowski, et al. 2000. Age-related changes of neuronal counts in the human pedunculopontine nucleus. *Neurosci Lett* 288: 195–198.

Rauchs, G., M. Schabus, S. Parapatics, et al. 2008. Is there a link between sleep changes and memory in Alzheimer's disease? *NeuroReport* 19: 1159–1162.

Ravassard, P., B. Pachoud, J. C. Comte, et al. 2009. Paradoxical (REM) sleep deprivation causes a large and rapidly reversible decrease in long-term potentiation, synaptic transmission, glutamate receptor protein levels, and ERK/MAPK activation in the dorsal hippocampus. *Sleep* 32: 227–240.

Redline, S., H. L. Kirchner, S. F. QuanF, D. J. Gottlieb, V. Kapur, and A. Newman. 2004. The effects of age, sex, ethnicity, and sleep-disordered breathing on sleep architecture. *Arch Intern Med* 164: 406–418.

Roodveldt, C., J. Christodoulou, and C. M. Dobson. 2008. Immunological features of alpha-synuclein in Parkinson's disease. *J Cell Mol Med* 12: 1820–1829.

Saper, C. B., and D. C. German. 1987. Hypothalamic pathology in Alzheimer's disease. *Neurosci Lett* 74: 364–370.

Saper, C. B., T. E. Scammell, and J. Lu. 2005. Hypothalamic regulation of sleep and circadian rhythms. *Nature* 437: 1257–1263.

Sawada, M., K. Imamura, and T. Nagatsu. 2006. Role of cytokines in inflammatory process in Parkinson's disease. *J Neural Transm* (Suppl) 70: 373–381.

Schabus, M., T. T. Dang-Vu, G. Albouy, et al. 2007. Hemodynamic cerebral correlates of sleep spindles during human non-rapid eye movement sleep. *Proc Natl Acad Sci USA* 104: 13164–13169.

Schmeichel, A. M., L. C. Buchhalter, P. A. Low, et al. 2008. Mesopontine cholinergic neuron involvement in Lewy body dementia and multiple system atrophy. *Neurology* 70: 368–373.

Schneider, J. A., Z. Arvanitakis, S. E. Leurgans, and D. A. Bennett. 2009. The neuropathology of probable Alzheimer disease and mild cognitive impairment. *Ann Neurol* 66: 200–208.

Schwartz, J. R., and T. Roth. 2008. Neurophysiology of sleep and wakefulness: Basic science and clinical implications. *Curr Neuropharmacol* 6: 367–378.

Sheng, J. G., S. H. Bora, G. Xu, D. R. Borchelt, D. L. Price, and V. E. Koliatsos. 2003. Lipopolysaccharide-induced-neuroinflammation increases intracellular accumulation of amyloid precursor protein and amyloid beta peptide in APPswe transgenic mice. *Neurobiol Dis* 14: 133–145.

Shin, H. K., P. B. Jones, M. Garcia-Alloza, et al. 2007. Age-dependent cerebrovascular dysfunction in a transgenic mouse model of cerebral amyloid angiopathy. *Brain* 130: 2310–2319.

Sotiropoulos, I., C. Catania, T. Riedemann, et al. 2008. Glucocorticoids trigger Alzheimer disease-like pathobiochemistry in rat neuronal cells expressing human tau. *J Neurochem* 107: 385–397.

Sparkman, N. L., and R. W. Johnson. 2008. Neuroinflammation associated with aging sensitizes the brain to the effects of infection or stress. *Neuroimmunomodulation* 15: 323–330.

Stamatakis, K. A., and N. M. Punjabi. 2010. Effects of sleep fragmentation on glucose metabolism in normal subjects. *Chest* 137: 95–101.

Steriade, M. 1999. Coherent oscillations and short-term plasticity in corticothalamic networks. *Trends Neurosci* 22: 337–345.

Sterpenich, V., G. Albouy, M. Boly, et al. 2007. Sleep-related hippocampo-cortical interplay during emotional memory recollection. *PLoS Biol* 5: e282.

Stickgold, R., and M. P. Walker. 2007. Sleep-dependent memory consolidation and reconsolidation. *Sleep Med* 8: 331–343.

Szymusiak, R., I. Gvilia, and D. McGinty. 2007. Hypothalamic control of sleep. *Sleep Med* 8: 291–301.

Tadavarty, R., T. K. Kaan, and B. R. Sastry. 2009. Long-term depression of excitatory synaptic transmission in rat hippocampal CA1 neurons following sleep-deprivation. *Exp Neurol* 216: 239–242.

Tarasiuk, A., S. Greenberg-Dotan, T. Simon-Tuval, A. Oksenberg, and H. Reuveni. 2008. The effect of obstructive sleep apnea on morbidity and health care utilization of middle-aged and older adults. *J Am Geriatr Soc* 56: 247–254.

Tartar, J. L., C. P. Ward, J. T. McKenna, et al. 2006. Hippocampal synaptic plasticity and spatial learning are impaired in a rat model of sleep fragmentation. *Eur J Neurosci* 23: 2739–2748.

Taylor, C. J., D. R. Ireland, I. Ballagh, et al. 2008. Endogenous secreted amyloid precursor protein-alpha regulates hippocampal NMDA receptor function, long-term potentiation and spatial memory. *Neurobiol Dis* 31: 250–260.

Terzaghi, M., E. Sinforiani, C. Zucchella, et al. 2008. Cognitive performance in REM sleep behaviour disorder: A possible early marker of neurodegenerative disease? *Sleep Med* 9: 343–351.

Thal, D. R., W. S. Griffin, R. A. de Vos, and E. Ghebremedhin. 2008. Cerebral amyloid angiopathy and its relationship to Alzheimer's disease. *Acta Neuropathol* 115: 599–609.

Thal, D. R., U. Rub, M. Orantes, and H. Braak. 2002. Phases of A beta-deposition in the human brain and its relevance for the development of AD. *Neurology* 58: 1791–1800.

Tiraboschi, P., D. P. Salmon, L. A. Hansen, R. C. Hofstetter, L. J. Thal, and J. Corey-Bloom. 2006. What best differentiates Lewy body from Alzheimer's disease in early-stage dementia? *Brain* 129: 729–735.

Truettner, J. S., T. Suzuki, and W. D. Dietrich. 2005. The effect of therapeutic hypothermia on the expression of inflammatory response genes following moderate traumatic brain injury in the rat. *Brain Res Mol Brain Res* 138: 124–134.

Uryu, K., X. H. Chen, D. Martinez, et al. 2007. Multiple proteins implicated in neurodegenerative diseases accumulate in axons after brain trauma in humans. *Exp Neurol* 208: 185–192.

Van Den Heuvel, C., E. Thornton, and R. Vink. 2007. Traumatic brain injury and Alzheimer's disease: A review. *Prog Brain Res* 161: 303–316.

Vassalli, A., and D. J. Dijk. 2009. Sleep function: current questions and new approaches. *Eur J Neurosci* 29: 1830–1841.

Vetrugno, R., M. Alessandria, R. D'Angelo, et al. 2009. Status dissociatus evolving from REM sleep behaviour disorder in multiple system atrophy. *Sleep Med* 10: 247–252.

Volicer, L., D. G. Harper, B. C. Manning, R. Goldstein, and A. Satlin. 2001. Sundowning and circadian rhythms in Alzheimer's disease. *Am J Psychiatry* 158: 704–711.

Walker, M. P. 2008. Cognitive consequences of sleep and sleep loss. *Sleep Med* 9 (Suppl 1): S29–34.

Walker, M. P. 2009. The role of sleep in cognition and emotion. *Ann NY Acad Sci* 1156: 168–197.

Walther, T., D. Albrecht, M. Becker, et al. 2009. Improved learning and memory in aged mice deficient in amyloid beta-degrading neutral endopeptidase. *PLoS One* 4: e4590.

Wasling, P., J. Daborg, I. Riebe, et al. 2009. Synaptic retrogenesis and amyloid-beta in Alzheimer's disease. *J Alzheimers Dis* 16: 1–14.

Wetter, T. C., C. Trenkwalder, O. Gershanik, and B. Hogl. 2001. Polysomnographic measures in Parkinson's disease: a comparison between patients with and without REM sleep disturbances. *Wien Klin Wochenschr* 113: 249–253.

Wisor, J. P., D. M. Edgar, J. Yesavage, et al. 2005. Sleep and circadian abnormalities in a transgenic mouse model of Alzheimer's disease: a role for cholinergic transmission. *Neuroscience* 131: 375–385.

Wurtman, R. J. 2006. Narcolepsy and the hypocretins. *Metabolism* 55: S36–39.

Yamamoto, M., T. Kiyota, M. Horiba, et al. 2007. Interferon-gamma and tumor necrosis factor-alpha regulate amyloid-beta plaque deposition and beta-secretase expression in Swedish mutant APP transgenic mice. *Am J Pathol* 170: 680–692.

Yamin, G. 2009. NMDA receptor-dependent signaling pathways that underlie amyloid beta-protein disruption of LTP in the hippocampus. *J Neurosci Res* 87: 1729–1736.

Yang, T. T., C. T. Hsu, and Y. M. Kuo. 2009. Cell-derived soluble oligomers of human amyloid-beta peptides disturb cellular homeostasis and induce apoptosis in primary hippocampal neurons. *J Neural Transm* 116: 1561–1569.

Yao, Y. Y., D. M. Liu, D. F. Xu, and W. P. Li. 2007. Memory and learning impairment induced by dexamethasone in senescent but not young mice. *Eur J Pharmacol* 574: 20–28.

Yehuda, S., B. Sredni, R. L. Carasso, and D. Kenigsbuch-Sredni. 2009. REM sleep deprivation in rats results in inflammation and interleukin-17 elevation. *J Interferon Cytokine Res* 29: 393–398.

Zhang, B., S. C. Veasey, M. A. Wood, et al. 2005. Impaired rapid eye movement sleep in the Tg2576 APP murine model of Alzheimer's disease with injury to pedunculopontine cholinergic neurons. *Am J Pathol* 167: 1361–1369.

Zhang, X., K. Zhou, R. Wang, et al. 2007. Hypoxia-inducible factor 1alpha (HIF-1alpha)-mediated hypoxia increases BACE1 expression and beta-amyloid generation. *J Biol Chem* 282: 10873–10880.

Zweig, R. M., W. R. Jankel, J. C. Hedreen, R. Mayeux, and D. L. Price. 1989. The pedunculopontine nucleus in Parkinson's disease. *Ann Neurol* 26: 41–46.

Chapter 9

Magnetic Resonance Spectroscopy: A Tool for Understanding Brain Chemical Changes in Dementias

Jacquelynn N. Copeland and
H. Randall Griffith

With the number of older adults in the United States projected to grow larger than ever over the next few decades, prevalence of dementia is also expected to rise. Therefore, early detection of neurodegenerative disease processes is a growing concern. In addition, more accurate diagnosis and treatment planning are imperative. *Neuroimaging* is a term describing different methods utilized to "visualize" changes in the brain. With the computer revolution over the past several decades, neuroimaging has become an important means of detecting and diagnosing neurological diseases, including those that cause dementias.

While all neuroimaging techniques help us to "see" some aspect of the brain, each technique provides distinct information about the brain, its function, and its dysfunction. Generally speaking, neuroimaging can be divided into two broad categories, structural and functional imaging. Structural imaging allows for the anatomy of the brain to be visualized, while functional imaging provides a means of seeing changes in blood flow, metabolism, or chemistry of the brain; both structural and functional neuroimaging have their place in research as well as clinical practice. Some types of neuroimaging that are used for dementia include structural imaging techniques such as magnetic resonance imaging (MRI), computed tomography (CT), and diffusion tensor imaging (DTI), along with functional imaging techniques including functional magnetic resonance imaging (fMRI), positron emission tomography (PET), single photon emission computed tomography (SPECT), and magnetic resonance spectroscopy (MRS).These techniques help identify abnormalities that may aid clinicians in making accurate diagnoses, prescribing the appropriate treatment, examining treatment response, and monitoring brain changes over time. The most common neuroimaging techniques used initially when a patient presents with cognitive impairment or dementia like symptoms are a CT scan or an MRI scan, which both show brain structure.

CT is less expensive and used primarily to rule out any potentially reversible causes of dementia such as brain tumor, stroke, bleeding, or normal-pressure hydrocephalus, a condition where excess fluid gradually builds up in the brain, resulting in dementia-like symptoms. In addition, CT can also reveal abnormal atrophy, or deterioration of brain volume, in general, or in particular regions of the brain (Petrella, Coleman, and Doraiswamy 2003; Scheltens et al. 2002). For instance, the medial temporal lobe and hippocampus, integral for learning and memory, along with other temporal and parietal regions and areas of the frontal lobe may be of particular importance to image for a patient with suspected dementia. A standard structural MRI is also sensitive to these conditions; in addition, an MRI can display different aspects regarding the makeup of the brain, such as the grey and white matter, and has the ability to detect other abnormalities such as white-matter hyperintensities, which show up on MRI as ultra-white patches, or lacunar infarcts, small areas of cell death caused by occlusion of small blood vessels in deeper parts of the brain, which both may contribute to a presentation of vascular dementia (Small et al. 2008).

Although CT and MRI are commonly used for dementia workups, they are particularly limiting when no structural changes are observable, like in early stages of dementia or mild cognitive impairment (MCI), a stage of cognitive difficulties between normal aging and dementia. In these cases, the neuropathological disease process, or the changes in the brain related to the course of the disease, may not have yet affected the overall structure of brain tissue; however, cognitive difficulties and symptoms may be present due to functional changes in brain tissue chemistry or metabolism that have yet to affect the structure of the brain that can be seen on MRI or CT. Thus, functional imaging can provide valuable information about biological and chemical changes occurring in the brain and can support clinicians in early detection and diagnosis of dementia when structural changes are absent. Furthermore, even when structural imaging reveals atrophy or other findings suggestive of dementia, functional imaging gives the doctors a way of understanding how the structural changes have affected the brain's working. However, it is important to remember that neuroimaging is only one piece of information that clinicians use when conducting a dementia workup, making a diagnosis, and providing treatment.

MAGNETIC RESONANCE SPECTROSCOPY

Magnetic resonance spectroscopy (MRS) is a functional imaging technique that provides information regarding different metabolites, or molecules that play important roles in the functioning of brain cells. MRS works by the same physical principles as does a standard MRI, that being the use of a strong magnetic field and radio-frequency signals. The primary difference between MRI and MRS is that in MRS scans the data obtained by the MR scanner is interpreted based upon the chemical composition of the area of the body being imaged, while in MRI the radio-frequency signal is reconstructed into an image. MRS works based upon the type of molecule that is being measured; of which several molecules can be "visualized," including those containing the ions hydrogen (^{1}H), phosphorus (^{31}P), carbon (^{13}C), and fluorine (^{18}F). The most common form of MRS measures brain chemicals based upon the presence and number of the hydrogen ions in different molecules (Minati, Grisali, and Bruzzone 2007), specifically referred to as proton magnetic resonance spectroscopy (^{1}H MRS) to define use of the hydrogen nucleus in contrast to other forms of MRS. Research supports the use of ^{1}H MRS with suspected dementia cases because of its accessibility, sensitivity to detection by an MR signal, and good spatial resolution (Jones and Waldman 2004; Ross and Bluml 2001). Before conducting an MRS scan, the clinician chooses a region of interest; these regions are usually areas of the brain where metabolic changes often occur, or in some instances can be a whole slice of the brain, similar to what one snapshot from an MRI scan would show.

The MRS scan then measures the concentrations of measurable brain chemicals in this region by sending in radio-frequency (RF) signals to vibrate the ions, which then respond back with their own identifiable RF, based upon the quantity of hydrogen ions in the molecules in that region. Instead of being constructed into an image as in an MRI, the data received from the scanner is plotted out into a fourier transform graph. This graph displays the relative concentrations, based on the RF signal intensity of the molecule, where higher signal intensity (peaks on the graph) indicates higher relative concentration of the brain chemicals, known as metabolites as they are the by-products of brain metabolism. Of note, concentrations are most often expressed as a ratio rather than absolute concentrations due to quantification and measurement difficulties. In addition, metabolites have different spectral patterns, such that some may have one peak, two peaks, or multiple peaks. The parameters of the the MRI RF scanning sequence, such as echo time (TE), also result in slightly different outputs, while increasing the magnetic strength of MRI scanner, such as doubling the magnet strength from 1.5 Tesla (or 30,000 times the strength of the Earth's magnetic field) to 3 Tesla (or 60,000 times the strength of the earth's magnetic field), helps separate the peaks and improves the ability to distinguish among metabolites.

Common metabolites measured in ^{1}H MRS include choline (Cho), creatine (Cr), glutamate-glutamine (Glx), myo-Inositol (mI), scyllo-Inositol (sI), and N-acetyleaspartate (NAA). Each metabolite is thought to represent a metabolic process (or processes) occurring in the brain, such as those associated with integrity of brain cells or breakdown of brain cell tissue. In the brain, most of these metabolites can be compared with the concentration of Cr, which is usually present at constant levels in all living tissue. Using these ratios, it is possible to establish levels of normal and abnormal concentration of metabolites in certain brain areas, such that abnormally low or high MRS ratios may indicate presence of brain diseases, such as Alzheimer's disease. Thus, MRS can measure biochemical information of a chosen area of the brain of a patient with suspected dementia, which can be compared directly to the typical metabolite ratios found in a same-age adult with no cognitive complaints or brain abnormalities. Abnormal metabolite ratios can serve as additional evidence supporting a specific diagnosis along with information collected from patient medical history, cognitive functioning, and structural imaging. Furthermore, MRS can be repeated over time and can be valuable to measure progression of the disease as well as response to potential medication treatments.

Advantages of MRS

The data provided by MRS is relatively unique and the technique is generally safe and readily available. Although other functional imaging techniques such as PET measure metabolic processes in the brain (such as use of glucose), MRS is the only technique that provides data concerning multiple metabolites within the same scan. Furthermore, MRS is particularly advantageous as it can be obtained within specified regions of the brain and is particularly useful when a specific area of the brain is commonly targeted by neuropathological disease processes, such as the posterior areas of the brain in Alzheimer's disease. MRS is noninvasive and does not require injection of radioactive materials or any surgical procedures. In many instances this type of data can be obtained along with a clinical MRI scan and does not add unreasonable time burdens on the patient. Thus, information regarding the brain's structure and function can be collected in one session and used together to evaluate disease. MRS can also be conducted on many of the clinically available MRI scanners, which means it has the potential to be utilized at many hospitals in the United States and worldwide.

Limitations of MRS

Most studies using MRS have measured metabolic ratios in specific regions of interest rather than examining whole brain ratios. Other functional imaging techniques may be more beneficial for examining overall brain functioning. Overall, low specificity is a main disadvantage of MRS. That is, information and interpretation of metabolites can be somewhat unclear because some metabolites are very close to one another on the spectrum, especially with lower magnetic strength scanners, such as 1.5 Tesla. Additionally, MRS is very susceptible to distortion by nonbrain-tissue signals, such as signals arising from bone and air in the sinuses and fat deposits in the scalp. Choosing the area of the brain from which the MRS signal will be measured thus requires avoiding areas close to the skull and scalp, as well as close to the base of the brain, where there is signal contamination from the sinuses. However, future advances in technology will likely address some of these limitations. In addition, MRS is currently considered a new and investigational technique, but has the potential to become more commonly used clinically to aid in dementia workups and diagnosis. In combination with other MRI imaging techniques, MRS has the potential to become an important adjunct in the clinical diagnosis of dementias.

COMPARISON OF MRS TO OTHER NEUROIMAGING TECHNIQUES

Comparison of MRS to Structural Techniques

MRS and structural MRI use the same hardware, a magnetic resonance scanner, and use similar RF sequences to excite or "pulse" molecules. The critical difference is in how the resulting RF signal from the body tissue being studied is compiled and analyzed. In structural MRI, RF signal data is constructed to display images of the brain's physical structures in high resolution, while MRS measures resonances of RF signal at different frequencies, which are "shifted" from the reference signal (most commonly the H_2O signal) depending on the concentration of metabolites. It is this "chemical shift," measured in parts-per-million (ppm), by which the metabolites are identified and quantified. Unlike MRS, which most often focuses on a region of interest, images created from an MRI typically (but not always) display the whole brain; however, images are created at different angles, called planes, each with a varying number of slices depending on the pulse sequence used during the MRI scan. Various anatomical structures can be identified depending on the particular slices examined and the plane of imaging. Furthermore, structural MRI analysis techniques can be used to measure volumes of particular structures using MRI images.

Another type of MR structural imaging, DTI, measures how water diffuses across membranes in the brain to create images of the nerve bundle pathways in the brain, which connect different parts of the brain to one another. DTI is useful for identifying these nerve bundle paths (or "white matter" paths, referred to because the fatty sheath that lines the nerves makes these tissues white compared to the brain cells, or neurons, which appear "grey" to the naked eye) because water diffuses along these white-matter paths in a uniform fashion, as compared to a random diffusion within the grey matter. Unlike MRI, which images both white and grey matter in the brain, DTI focuses solely on white-matter tracts and supplies information regarding their integrity and orientation. Thus, in contrast to MRS, which can reveal abnormal metabolite ratios in a chosen area of the brain, DTI provides information regarding changes in connectivity in the brain, which may indicate less efficiency or diminished ability for communication between various aspects of the brain. However, structural MRI and DTI only provide information about structure, and cannot provide information regarding brain function.

MRS Compared to Functional Imaging Techniques

In addition to MRS, another functional technique that utilizes MR hardware is called fMRI. Although fMRI and MRS both utilize magnetic fields to supply information regarding the brain's functioning, fMRI measures changes in signal intensity to represent changes in oxygen content of the blood as it is used by the brain cells. fMRI mostly is obtained while an active cognitive task is completed within the scanner so the difference in blood oxygenation concentration can be compared when the brain is engaged in a cognitive task versus when at "rest." Areas of the brain that show more oxygen use during a task are considered to be "activated." Like MRS, though, fMRI has the ability to potentially identify functional abnormalities not seen on standard structural imaging. Finally, practical difficulties caused by the cognitive paradigms used during fMRI make it somewhat difficult for patients with dementias to maintain focus during the long periods required to complete a full fMRI scanning session. Recent advances in resting fMRI may obviate the need to use cognitive tasks within the scanner and may be able to provide information regarding changes in the efficiency of brain function. When used clinically, fMRI is potentially less expensive and is less invasive than PET (Small et al. 2008).

PET, on the other hand, applies a different type of functional neuroimaging technology that requires intravenous injection of a radioactive tracer and imaging of this tracer in the brain, such that cerebral blood flow, utilization of glucose, or other metabolic processes can be measured. PET imaging can employ various types of radioactive tracers. A commonly used tracer in clinical practice, flourodeoxyglucose (FDG)-PET, identifies regional glucose metabolism in the brain, indirectly representing activity of neurons in the grey matter. However, other types of PET can examine specific aspects of the brain or brain pathology. For instance, PiB-PET has been developed to examine amyloid plaques, one of the neuropathological markers of Alzheimer's disease (for a review, see Noble and Scarmeas 2009). Therefore, in contrast to MRS, PET cannot provide information concerning several metabolites at one time as in MRS, but PET can detect significant changes in brain neurochemical activity, including hypometabolism, which can signify underactivity in particular regions of the brain. In addition, the invasive and radioactive nature of injected tracers, along with limited availability of the equipment needed to make these radioisotopes on site, are some current disadvantages of PET imaging.

Another functional imaging technology, SPECT, measures blood flow in the brain by detecting an intravenously injected single-photon radioactive tracer. This technology indirectly reveals brain activity by examining blood flow in the brain; it is less expensive and the tracer is more readily available than PET. Nevertheless, similar disadvantages in PET apply to SPECT when comparing MRS; it is more invasive and requires additional technology. In further contrast to MRS, SPECT can only provide information about one biochemical at a time and cannot provide comparative information on metabolism as in MRS.

RESEARCH WITH ^{1}H MRS IN DEMENTIA AND MILD COGNITIVE IMPAIRMENT

Main Metabolites of Interest

The following metabolites are the most commonly used in dementia research.

N-Acetyleaspartate

N-acetyleaspartate (NAA), resonating at 2.02 parts per million (ppm), represents the highest peak on a normal spectrum, due to its high proton metabolic concentration in the brain (Kwock 1998; Valenzuela and Sachdev 2001). NAA is found primarily in the main cell body of neurons, the primary signaling cell of the brain, and their axons, the processes of neurons that send information from cell to cell. Furthermore, NAA is present throughout the brain and, due to its location in neurons and axons, found in both grey and white matter. Although the exact function of NAA is unknown, this metabolite serves as a neuronal marker, signifying the density, integrity, and viability of neurons. Measuring NAA in MRS contributes information regarding the number of functioning brain cells; thus, lower concentration ratios of NAA are considered an indication of less neuronal viability and integrity, presumably caused by neuronal death, or loss or injury of axons and dendrites (Birken and Oldendorf 1989).

Choline

With a peak at 3.22 ppm, choline (Cho) metabolite ratios represent several related neurochemicals in the brain containing choline, such as free Cho, phosphorylcholine, and glycerophosphorylcholine, and to a small extent acetylcholine (Firbank, Harrison, and O'Brien 2002; Kantarci 2007; Valenzuela and Sachdev 2001). The greatest amount of choline in the brain is found in the phospholipids of cellular membranes (Kantarci 2007), which is the outmost layer of a cell that serves as a selective barrier; in addition, choline molecules are related to synthesis and turnover of these membranes (Minati, Grisoli, and Bruzzone 2007). Therefore, metabolite ratios in MRS are considered a crude metabolic marker of membrane density, integrity, and turnover. Furthermore, in ^{1}H MRS the Cho peak can signify inflammation (Mueller, Schuff, and Weiner 2006).

Creatine

Resonating at 3.02 ppm, creatine (Cr) includes both creatine and phosphocreatine. In short, these metabolites represent the energy metabolism or storage of energy in a cell (Minati, Grisoli, and Bruzzone 2007; Valenzuela and Sachdev 2001). Since creatine concentrations are relatively stable across individuals, they are considered constant and used to calculate ratio concentrations (i.e., NAA/Cr; Cho/Cr).

Myo-Inositol

A naturally occurring sugar alcohol found in the brain, the myo-inositol (mI) peak resonates at 3.56 ppm. Not occurring in neurons, the main signaling cell of the brain, mI is found in higher concentrations in glial cells, brain cells that support and protect neurons. Thus, the mI peak is presumed a glial marker (Castillo et al. 1998; Downes and Macphee 1990; Garcia-Perez and Burg 1991) An increase in mI ratio concentrations may reflect an increase in the amount of glial cells or increased cell size, which is thought to represent inflammation or gliosis, an accumulation of cells as a response to damaged neurons (Brand, Richter-Landsberg, and Leibfritz 1993; Rosen and Lenkinski 2007; Strange et al. 1994; Valenzuela and Sachdev 2001).

Scyllo-Inositol

In addition to mI, scyllo-inositol, a related metabolite resonating at 3.342 ppm is also presented as a peak on normal MRS spectrum. Less is known about sI's chemical functions in the brain and how it differs from mI; however, sI is a product of mI metabolism (McLaurin et al. 2000).

Glutamate-Glutamine

The GLX peak (2.1–2.4 ppm) includes both metabolites: glutamate (Glu) and glutamine (Gln) since the concentration of each substance cannot be separated on lower magnetic strength scanners, such as a 1.5 Tesla. However, improved differentiation of Glu and Gln and their specific concentrations may be revealed using a higher field strength scanner, like a 3 Tesla (Kantarci et al. 2003; Kantarci 2007; Schubert et al. 2004). Glu is the most abundant excitatory neurotransmitter in the brain, thus it is a chemical that is transferred from neuron to another to increase signaling and activity between cells.

As a precursor of Glu, Gln is believed to have an important neurobiological function related to the detoxification and regulation of Glu (Valenzuela and Sachdev 2001). Glu and Gln are involved in neuronal function, metabolism, and plasticity (Antuono et al. 2001); thus, these metabolites are related to efficient transmission of information, energy production, and adaptability and repair of the brain.

¹H MRS Findings in Alzheimer's Disease

Alzheimer's disease (AD) is the most common cause of dementia affecting older adults (McMurtray et al. 2006). The disease is characterized by two particular abnormal findings in the brain called amyloid plaques and neurofibrillary tangles. Amyloid plaques are accumulations of beta amyloid protein that occur outside of neurons in the brain, and neurofibrillary tangles refer to twisted and tangled protein fibers that make up a neuron. Both result in death of neurons in the brain, particularly in a pattern with early involvement of areas very important for memory, the medial temporal lobes and hippocampus, but also with further spread into other regions of the brain related to additional cognitive abilities (Braak and Braak 1991). However, examination of the brain at the cellular level is needed for identification of these hallmark brain abnormalities, thus a definitive diagnosis of AD can usually only be made after death (Cummings et al. 1998). Therefore, MRS may help display a specific pattern of abnormal concentrations of metabolites that may represent the cellular changes occurring because of the underlying brain disease in AD, and has the potential to aid in differentiating this pattern from other types of dementias (Kantarci et al. 2008).

In studies examining Alzheimer's disease, the most common finding is reduction of NAA ratio concentrations (Adalsteinsson et al. 2000; Chantal et al. 2002; Christiansen, Schlosser, and Henriksen 1995; Ernst et al. 1997; Heun et al. 1997; Parnetti et al. 1997; Rose et al. 1999; Schuff et al. 1997; Watanabe et al. 2002). In research where a particular region of interest was examined in patients with AD, decreased NAA/Cr ratios were consistently found in many studies in the hippocampus and medial temporal lobe (Chantal et al. 2002, 2004; Dixon et al. 2002; Jessen et al. 2000; Schuff et al. 1997; Watanabe et al. 2002), along with other specific areas of the temporal lobes (Frederick et al. 1997; Kantarci et al. 2000; Herminghaus et al. 2003; Parnetti et al. 1997) and parietal lobes (Antuono et al. 2001; Griffith, den Hollander, et al. 2007; Hattori et al. 2002; Herminghaus et al. 2003; Kantarci et al. 2000; Kantarci, Xu, et al. 2002; Kantarci, Smith, et al. 2002; Kantarci et al. 2003; Martinez-Bisbal et al. 2004; Rose et al. 1999).

Furthermore, other regions of the brain including the occipital lobes (Kantarci et al. 2000; Moats et al. 1994; Shonk et al. 1995; Waldman et al. 2002; Watanabe et al. 2002; Weiss et al. 2003) and frontal lobes (Chantal et al. 2002, 2004; Christiansen, Schlosser, and Henriksen 1995; Herminghaus et al. 2003; Parnetti et al. 1997) showed similar findings of depleted NAA/Cr. Many studies have also displayed NAA reductions in white matter (Catani et al. 2001; Hattori et al. 2002; Herminghaus et al. 2003; Heun et al. 1997; Meyerhoff et al. 1994; Moats et al. 1994); however, a few studies did not find these results (Catani et al. 2002; Watanabe et al. 2002). Additionally, research using MRS techniques to examine larger areas of the brain or whole brain metabolites generally demonstrate a reduction of NAA in AD (Adalsteinsson et al. 2000; Pfefferbaum et al. 1999). Thus, MRS studies in AD seem to support NAA as a marker of both functioning ability of neurons (grey matter) and their axons (white matter). Overall, widespread reductions in NAA are consistent with disease progression and the neurofibrillary tangles present in AD, which may first occur in early stages of the disease in the medial temporal lobes and hippocampus but then spread to areas responsible for vision, sensory, and motor abilities such as the occipital lobe and parietal lobes in later stages of the disease (Braak and Braak 1991).

So far, only a few studies have investigated changes in NAA ratios in AD over time. Four studies examined NAA ratios in patients with AD over a one-year period; two of them generally found NAA decreases over time (Adalsteinsson et al. 2000; Kantarci et al. 2007) in individuals with AD, while two other studies did not show declines (Dixon et al. 2002; Jessen et al. 2001). However, in one of the studies with negative results, patients with AD displayed lower ratios of NAA than older controls at both time points (Dixon et al. 2002). Thus, there is a possibility that greater reductions in NAA may indicate later stages of AD and may signify greater amount of brain abnormalities over time due to the disease; nonetheless, more studies are needed to support these results and further examine NAA ratios over longer amounts of time.

Abnormalities in the Cho peak have been documented in some studies (Chantal et al. 2002,. 2004; Jessen et al. 2000; Kantarci et al. 2000, 2003; Lazeyras et al. 1998; MacKay et al. 1996; Meyerhoff et al. 1994); however, results have been conflicting. When comparing patients with AD to control participants, some studies find elevations of Cho (Lazeyras et al. 1998; MacKay et al. 1996; Meyerhoff et al. 1994), while others displayed reductions in Cho levels (Chantal et al. 2002, 2004; Jessen et al. 2000; Kantarci et al. 2000, 2003). The meaning behind these inconsistent results is unknown, although there are several hypotheses. Higher levels of Cho may be the result of the loss of functioning neurons during AD resulting in increased membrane turnover, or could be related to an increase in the response to help compensate for reduced acetycholine levels seen in AD (Kantarci et al. 2007). There is also the possibility that common medications for AD that are cholinergic, like donapezil, may indirectly result in abnormal Cho levels found in MRS (Griffith et al. 2008; Kantarci et al. 2007). Alternatively, variable results across studies could also be due to differences between methods using ^{1}H MRS, such that variations in length of echo times or particular areas of interest chosen may influence the chance of finding increased or decreased Cho levels (Griffith, Stewart, and den Hollander 2009).

Abnormal mI elevations have been found in areas consistent with regions of the brain most affected by the plaques and tangles and neuronal loss in AD, including aspects of the brain such as the temporal-parietal area (Chantal et al. 2002, 2004; Ernst et al. 1997; Parnetti et al. 1996), posterior cingulate gyrus/mesial parietal lobe (Griffith, den Hollander, et al. 2007; Herminghaus et al. 2003; Kantarci et al. 2000, 2003; Kantarci, Xu, et al. 2002; Lazeyras et al. 1998; Martinez-Bisbal et al. 2004; Rose et al. 1999; Waldman and Rai 2003), parietal white matter (Herminghaus et al. 2003; Moats et al. 1994), and occipital lobes (Moats et al. 1994; Shonk et al. 1995; Waldman et al. 2002). Furthermore, frontal lobes (Chantal et al. 2002, 2004; Herminghaus et al. 2003; Parnetti et al. 1997) and subcortical regions (Catani et al. 2001, 2002; Hattori et al. 2002; Heun et al. 1997), which are less commonly affected by the disease, less often display abnormal mI levels. Along with decreased NAA concentrations, increased mI levels are one of the most prominent and consistent findings in ^{1}H MRS among AD patients. Thus, both metabolites seem to serve as separate indicators of the effects of AD on the brain's functioning with NAA serving as a neuronal marker and mI representing as a glial marker.

Cr, sI, and Glx have been less explored in ^{1}H MRS studies with patients who have AD. Cr is consistently used as the denominator of ratios because of its suggested stability even in brain disease (Valenzuela and Sachdev 2001); moreover, AD patients generally show stable Cr levels compared to controls (Ernst et al. 1997; Pfefferbaum et al. 1999; Schuff et al. 1997). Investigation of sI has also been less common; one study revealed sI/Cr elevations in AD patients (Griffith et al. 2006), while another study showed raised concentrations in the normal aging brain (Kaiser et al. 2005). Elevations in sI may occur for the same reasons mI concentrations are increased since they are directly related; however, more research needs to be conducted on sI to support these findings and their possible explanation for elevations. Overall, findings regarding Glx in AD patients using ^{1}H MRS are inconsistent. Some studies have shown decreased Glx levels in specific posterior aspects of the brain (Antuono et al. 2001; Hattori et al. 2002) and specific regions in the temporal lobe (Herminghaus et al. 2003) and occipital lobe (Moats et al. 1994).

Further research has been conducted to examine the ability for studies using ^{1}H MRS to distinguish patients diagnosed with probable AD from healthy older adults. Several studies have demonstrated that NAA levels can aid in discrimination of normal controls from AD patients (Antuono et al. 2001; Schuff et al. 1997; Shonk et al. 1995). Furthermore, the addition of NAA metabolite levels can improve discrimination of AD patients when information from structural imaging is available (Dixon et al. 2002; Ernst et al. 1997; Kantarci, Xu, et al. 2002; MacKay et al. 1996). Using an NAA/mI ratio, in contrast to other metabolite ratios, seems to best discriminate AD patients from normal controls (Kantarci et al. 2007).

Research has also been performed to investigate how cognitive abilities, everyday functioning, and brain abnormalities observed after death relate to ^{1}H MRS findings in AD. The majority of studies have found correlations between ^{1}H MRS and scores on a common mental status screening, the Mini Mental Status Examination (MMSE) (Antuono et al. 2001; Dixon et al. 2002; Doraiswamy, Charles, and Krishnan 1998; Ernst et al. 1997; Heun et al. 1997; Jessen et al. 2000, 2001; Parnetti et al. 1997; Rose et al. 1999; Waldman and Rai 2003). The ability to perform everyday activities, like finances, has also been related to metabolite ratios found in ^{1}H MRS (Griffith, Okonkwo, et al. 2007). Finally, NAA and mI findings from patients with probable AD using ^{1}H MRS before and after death have been found to relate to the extent of damage seen in the brain as a result of senile plaques and neurofibrillary tangles after death (Kantarci et al. 2008).

^{1}H MRS Findings in Frontotemporal Dementia

Frontotemporal dementia (FTD) is a broad term that refers to a varied group of clinical syndromes that involve deterioration primarily of the frontal and/or temporal lobes of the brain by processes such as neuronal loss and gliosis. Moreover, FTD is characterized by early personality changes and behavior changes including apathy and disinhibition (Coulthard et al. 2006; Ernst et al. 1997).

^{1}H MRS studies with FTD patients have revealed metabolic abnormalities in several regions of the brain. Lower NAA/Cr ratios in the primarily diseased regions of the brain, the temporal and frontal lobes, was found in one study. In addition, mI/Cr ratios were increased in the frontal lobe region of interest; however, no metabolic abnormalities were present on the ^{1}H MRS of a selected parietal lobe region (Coulthard et al. 2006). Furthermore, other research comparing FTD and AD patients supports differing regional patterns of metabolite abnormalities. That is, areas primarily more susceptible to reduced functioning and neuronal death in each disease may show abnormalities on the metabolite spectrum, such that findings in particular regions, such as the midfrontal grey matter in FTD and the temporoparietal grey matter in AD, may help distinguish between these two types of dementia (Ernst et al. 1997; Mihara et al. 2006). Moreover, clinical and cognitive features, such as severity of dementia using the Clinical Dementia Rating and global mental status measured by MMSE scores, were also associated with metabolic abnormalities in the frontal region and temporoparietal regions in a group of FTD, AD, and healthy controls (Ernst et al. 1997).

^{1}H MRS Findings in Vascular Dementia

Another common form of dementia, vascular dementia (VaD), pertains to a syndrome related to one or more cerebrovascular mechanisms, those which are related to the blood supply to the brain, that cause neuronal death and deterioration of brain functioning. Types of cerebrovascular problems in VaD include infarcts, which are areas of dead neurons and tissue due to deprivation of blood supply and oxygen, white matter lesions, which refer to areas of dead axons, and consequently, atrophy, or shrinkage of the brain (Wiederkehr et al. 2008). Because of VaD's various causes, different presentation of symptoms, and high co-occurrence with characteristics of AD, diagnosis is particularly difficult (Holmes et al. 1999; Jones and Waldman 2004). Thus, ^{1}H MRS may be useful clinically to distinguish VaD from other dementias, if a pattern of abnormal metabolite findings could be established in research.

Research studies using ^{1}H MRS in VaD have demonstrated widespread metabolite abnormalities. For instance, Herminghaus et al. (2003) explored metabolite ratios in five regions of interest including grey and white matter in the mid-parietal, mid-frontal and temporal gyrus. In contrast to controls, NAA/Cr ratios were reduced in all five regions of interests suggesting global areas of neuronal death. Furthermore, elevations of mI/Cr ratios were found in the parietal grey and white matter, frontal white matter, and the temporal lobe, while Glx ratios were also abnormally elevated in parietal grey matter and temporal lobe (Herminghaus et al. 2003). Results from a study by Kantarci et al. (2004) also displayed lower ratios of NAA/Cr in patients with VaD, although these reductions were found in the posterior cingulate region of the brain. However, mI/Cr and Cho/Cr ratios were comparable to healthy controls in this brain area (Kantarci et al. 2004). Together, the pervasive abnormal metabolite findings suggest many brain regions directly related and indirectly related to those involved in vascular pathology, such as infarcts and white matter lesions, are disrupted in VaD. Moreover, the NAA/Cr decreases and mI/Cr elevations suggest that both neuronal dysfunction/death and damage to axons are occurring along with gliosis. Finally, abnormal NAA findings in regions such as the posterior cingulate, far away from areas with vascular pathology, are hypothesized to be indirectly related to the degeneration of neurons in these areas with vascular infarcts and lesions (Kantarci et al. 2004).

¹H MRS Findings in Dementia with Lewy Bodies

Dementia with Lewy Bodies (DLB) is named for the abnormal protein formations, Lewy bodies, which develop in neurons and are found at the cellular level when examining the brain after death. This type of dementia is characterized by worsening of cognitive dysfunction over time, accompanied by fluctuations in alertness and attention. Furthermore, visual hallucinations and motor symptoms like those seen in Parkinson's disease, such as stiffness and rigidity or loss of the ability to initiate and maintain movement, are also main features of DLB (McKeith et al. 2005).

Overall, less research has focused on ¹H MRS in DLB; furthermore, findings from these studies are generally inconsistent at this time. Molina et al. (2002) found decreased NAA/Cr, Cho/Cr, and Glx/Cr ratios in patients with DLB compared to controls in one region of white matter, but did not find differences in grey matter in the mid-parietal lobe. Moreover, clinical, cognitive, and motor measures were not related to any of these abnormal metabolite findings (Molina et al. 2002). Studies examining other regions of the brain such as the hippocampus and posterior cingulate gyrus in patients with DLB revealed contradicting results. That is, in one study elevated NAA/Cr ratios were found in the hippocampi of DLB patients in contrast with controls; however, Cho/Cr ratios did not show group differences (Xuan, Ding, and Gong 2008). While another study showed Cho/Cr elevations in the posterior cingulate gyrus but no group differences in NAA/Cr or mi/Cr ratios of DLB patients versus healthy controls (Kantarci et al. 2004).

Several explanations could explain variability of ¹H MRS findings in patients with DLB. First of all, only a few studies have been conducted, and their methods vary considerably; thus differences in patient characteristics or imaging methods may have an effect on the data obtained.

However, studies examining damage and loss of neurons in patients with DLB after death have also been inconsistent (Cordato et al. 2000; Gomez-Isla et al. 1999). Thus, the nature of DLB, itself, and the way it affects the brain may vary, such that it produces different results.

^{1}H MRS Findings in Parkinson's Disease Dementia

Parkinson's disease, primarily categorized as a movement disorder, many times also involves cognitive changes which may later develop into dementia. Parkinson's disease dementia (PDD) is a specific dementia in patients with Parkinson's disease which involves onset of worsening cognition and functional impairment after at least one year after initial onset of the movement disorder (McKeith et al. 2005). PDD is thought of as a separate dementia with characteristics that can be distinguished from patients with DLB (Benecke 2003) and AD with late motor complications (Dickson 2000).

Many studies examining PDD use two comparison groups: a nondemented PD group and a healthy control group. Overall, ^{1}H MRS findings displayed abnormal brain metabolism in PDD patients when compared to both groups. Metabolite levels were first examined in the occipital cortex in PDD patients, where NAA levels were reduced when compared to non-demented PD patients, but not healthy controls (Summerfield et al. 2002). The posterior cingulate gyrus in PDD patients has displayed cellular changes and damage in brains when examined after death (Braak et al. 2004), in addition to abnormal blood flow (Osaki et al. 2005) and neurochemical changes (Brooks and Piccini 2006) in functional imaging studies. Because of these abnormalities, this region of interest was examined in a recent ^{1}H MRS study. Providing further evidence of abnormal chemical changes in the brain, PDD patients displayed reduced NAA/Cr ratios when compared to healthy controls and nondemented PD patients. Furthermore, Glu/Cr ratios were also reduced compared to healthy controls (Griffith et al. 2008). Low NAA levels are thought to signify limited ability for neurons in the cingulate gyrus and occipital lobes to function in PDD, while Glu reductions could possibly relate to other disease processes. This pattern of metabolic abnormalities obtained from ^{1}H MRS in the posterior cingulate gyrus seems to distinguish PDD patients with dementia from those without. In addition, the reduction of NAA/Cr ratios seems to not only discriminate PDD from PD without dementia, but also from normal healthy controls. Furthermore, mental status and cognitive function as measured by the MMSE and Dementia Rating Scale (DRS), also seem to be related to both NAA and Glu levels (Griffith et al. 2008). Ultimately,

^{1}H MRS studies examining brain metabolic abnormalities over time in patients with PD who may or may not develop dementia will need to be conducted to understand more about when these brain changes occur in comparison to clinical symptoms.

^{1}H MRS Findings in Amnestic Mild Cognitive Impairment

Amnestic Mild Cognitive Impairment (MCI) is a classification used to diagnose a stage of cognitive difficulties between normal cognition with aging and AD. There are specific criteria that need to be met for a diagnosis of amnestic MCI, which include: (1) complaints of memory loss by the patient, if possible confirmed by others; (2) impairment on memory testing when compared to performance of adults with the same age and education; (3) generally, normal performance on tests in other domains of cognition; and (4) overall, maintained ability to function in activities of daily living (Petersen et al. 2001). Furthermore, individuals diagnosed with MCI have a higher yearly rate of developing probable AD than cognitively normal peers (Ganguli et al. 2004; Petersen et al. 2001).

Overall, ^{1}H MRS studies examining patients with amnestic MCI cross-sectionally (i.e., at only one period in time) have found consistent metabolic brain abnormalities between the levels seen with normal healthy controls and AD. For instance, one study found that mI/Cr ratios in the posterior cingulate in patients with MCI were significantly increased compared to controls; however, mI/Cr was significantly lower in MCI patients in contrast to patients with AD. Thus, increased ratios of mI in patients with MCI may have reflected early brain changes, such as gliosis, occurring before indication of neuronal damage or loss as usually seen by decrements in NAA (Kantarci et al. 2000). Additional studies have also found mI elevations in patients with MCI compared to controls in the posterior cingulate (Kantarci et al. 2003; Rami et al. 2007), left hippocampus (Franczak et al. 2007), and other areas of the brain including white matter (Catani et al. 2001) and the parietotemporal cortex (Chantal et al. 2004; Rami et al. 2007). However, some studies have not found differences between mI levels in AD and MCI (Catani et al. 2001; Chantal et al. 2004; Garcia Santos et al. 2008; Kantarci et al. 2003).

mI elevations are not the only abnormal metabolite findings in cross-sectional studies with MCI. Some studies have also found NAA and Cho abnormalities. Cho was found significantly increased in the right frontal cortex and posterior cingulate, but decreased levels of Cho and NAA were discovered in the left medial temporal lobe in patients with MCI (Chantal et al. 2004; Kantarci et al. 2003). More specifically, NAA decreases were seen in the right hippocampus of a small sample of MCI patients (Franc-zak et al. 2007), and NAA/Cr was found to be as equally reduced in the hippocampus of MCI patients and AD patients in another study (Ackl et al. 2005). In contrast, when the posterior cingulate region was examined MCI patients showed abnormal reduction in NAA, but not as severe as declines seen in AD in one study (Ackl et al. 2005; Kantarci et al. 2003), while in another, only NAA abnormalities were seen in AD patients (Ackl et al. 2005). Some studies have found no evidence of NAA changes in MCI (Garcia Santos et al. 2008; Kantarci, Smith, et al. 2002). However, the over-all findings from ¹H MRS cross-sectional studies generally suggest that abnormal metabolite ratios found in patients with MCI reflects the tran-sitional phase between normal cognitive aging and Alzheimer's disease. That is, MCI patients, in general, do not display the normal metabolism seen in healthy older adults but also do not exhibit as severe abnormalities as found in studies with AD. This conclusion is further supported by find-ings concerning early cellular brain changes seen in AD (Braak and Braak 1991; Markesbery et al. 2006).

In contrast with cross-sectional studies, very few ¹H MRS studies have investigated metabolic changes over time in patients with MCI. One such study reported NAA/Cr decreases in the posterior cingulate region of the brain in MCI and AD patients one year later. Furthermore, MCI patients who converted to AD and those who did not convert to AD showed a similar rate of decline in NAA, while interestingly, Cho/Cr levels only declined in the nonconverters. Thus, it was hypothesized that some sort of cholinergic mechanism may have been functioning to help compensate for neuronal damage in MCI patients who remained stable. Of note, no mI/Cr abnormalities were found (Kantarci et al. 2007). Quite the oppo-site results were found by Bartnik Olson et al. (2008), where the poste-rior cingulate gyrus of MCI patients showed increased mI concentrations but no change in NAA or Cho concentrations approximately 11 months later. These diverging results may be due to different methodological tech-niques for measuring abnormal metabolite concentrations; nevertheless, they demonstrate the need for more longitudinal ¹H MRS studies in MCI patients to better understand the chemical brain changes occurring in this particular stage of cognitive dysfunction.

¹H MRS studies have also explored relationship between abnormal metabolite findings and cognition in MCI patients. Posterior cingulate ¹H MRS ratios in MCI have been found to correlate with different cogni-tive abilities, such as global cognition and learning (Kantarci, Smith, et al. 2002), and hippocampal NAA/Cr in MCI patients was related to verbal fluency and naming ability (Ackl et al. 2005). Furthermore, the ability to

predict "conversion," or worsening of diagnosis from MCI to dementia, from ¹H MRS findings has also been investigated. In general, NAA/Cr baseline ratios and reductions show the most promise in predicting conversion from MCI to dementia (Metastasio et al. 2006; Modrego, Fayed, and Pina 2005); nevertheless, more research needs to be conducted using similar diagnostic criteria and methodological techniques to examine MCI participants and the chemical brain changes that occur over time in converters and nonconverters.

CLINICAL APPLICATIONS OF MRS

One of the most important purposes for conducting research is to eventually apply the findings to individual patients in clinical situations. Although MRS is still considered experimental and investigational at this point in time, research has expanded our knowledge of abnormal metabolite patterns associated with different dementia types. Future studies using ¹H MRS with dementia and MCI patients can confirm results and provide further evidence for the utility of MRS when conducting dementia evaluations in clinical situations. Potentially, consistent metabolite patterns found in research with dementias could possibly serve as a clinical biomarker for the type of neurodegenerative disease in the future. Furthermore, with technological advances such as stronger magnetic field strength of scanners, MRS may become more powerful and more commonly used clinically. Although the prospect of applying MRS clinically is very hopeful, MRS will only be one of many techniques used for information gathering for a dementia evaluation. MRS findings will be considered only an additional tool in an extensive dementia assessment that will supplement other structural and functional imaging results, patient medical history, report of cognitive and functional difficulties, and so on.

In addition to its use in initial dementia evaluations and establishing a diagnosis, MRS also has the possibility to aid in monitoring of disease progression in those with a probable or suspected diagnosis of dementia. As more longitudinal research is conducted, more evidence will demonstrate types of changes in metabolites over time. Consistent patterns of abnormalities may develop that will give patients and their families a better idea of the course and progression of the disease and the accompanied brain changes. Since MRS is not intrusive and does not include exposure to radiation, it is easily repeatable over time. In our experience, it is also well tolerated by patients with dementias in the mild and moderate stages, and in those with movement disorders. Moreover, MRS also has further potential to act as a treatment indicator, to help clinicians monitor the value and effectiveness of different medications. That is, MRS could help track the patient's response to certain medications by examining the chemical changes occurring in the brain to see if the disease process may have slowed or stabilized over time.

Because of the widespread commercial availability of MRI scanners from which MRS data can potentially be obtained, MRS has the possibility to provide information to clinicians that could greatly benefit many future patients with dementia. More ^{1}H MRS studies in patients with MCI and different dementias will hopefully establish better discrimination between converters and non-converters and between different types of dementia. Thus, future research advances in MRS and dementia studies may provide unique information to facilitate diagnosis and treatment of dementia in the 21st century.

REFERENCES

Ackl, N., M. Ising, Y. A. Schreiber, M. Atiya, A. Sonntag, and D. P. Auer. 2005. Hippocampal metabolic abnormalities in mild cognitive impairment and Alzheimer's disease. *Neurosci Lett* 384 (1–2): 23–28.

Adalsteinsson, E., E. V. Sullivan, N. Kleinhans, D. M. Spielman, and A. Pfefferbaum. 2000. Longitudinal decline of the neuronal marker N-acetyl aspartate in Alzheimer's disease. *Lancet* 355 (9216): 1696–1697.

Antuono, P. G., J. L. Jones, Y. Wang, and S. J. Li. 2001. Decreased glutamate + glutamine in Alzheimer's disease detected in vivo with ^{1}H-MRS at 0.5 T. *Neurology* 56 (6): 737–742.

Bartnik Olson, B. L., B. A. Holshouser, W. Britt III, C. Mueller, W. Baqai, S. Patra, F. Petersen, and W. M. Kirsch. 2008. Longitudinal metabolic and cognitive changes in mild cognitive impairment patients. *Alzheimer Dis Assoc Disord* 22 (3): 269–277.

Birken, D. L., and W. H. Oldendorf. 1989. N-acetyl-L-aspartic acid: A literature review of a compound prominent in 1H-NMR spectroscopic studies of brain. *Neurosci Biobehav Rev* 13 (1): 23–31.

Benecke, R. 2003. Diffuse Lewy body disease—a clinical syndrome or a disease entity? *J Neurol* 250 (Suppl 1): I39–42.

Braak, H., and E. Braak. 1991. Neuropathological stageing of Alzheimer-related changes. *Acta Neuropathol (Berl)* 82 (4): 239–259.

Braak, H., E. Ghebremedhin, U. Rub, H. Bratzke, and K. Del Tredici. 2004. Stages in the development of Parkinson's disease–related pathology. *Cell Tissue Res* 318 (1): 121–134.

Brand, A., C. Richter-Landsberg, and D. Leibfritz. 1993. Multinuclear NMR studies on the energy metabolism of glial and neuronal cells. *Dev Neurosci* 15 (3–5): 289–298.

Brooks, D. J., and P. Piccini. 2006. Imaging in Parkinson's disease: The role of monoamines in behavior. *Biol Psychiatry* 59 (10): 908–918.

Castillo, M., L. Kwock, J. Scatliff, and S. K., Mukherji. 1998. Proton MR spectroscopy in neoplastic and non-neoplastic brain disorders. *Magn Reson Imaging Clin N Am* 6: 1–20.

Catani, M., A. Cherubini, R. Howard, R. Tarducci, G. P. Pelliccioli, M. Piccirilli, G. Gobbi, U. Senin, and P. Mecocci. 2001. (1)H-MR spectroscopy differentiates mild cognitive impairment from normal brain aging. *NeuroReport* 12 (11): 2315–2317.

Catani, M., P. Mecocci, R. Tarducci, R. Howard, G. P. Pelliccioli, E. Mariani, A. Metastasio, C. Benedetti, U. Senin, and A. Cherubini. 2002. Proton magnetic resonance spectroscopy reveals similar white matter biochemical changes in patients with chronic hypertension and early Alzheimer's disease. *J Am Geriatr Soc* 50 (10): 1707–1710.

Chantal, S., C. M. Braun, R. W. Bouchard, M. Labelle, and Y. Boulanger. 2004. Similar ^{1}H magnetic resonance spectroscopic metabolic pattern in the medial temporal lobes of patients with mild cognitive impairment and Alzheimer disease. *Brain Res* 1003 (1–2): 26–35.

Chantal, S., M. Labelle, R. W. Bouchard, C. M. Braun, and Y. Boulanger. 2002. Correlation of regional proton magnetic resonance spectroscopic metabolic changes with cognitive deficits in mild Alzheimer disease. *Arch Neurol* 59 (6): 955–962.

Christiansen, P., A. Schlosser, and O. Henriksen. 1995. Reduced N-acetylaspartate content in the frontal part of the brain in patients with probable Alzheimer's disease. *Magn Reson Imaging* 13 (3): 457–462.

Cordato, N. J., G. M. Halliday, A. J. Harding, M. A. Hely, and J. G. Morris. 2000. Regional brain atrophy in progressive supranuclear palsy and Lewy body disease. *Ann Neurol* 47 (6): 718–728.

Coulthard, E., M. Firbank, P. English, J. Welch, D. Birchall, J. O'Brien, and T. D. Griffiths. 2006. Proton magnetic resonance spectroscopy in frontotemporal dementia. *J Neurol* 253 (7): 861–868.

Cummings, J. L., H. V. Vinters, G. M. Cole, and Z. S. Khachaturian. 1998. Alzheimer's disease: Etiologies, pathophysiology, cognitive reserve, and treatment opportunities. *Neurology* 51 (1 Suppl 1): S2–S17; discussion S65–S67.

Dickson, D. 2000. Alzheimer-Parkinson disease overlap: neuropathology. In *Neurodegenerative dementias*, ed. C. Clark and J. Trojanowski, 247–259. New York: McGraw-Hill.

Dixon, R. M., K. M. Bradley, M. M. Budge, P. Styles, and A. D. Smith. 2002. Longitudinal quantitative proton magnetic resonance spectroscopy of the hippocampus in Alzheimer's disease. *Brain* 125 (Pt 10): 2332–2341.

Doraiswamy, P. M., H. C. Charles, and K. R. Krishnan. 1998. Prediction of cognitive decline in early Alzheimer's disease. *Lancet* 352 (9141): 1678.

Downes, C. P., and C. H. Macphee. 1990. Myo-inositol metabolites as cellular signals. *Eur J Biochem* 193 (1): 1–18.

Ernst, T., L. Chang, R. Melchor, and C. M. Mehringer. 1997. Frontotemporal dementia and early Alzheimer disease: differentiation with frontal lobe H-1 MR spectroscopy. *Radiology* 203 (3): 829–836.

Firbank, M. J., R. M. Harrison, and J. T. O'Brien. 2002. A comprehensive review of proton magnetic resonance spectroscopy studies in dementia and Parkinson's disease. *Dement Geriatr Cogn Disord* 14 (2): 64–76.

Franczak, M., R. W. Prost, P. G. Antuono, L. P. Mark, J. L. Jones, and J. L. Ulmer. 2007. Proton magnetic resonance spectroscopy of the hippocampus in patients with mild cognitive impairment: A pilot study. *J Comput Assist Tomogr* 31 (5): 666–670.

Frederick, B. B., A. Satlin, D. A. Yurgelun-Todd, and P. F. Renshaw. 1997. In vivo proton magnetic resonance spectroscopy of Alzheimer's disease in the parietal and temporal lobes. *Biol Psychiatry* 42 (2): 147–150.

Ganguli, M., H. H. Dodge, C. Shen, and S. T. DeKosky. 2004. Mild cognitive impairment, amnestic type: An epidemiological study. *Neurology* 63: 115–121.

Garcia Santos, J. M., D. Gavrila, C. Antunez, M. J. Tormo, D. Salmeron, R. Carles, J. Jimenez Veiga, et al. 2008. Magnetic resonance spectroscopy performance for detection of dementia, Alzheimer's disease and mild cognitive impairment in a community-based survey. *Dement Geriatr Cogn Disord* 26 (1): 15–25.

Garcia-Perez, A., and M. B. Burg. 1991. Renal medullary organic osmolytes. *Physiol Rev.* 71 (4): 1081–1115.

Gomez-Isla, T., W. B. Growdon, M. McNamara, K. Newell, E. Gomez-Tortosa, E. T. Hedley-Whyte, and B. T. Hyman. 1999. Clinicopathologic correlates in temporal cortex in dementia with Lewy bodies. *Neurology* 53 (9): 2003–2009.

Griffith, H. R., J. A. den Hollander, O. C. Okonkwo, T. O'Brien, R. L. Watts, and D. C. Marson. 2008. Brain N-acetylaspartate is reduced in Parkinson disease with dementia. *Alzheimer Dis Assoc Disord* 22 (1): 54–60.

Griffith, H. R., J. A. den Hollander, C. C. Stewart, W. T. Evanochko, S. D. Buchthal, L. E. Harrell, E. Y. Zamrini, J. C. Brockington, and D. C. Marson. 2007. Elevated brain scyllo-inositol concentrations in patients with Alzheimer's disease. *NMR Biomed* 20: 709–716.

Griffith, H. R., O. C. Okonkwo, J.A. den Hollander, K. Belue, S. Lanza, L.E. Harrell, J.C. Brockington, D. G. Clark, and D. C. Marson. 2007. Brain proton MRS is correlated with financial abilities in patients with Alzheimer's disease. *Brain Imaging and Behavior* 1: 23–29.

Griffith, H. R., C. C. Stewart, and J. A. den Hollander. 2009. Proton magnetic resonance spectroscopy in dementias and mild cognitive impairment. *Int Rev Neurobiol* 84: 105–131.

Griffith, H. R., C. C. Stewart, J. A. den Hollander, W. T. Evanochko, S. D. Buchthal, L. E. Harrell, E. Y. Zamrini, J. C. Brockington, and D. C. Marson. 2006. In-vivo 3T 1H magnetic resonance spectroscopy of the brain reveals elevated scyllo-inositol in patients with mild Alzheimer's disease. Paper read at

Proceedings of the International Society of Magnetic Resonance in Medicine, at Seattle, WA.

Hattori, N., K. Abe, S. Sakoda, and T. Sawada. 2002. Proton MR spectroscopic study at 3 Tesla on glutamate/glutamine in Alzheimer's disease. *NeuroReport* 13 (1): 183–186.

Herminghaus, S., L. Frolich, C. Gorriz, U. Pilatus, T. Dierks, H. J. Wittsack, H. Lanfermann, K. Maurer, and F. E. Zanella. 2003. Brain metabolism in Alzheimer disease and vascular dementia assessed by in vivo proton magnetic resonance spectroscopy. *Psychiatry Res* 123 (3): 183–190.

Heun, R., S. Schlegel, M. Graf-Morgenstern, J. Tintera, J. Gawehn, and P. Stoeter. 1997. Proton magnetic resonance spectroscopy in dementia of Alzheimer type. *Int J Geriatr Psychiatry* 12 (3): 349–358.

Holmes, C., N. Cairns, P. Lantos, and A. Mann. 1999. Validity of current clinical criteria for Alzheimer's disease, vascular dementia and dementia with Lewy bodies. *Br J Psychiatry* 174: 45–50.

Jessen, F., W. Block, F. Traber, E. Keller, S. Flacke, R. Lamerichs, H. H. Schild, and R. Heun. 2001. Decrease of N-acetylaspartate in the MTL correlates with cognitive decline of AD patients. *Neurology* 57 (5): 930–932.

Jessen, F., W. Block, F. Traber, E. Keller, S. Flacke, A. Papassotiropoulos, R. Lamerichs, R. Heun, and H. H. Schild. 2000. Proton MR spectroscopy detects a relative decrease of N-acetylaspartate in the medial temporal lobe of patients with AD. *Neurology* 55 (5): 684–688.

Jones, R. S., and A. D. Waldman. 2004. 1H-MRS evaluation of metabolism in Alzheimer's disease and vascular dementia. *Neurol Res* 26 (5): 488–495.

Kaiser, L. G., N. Schuff, N. Cashdollar, and M. W. Weiner. 2005. Scyllo-inositol in normal aging human brain: [1]H magnetic resonance spectroscopy study at 4 Tesla. *NMR Biomed* 18 (1): 51–55.

Kantarci, K. 2007. [1]H Magnetic resonance spectroscopy in dementia. *Br J Radiol* 80: S146–S152.

Kantarci, K., C. R. Jack Jr., Y. C. Xu, N. G. Campeau, P. C. O'Brien, G. E. Smith, R. J. Ivnik, et al. 2000. Regional metabolic patterns in mild cognitive impairment and Alzheimer's disease: A ^{1}H MRS study. *Neurology* 55 (2): 210–217.

Kantarci, K., D. S. Knopman, D. W. Dickson, J. E. Parisi, J. L. Whitwell, S. D. Weigand, K. A. Josephs, B. F. Boeve, R. C. Petersen, and C. R. Jack Jr. 2008. Alzheimer disease: Postmortem neuropathologic correlates of antemortem 1H MR spectroscopy metabolite measurements. *Radiology* 248 (1): 210–220.

Kantarci, K., R. C. Petersen, B. F. Boeve, D. S. Knopman, D. F. Tang-Wai, P. C. O'Brien, S. D. Weigand, et al. 2004. [1]H MR spectroscopy in common dementias. *Neurology* 63 (8): 1393–1398.

Kantarci, K., G. Reynolds, R. C. Petersen, B. F. Boeve, D. S. Knopman, S. D. Edland, G. E. Smith, R. J. Ivnik, E. G. Tangalos, and C. R. Jack Jr. 2003. Proton MR spectroscopy in mild cognitive impairment and Alzheimer disease: comparison of 1.5 and 3 T. *AJNR Am J Neuroradiol* 24 (5): 843–849.

Kantarci, K., G. E. Smith, R. J. Ivnik, R. C. Petersen, B. F. Boeve, D. S. Knopman, E. G. Tangalos, and C. R. Jack Jr. 2002. ¹H magnetic resonance spectroscopy, cognitive function, and apolipoprotein E genotype in normal aging, mild cognitive impairment and Alzheimer's disease. *J Int Neuropsychol Soc* 8 (7): 934–942.

Kantarci, K., S. D. Weigand, R. C. Petersen, B. F. Boeve, D. S. Knopman, J. Gunter, D. Reyes, et al. 2007. Longitudinal ¹H MRS changes in mild cognitive impairment and Alzheimer's disease. *Neurobiol Aging* 28 (9): 1330–1339.

Kantarci, K., Y. Xu, M. M. Shiung, P. C. O'Brien, R. H. Cha, G. E. Smith, R. J. Ivnik, et al. 2002. Comparative diagnostic utility of different MR modalities in mild cognitive impairment and Alzheimer's disease. *Dement Geriatr Cogn Disord* 14 (4): 198–207.

Kwock, L. 1998. Localized MR spectroscopy: Basic principles. *Neuroimaging Clin N Am* 8 (4): 713–731.

Lazeyras, F., H. C. Charles, L. A. Tupler, R. Erickson, O. B. Boyko, and K. R. Krishnan. 1998. Metabolic brain mapping in Alzheimer's disease using proton magnetic resonance spectroscopy. *Psychiatry Res* 82 (2): 95–106.

MacKay, S., F. Ezekiel, V. Di Sclafani, D. J. Meyerhoff, J. Gerson, D. Norman, G. Fein, and M. W. Weiner. 1996. Alzheimer disease and subcortical ischemic vascular dementia: Evaluation by combining MR imaging segmentation and H-1 MR spectroscopic imaging. *Radiology* 198 (2): 537–545.

Markesbery, W. R., F. A. Schmitt, R. J. Kryscio, D. G. Davis, C. D. Smith, and D. R. Wekstein. 2006. Neuropathologic substrate of mild cognitive impairment. *Arch Neurol* 63 (1): 38–46.

Martinez-Bisbal, M. C., E. Arana, L. Marti-Bonmati, E. Molla, and B. Celda. 2004. Cognitive impairment: Classification by 1H magnetic resonance spectroscopy. *Eur J Neurol* 11 (3): 187–193.

McKeith, I. G., D. W. Dickson, J. Lowe, M. Emre, J. T. O'Brien, H. Feldman, J. Cummings, et al. 2005. Diagnosis and management of dementia with Lewy bodies: Third report of the DLB Consortium. *Neurology* 65 (12): 1863–1872.

McLaurin, J., R. Golomb, A. Jurewicz, J. P. Antel, and P. E. Fraser. 2000. Inositol stereoisomers stabilize an oligomeric aggregate of Alzheimer amyloid beta peptide and inhibit abeta -induced toxicity. *J Biol Chem* 275 (24): 18495–18502.

McMurtray, A., D. G. Clark, D. Christine, and M. F. Mendez. 2006. Early-onset dementia: Frequency and causes compared to late-onset dementia. *Dement Geriatr Cogn Disord* 21 (2): 59–64.

Metastasio, A., P. Rinaldi, R. Tarducci, E. Mariani, F. T. Feliziani, A. Cherubini, G. P. Pellicciioli, G. Gobbi, U. Senin, and P. Mecocci. 2006. Conversion of MCI to dementia: Role of proton magnetic resonance spectroscopy. *Neurobiol Aging* 27 (7): 926–932.

Meyerhoff, D. J., S. MacKay, J. M. Constans, D. Norman, C. Van Dyke, G. Fein, and M. W. Weiner. 1994. Axonal injury and membrane alterations in Alzheimer's disease suggested by in vivo proton magnetic resonance spectroscopic imaging. *Ann Neurol* 36 (1): 40–47.

Mihara, M., N. Hattori, K. Abe, S. Sakoda, and T. Sawada. 2006. Magnetic resonance spectroscopic study of Alzheimer's disease and frontotemporal dementia/ Pick complex. *NeuroReport* 17 (4): 413–416.

Minati, L., M. Grisoli, and M. G. Bruzzone. 2007. MR spectroscopy, functional MRI, and diffusion-tensor imaging in the aging brain: A conceptual review. *J Geriatr Psychiatry Neurol* 20 (1): 3–21.

Moats, R. A., T. Ernst, T. K. Shonk, and B. D. Ross. 1994. Abnormal cerebral metabolite concentrations in patients with probable Alzheimer disease. *Magn Reson Med* 32 (1): 110–115.

Modrego, P. J., N. Fayed, and M. A. Pina. 2005. Conversion from mild cognitive impairment to probable Alzheimer's disease predicted by brain magnetic resonance spectroscopy. *Am J Psychiatry* 162 (4): 667–675.

Molina, J. A., J. M. Garcia-Segura, J. Benito-Leon, C. Gomez-Escalonilla, T. del Ser, V. Martinez, and J. Viano. 2002. Proton magnetic resonance spectroscopy in dementia with Lewy bodies. *Eur Neurol* 48 (3): 158–163.

Mueller, S. G., N. Schuff, and M. W. Weiner. 2006. Evaluation of treatment effects in Alzheimer's and other neurodegenerative diseases by MRI and MRS. *NMR Biomed* 19 (6): 655–668.

Noble, J. M. and N. Scarmeas. 2009. Application of pet imaging to diagnosis of Alzheimer's disease and mild cognitive impairment. *Int Rev Neurobiol.* 84: 133–149.

Osaki, Y., Y. Morita, M. Fukumoto, N. Akagi, S. Yoshida, and Y. Doi. 2005. Three-dimensional stereotactic surface projection SPECT analysis in Parkinson's disease with and without dementia. *Mov Disord* 20 (8): 999–1005.

Parnetti, L., D. T. Lowenthal, O. Presciutti, G. P. Pelliccioli, R. Palumbo, G. Gobbi, P. Chiarini, B. Palumbo, R. Tarducci, and U. Senin. 1996. ^{1}H-MRS, MRI-based hippocampal volumetry, and 99mTc-HMPAO-SPECT in normal aging, age-associated memory impairment, and probable Alzheimer's disease. *J Am Geriatr Soc* 44 (2): 133–138.

Parnetti, L., R. Tarducci, O. Presciutti, D. T. Lowenthal, M. Pippi, B. Palumbo, G. Gobbi, G. P. Pelliccioli, and U. Senin. 1997. Proton magnetic resonance spectroscopy can differentiate Alzheimer's disease from normal aging. *Mech Ageing Dev* 97 (1): 9–14.

Petersen, R. C., R. Doody, A. Kurz, R. C. Mohs, J. C. Morris, P. V. Rabins, K. Ritchie, M. Rossor, L. Thal, and B. Winblad. 2001. Current concepts in mild cognitive impairment. *Arch Neurol* 58 (12): 1985–1992.

Petrella, J. R., R. E. Coleman, and P. M. Doraiswamy. 2003. Neuroimaging and early diagnosis of Alzheimer disease: A look to the future. *Radiology* 226 (2): 315–336.

Pfefferbaum, A., E. Adalsteinsson, D. Spielman, E. V. Sullivan, and K. O. Lim. 1999. In vivo brain concentrations of N-acetyl compounds, creatine, and choline in Alzheimer disease. *Arch Gen Psychiatry* 56 (2): 185–192.

Rami, L., B. Gomez-Anson, B. Bosch, R. Sanchez-Valle, G. C. Monte, A. Villar, and J. L. Molinuevo. 2007. Cortical brain metabolism as measured by proton spectroscopy is related to memory performance in patients with amnestic mild cognitive impairment and Alzheimer's disease. *Dement Geriatr Cogn Disord* 24 (4): 274–279.

Rose, S. E., G. I. de Zubicaray, D. Wang, G. J. Galloway, J. B. Chalk, S. C. Eagle, J. Semple, and D. M. Doddrell. 1999. A 1H MRS study of probable Alzheimer's disease and normal aging: implications for longitudinal monitoring of dementia progression. *Magn Reson Imaging* 17 (2): 291–299.

Rosen, Y., and R. E. Lenkinski. 2007. Recent advances in magnetic resonance neurospectroscopy. *Neurotherapeutics* 4 (3): 330–345.

Ross, B., and S. Bluml. 2001. Magnetic resonance spectroscopy of the human brain. *The Anatomical Record* 265 (2): 54–84.

Scheltens, P., N. Fox, F. Barkhof, and C. De Carli. 2002. Structural magnetic resonance imaging in the practical assessment of dementia: Beyond exclusion. *Lancet Neurol* 1 (1): 13–21.

Schubert, F., J. Gallinat, F. Seifert, and H. Rinneberg. 2004. Glutamate concentrations in human brain using single voxel proton magnetic resonance spectroscopy at 3 Tesla. *NeuroImage* 21 (4): 1762–1771.

Schuff, N., D. Amend, F. Ezekiel, S. K. Steinman, J. Tanabe, D. Norman, W. Jagust, et al. 1997. Changes of hippocampal N-acetyl aspartate and volume in Alzheimer's disease. A proton MR spectroscopic imaging and MRI study. *Neurology* 49 (6): 1513–1521.

Shonk, T. K., R. A. Moats, P. Gifford, T. Michaelis, J. C. Mandigo, J. Izumi, and B. D. Ross. 1995. Probable Alzheimer disease: Diagnosis with proton MR spectroscopy. *Radiology* 195 (1): 65–72.

Small, G. W., S. Y. Bookheimer, P. M. Thompson, G. M. Cole, S. C. Huang, V. Kepe, and J. R. Barrio. 2008. Current and future uses of neuroimaging for cognitively impaired patients. *Lancet Neurol* 7 (2): 161–172.

Strange, K., F. Emma, A. Paredes, and R. Morrison. 1994. Osmoregulatory changes in myo-inositol content and Na+/myo-inositol cotransport in rat cortical astrocytes. *Glia* 12 (1): 35–43.

Summerfield, C., B. Gomez-Anson, E. Tolosa, J. M. Mercader, M. J. Marti, P. Pastor, and C. Junque. 2002. Dementia in Parkinson disease: A proton magnetic resonance spectroscopy study. *Arch Neurol* 59 (9): 1415–1420.

Valenzuela, M. J., and P. Sachdev. 2001. Magnetic resonance spectroscopy in AD. *Neurology* 56 (5): 592–598.

Waldman, A. D., and G. S. Rai. 2003. The relationship between cognitive impairment and in vivo metabolite ratios in patients with clinical Alzheimer's disease and vascular dementia: A proton magnetic resonance spectroscopy study. *Neuroradiology* 45 (8): 507–512.

Waldman, A. D., G. S. Rai, J. R. McConnell, M. Chaudry, and D. Grant. 2002. Clinical brain proton magnetic resonance spectroscopy for management of Alzheimer's and sub-cortical ischemic vascular dementia in older people. *Arch Gerontol Geriatr* 35 (2): 137–142.

Watanabe, T., I. Akiguchi, H. Yagi, K. Onishi, T. Kawasaki, A. Shiino, and T. Inubushi. 2002. Proton magnetic resonance spectroscopy and white matter hyperintensities on magnetic resonance imaging in patients with Alzheimer's disease. *Ann NY Acad Sci* 977: 423–429.

Weiss, U., R. Bacher, H. Vonbank, G. Kemmler, A. Lingg, and J. Marksteiner. 2003. Cognitive impairment: Assessment with brain magnetic resonance imaging and proton magnetic resonance spectroscopy. *J Clin Psychiatry* 64 (3): 235–242.

Wiederkehr, S., M. Simard, C. Fortin, and R. van Reekum. 2008. Comparability of the clinical diagnostic criteria for vascular dementia: A critical review. Part I. *J Neuropsychiatry Clin Neurosci* 20 (2): 150–161.

Xuan, X., M. Ding, and X. Gong. 2008. Proton magnetic resonance spectroscopy detects a relative decrease of N-acetylaspartate in the hippocampus of patients with dementia with Lewy bodies. *J Neuroimaging* 18 (2): 137–141.

About the Contributors

PAUL M. BUTLER, MTS, is an MD-PhD candidate at Boston University School of Medicine. His research interests and publications include topics at the interstices of evolution, medicine, and the humanities.

JACQUELYNN N. COPELAND is a graduate student in the University of Alabama at Birmingham's Medical/Clinical Psychology doctoral program. She received her Bachelor of Science degree in psychology and graduated summa cum laude from the University of Florida in 2006. Her main area of interest is geriatric neuropsychology, with particular focus on dementia and aging.

Dr. PETER ENGEL is Geriatric Internist and currently a staff physician in the Geriatric Research, Education and Clinical Center of the VA Boston Healthcare System. Dr. Engel has appointments as Lecturer on Medicine at Harvard Medical School and Adjunct Instructor in Medicine, Boston University. He has a long-standing interest in dementia and degenerative brain disorders of late life. Previously, he was an Associate Professor of Medicine, Albany Medical College, Director of the Memory Clinic at the Albany VA, and co-director of the Partners in Dementia Care Project of the Upstate New York VA Healthcare System. Dr. Engel moved to Boston in 2009.

MARIANA KNEESE FLAKS graduated from the Pontific Catholic University of São Paulo, São Paulo, Brazil, with a bachelor's degree in psychology and clinical psychology license in 2000. From 2002 to 2004, she attended a hospital psychology specialization on neuropsychology and personality evaluation at the Psychiatry Institute of the Faculty of Medicine of the

University of São Paulo. Since 2003, she has dedicated herself to scientific research in the field of cognitive effects of aging and the differential diagnosis to detect, at the very beginning, cases that are turning into mild cognitive impairment or dementia. She pursued her doctoral degree in science at the same institution between 2004 and 2008, focusing on validation and diagnosis properties of cognitive screening tests for attention and memory. In 2009 she initiated her postdoctoral studies on neuropsychological factors associated with resilience and vulnerability to post-traumatic stress disorder at the Federal University of São Paulo.

LAURA FRATIGLIONI is the director of the Aging Research Center (ARC) and currently employed as a professor at the Karolinska Institutet. She is a medical doctor, specialized in both neurology and epidemiology. She has scientific, clinical, and pedagogic commitments. Under her supervision, 11 PhD students and two postdocs have completed their studies since 1996. She is currently supervising four PhD students. She regularly serves as a reviewer for various clinical and epidemiological journals. Since 1996, as principal investigator, she has regularly received grants from several of the major research councils in Sweden. She has been awarded the Luigi Amaducci Award by the Italian Neurological Association and has been recognized by the Swedish Society of Medicine. She is the scientific coordinator of the Kungsholmen Project on Aging and Dementia, co-investigator for the project "Harmony: A Twin Study on Dementia," and the principal investigator for the SNAC-Kungsholmen population study. Her scientific production has led to 161 original publications, 31 review articles in peer-reviewed journals, 17 chapters in edited volumes, and eight reports.

H. RANDALL GRIFFITH, PhD, is a clinical neuropsychologist in a private practice in Birmingham, Alabama. He received his PhD in psychology from Rosalind Franklin University/Chicago Medical School and completed a postdoctoral fellowship in the University of Alabama (UAB) Department of Neurology where he worked for several years with the UAB Alzheimer's Center. His research interests include using neuroimaging to better understand changes in cognition and changes in everyday activities of persons with neurodegenerative dementias.

HANS-HELMUT KÖNIG, MD, MPH, is Professor of Health Services Research and Health Economics, and co-chair of the Department of Medical Sociology and Health Economics at the University Medical Centre Hamburg-Eppendorf. Before joining the faculty of the University of Hamburg in 2010, he was Professor of Health Economics at the University of Leipzig. Hans-Helmut König studied medicine at the Universities of Tübingen, London and Oxford, received his doctoral degree from the University of Tübingen in 1993 and a master's degree in public health from Yale University in 1995. His main research fields are cost-of-illness studies, and empirical and model-based cost-effectiveness analyses, as well as the measurement of preferences for health and health care, with a special focus on mental health care.

HANNA LEICHT is a research associate at the Department of Medical Sociology and Health Economics at the University Medical Centre Hamburg-Eppendorf. She completed a BA in philosophy, politics and economics at Oxford University in 2000 and graduated from the University of Potsdam with a diploma in psychology in 2006. She has worked as a research assistant at the University of Leipzig at the Department of Psychiatry, studying insight into illness in Alzheimer's disease patients for a dissertation on this subject and at the Health Economics Research Unit. Her publications cover both issues from her dissertation work and topics in cost-of-illness analysis.

MELANIE LUPPA is a research fellow at the Department of Psychiatry and Psychotherapy, University of Leipzig (Public Health Research Unit). She holds a degree in medical sciences and is about to complete her graduate diploma of psychotherapy (CBT). She studied psychology at the University of Leipzig, where she graduated in 1998. Her primary expertise lies in the field of epidemiology and health economics of mental disorders.

Dr. LAURA E. MIDDLETON's work is motivated by the goal of decreasing the risk of cognitive impairment and dementia in old age. Her research has focused on the identification of modifiable lifestyle risk factors for dementia. She is particularly interested in empowering people to decrease their own risk of cognitive impairment outside of the health care system. Dr. Middleton's PhD (Dalhousie University, Halifax, NS, Canada) and postdoctoral fellowship (University of California, San Francisco) examined the relationship between physical activity and cognitive change in old age. It appears that physical activity not only decreases the risk of dementia but also increases the chance of improved cognition in old age. One of her recent studies indicated that being physically active in teenage years reduced the likelihood of cognitive impairment in old age. She is currently conducting studies evaluating the relationship between daily activity (exercise, chores and other movement) and cognition. In addition, she is evaluating how rehabilitation programs might be able to improve cognitive and physical outcomes in patients who have mild cognitive impairment or who have suffered a ministroke.

FERNANDA SPEGGIORIN PEREIRA graduated with a bachelor's degree in psychology from the University of Santa Catarina, Santa Catarina, Brazil, in 2002. She has been a neuropsychology specialist since 2004, and in March 2010 she completed her doctoral degree in psychiatry. Her studies, under the supervision of Dr. Orestes Forlenza and Dr. Mônica Yassuda at the Laboratory of Neuroscience at the University of São Paulo, focused on executive functions and functionality in the context of normal and pathological aging. She was then particularly interested in the relationship of executive dysfunction and instrumental activities of daily living. She teaches and conducts research on topics related to cross-cultural validation of neuropsychological instruments, cognitive and functional assessment and rehabilitation of the elderly.

CHENGXUAN QIU, MD, PhD, a research scientist, received his medical degree from Shandong Medical University (China, 1980–1985), master's degree in medical epidemiology from Tianjin Medical University (China, 1987–1990), and doctoral degrees (PhD) in epidemiology and biostatistics from Tongji Medical University (China, 1996–1999) and in geriatric epidemiology from Karolinska Institutet (Sweden, 2001–2004). He completed research training as a post-doctoral fellow and visiting scientist at the National Institute on Aging (NIA)/National Institutes of Health (NIH) (2005–2006, 2008), USA. He is currently employed as a research scientist by Karolinska Institutet. Since 1999 Dr. Qiu has been with Karolinska Institutet focusing on epidemiology of dementia and brain aging. His research is based on several population-based databases, for example, the Kungsholmen Project, the Swedish National Study on Aging and Care (SNAC) in Kungsholmen, and the Swedish Brain Power Initiatives. Dr. Qiu's research topics include the genetic (e.g., APOE genotype and familial aggregation), environmental (education, occupational exposures, and lifestyle factors), and biological (blood pressure, diabetes, and heart disease) factors and their interactions for dementia, Alzheimer's disease, and brain lesions (brain regional atrophy, infarcts, white matter changes, and cerebral microbleeds). Dr. Qiu's research also involves collaboration with the U.S. NIA/NIH (Project: The Age, Gene/Environment Susceptibility-Reykjavik Study) and the National Institute for Health and Welfare in Helsinki, Finland (Project: The Cardiovascular Risk Factors in Dementia).

WILM QUENTIN is a research fellow at the Department of Health Care Management at Berlin Technical University. He is a medical doctor and completed an MSc in health policy, planning and financing at the London School of Hygiene and Tropical Medicine and the London School of Economics in September 2009. He studied medicine and political sciences in Würzburg, Munich, Madrid, Leipzig, and Marburg, where he graduated in 2007. He has worked as a research assistant at the department of Health Economics of the University of Leipzig and published articles on a broad range of topics ranging from tobacco control policies over costs of HIV/AIDS treatment to cost-of-illness of dementia.

STEFFI G. RIEDEL-HELLER is working as a professor for public health at the University of Leipzig. She is a physician, specialized in psychiatry and psychotherapy, and obtained her master of public health degree from Johns Hopkins University, Baltimore, Maryland. Her scientific interest lies in the interface of public health and psychiatry, especially in the field of epidemiology of mental disorders in old age and health service research. She has profound experience in conducting cohort studies in old age. She is also chief editor of a German scientific journal, *Psychiatrische Praxis*.

Dr. MICHAEL J. VALENZUELA is a Research Fellow in Regenerative Neuroscience at the School of Psychiatry, University of New South Wales (UNSW). His background is in psychology, clinical medicine, and neuroscience research. Dr. Valenzuela's PhD focused on the topic of brain reserve and for this work he was awarded the prestigious Eureka Prize for Medical Research in 2006. Dr. Valenzuela's current research interests are aimed at understanding the competing forces of brain plasticity and degeneration in the human brain. In particular, he is interested in how we can use the science of neuroplasticity to help prevent dementia in the first place. He has published over 30 scientific papers, gained over $1 million in research funds, and is the author of the best-selling popular science book *It's Never Too Late to Change Your Mind*, which details the latest medical thinking about what you can do to avoid dementia (ABC Books, 2009).

Dr. ART WALASZEK is a board-certified geriatric psychiatrist and Associate Professor of Psychiatry at the University of Wisconsin School of Medicine and Public Health. He received his medical degree from Northwestern University Medical School, completed psychiatry training at the University of Washington, and completed a fellowship in geriatric psychiatry at

Northwestern Memorial Hospital in Chicago. Dr. Walaszek is currently the Director of Psychiatry Residency Training at the University of Wisconsin Hospital and Clinics. He directs the CME activities of the University of Wisconsin Department of Psychiatry and is the chair of the CME Committee of the Wisconsin Psychiatric Association. He is a member of the editorial board of *Academic Psychiatry* and is on the executive council of the American Association of Directors of Psychiatry Residency Training. The Association for Academic Psychiatry has recognized Dr. Walaszek's educational contributions with the 2007 AAP/Forest Junior Faculty Career Award. As a member of the Wisconsin Geriatric Psychiatry Initiative, he speaks extensively on geriatric topics in various medical and nonmedical settings across the state. He has coauthored articles and book chapters on late-life emotional and behavioral problems, anxiety disorders in long-term care, and late-life depression. His clinical practice involves caring for primarily older adults with depressive disorders, anxiety disorders, and dementia, and their families.

MÔNICA SANCHES YASSUDA graduated from the University of São Paulo, São Paulo, Brazil, with a bachelor's degree in clinical psychology in 1990. She later moved to Gainesville, Florida, where she pursued her master's and doctoral degrees in developmental psychology. Her studies, under the supervision of Dr. Robin Lea West, focused on metamemory and memory training in the context of normal cognitive aging. She was then particularly interested in investigating the possibility of changing negative beliefs about cognition and aging and developing techniques for memory improvement among healthy seniors. Since 2005 she has been an assistant professor at the University of São Paulo. She teaches and conducts research in topics related to neuropsychological markers of pathological cognitive decline, memory interventions, frailty, and cognition.

About the Series Editor

PATRICK MCNAMARA, PhD, is Associate Professor of Neurology and Psychiatry at Boston University School of Medicine (BUSM) and is Director of the Evolutionary Neurobehavior Laboratory in the Department of Neurology at the BUSM and the VA New England Healthcare System. Upon graduating from the Behavioral Neuroscience Program at Boston University in 1991, he trained at the Aphasia Research Center at the Boston VA Medical Center in neurolinguistics and brain-cognitive correlation techniques. He then began developing an evolutionary approach to problems of brain and behavior and currently is studying the evolution of the frontal lobes, the evolution of the two mammalian sleep states (REM and NREM) and the evolution of religion in human cultures.

Index